Examine Your Life Through the Carpet Weaver of the Night

Basic Concepts of Dream Interpretation
in the Homeopathic Practice

Luc De Schepper, M.D., Lic. Ac.

FULL OF LIFE PUBLISHING • SANTA FE, NM

DISCLAIMER

The information in this book is presented for informational purposes only. All therapies, treatments, or energetic interventions of any nature should be undertaken only under the direct guidance and care of a properly trained and legally qualified healthcare professional specializing in the service rendered. Nothing described in this book should be construed by any reader or any other person to be a diagnosis or treatment for any disease or condition. Neither the author nor the publisher can accept any responsibility for any ill effects resulting from the use or misuse of the information contained herein. Any uses or misuses of the information presented here for educational purposes are the responsibility of the reader. The names and other identifying characteristics of the persons included in this book have been changed.

CONTACTING THE AUTHOR

The author welcomes feedback from the readers mailed to the publisher's address below. To order other books by Dr. Luc, please visit his website at drluc.com

---

Printed in the United States of America
Full of Life Publishing
P.O. Box 31025
Santa Fe, NM 87594
ISBN 978-0-942501-16-2

Editing: Tricia Feijo

Copyediting: Sasha Smith

Art Direction and Cover Image: Yolanda De Schepper

(photo taken in Istanbul, Turkey)

Cover Art Direction and Design Execution: Marguerite Theuret and Moonlit Fox Design

Back Cover Photo: Dr. Luc De Schepper with his wife Yolanda

To my wife Yolanda,
whose inner beauty equals her outer beauty

ACKNOWLEDGMENTS

Being one of my best students worldwide, I could not have found a better person than Tricia Feijo to assist me in bringing this complex subject to the homeopathic community. With a great mind and compassion that is extended not only to her fellow homeopaths but to all her patients, she was the ideal person for me to make the text fluent and easily readable. Her enthusiasm and love for the subject always supported me in this long-lasting project as it brought as much pleasure to her as to me.

Sasha Smith was my excellent copyeditor. She added polish with her conscientious eye for detail and mastery of the English language, and was also a joy to work with.

Marguerite Theuret once again helped to design the beautiful cover, truly a great gift to me for which I am ever grateful.

CONTENTS

SECTION FOUR: BIRTH OF THE CYBER DELUSION (CD) AND DIRECTION OF CURE

INTRODUCTION

> *"I woke up in a cold sweat and was filled with rage. My dream finally told me what I so long suspected: I saw my husband seducing another woman. Upon awakening, I did not hesitate to confront him immediately, and from the surprised look on his face, I knew I had caught him in the crime of deception. The more I insisted on hearing the truth, the more flustered and confused he became, stammering that I had been caught with a whiff of insanity. The more he pleaded, the more he was signaling to me that there was no doubt! He was possessed of the spirit of the crazed Rasputin, the demonic confidant of Czar Nicholas II and Tsaritsa Alexandria in the early 1900s. Guilty as charged!"*

I often wonder how such incredible stories have sown thorns in mankind's garden of love, and to what extent disastrous results have occurred. More than likely, emotions of jealousy, suspicion, and rage have descended with tsunami-like forces on the Self of the dreamer: the Self being the center of the *total personality, the total psychological being of man, conscious and uncon-*

scious, versus the ego, defined as the center of the conscious personality. And who has not shuddered in the middle of a nightmare, when feeling hurled headlong to the bottom of an abyss? During sleep, we all regularly have the same experiences as madmen do when awake—indeed sometimes even more improbable ones. Who has never dreamed of being chased by ferocious animals or gangsters? Of being lost in a city, or stranded on an island … of drowning in a pool, being a king among paupers, or being ill-prepared for an examination?

Weird and tragic stories happen all the time at night, as if the dreamer is different from the daytime person. Sometimes there are nights of sheer terror and despair, or nights charged with the vices of life. Each night we fail to recognize the warnings and messages and say to ourselves, relieved in the morning, "It was just a dream." It seems that these nightly messages cannot stand the daylight, and instead fade and disappear in the splendor of the day. The day might give us cheer and peace, but the night appears to be a joker who often brings nothing but nonsense, disarray, and even cruel stories. The human mind never stops, instead reaching in many directions—creating, musing, always engaged—and even carries on during the dream phase of sleep, never pausing, as the dance of life continues. But who really wants to understand dreams? Most people don't want to know that most of our troubles are to be found entirely within our own nature, preferring to laugh at the dream messages because we don't understand them. Yet they are the first step to self-awareness!

To whom, then, can one look for their explanation? To the long-trusted family physician, who speaks with dignified joviality and a trusted voice so common to family doctors (especially when they attain a certain familiarity as strong as your furniture)? They all eventually acquire the same tone of voice, as if it's a common biological characteristic of that professional status. He will reassure you with a wink and a gentle touch on your shoulder: "You know that these dreams are all nonsense, absurd and ludicrous!" "Trust me," he says, with a soothing fatherly voice reinforced with the perfect, current medical knowledge of man's bodily and mental expressions. When you leave, you close his office door with great deference, as if the doctor, simply by touching the doorknob, has left a healing potion on it. You still hear his laughing voice, "All will be well," when you hurry to the next savior you hope will release you from the clutches of nightmarish "fables" and morass of jumbled images. You then are referred to the psychiatrist, the physician who deals with derangements of the mind. Certainly, the reaction of the dreamer and the created story in the dream look like the handiwork of a delusional person and the creation of an evil genius, respectively. But after examining the state of your married life, the stress at work, and the negative influence of your extended family, he throws his hands up and declares you "sane"—yet possibly still prescribes those unnecessary, readily available allopathic "wonder" drugs to restore the out-of-balance neurotransmitters. Most physicians use the latter handy metaphor, which is only a kind of bumper-sticker phrase to buy time, considering the patient as a self contained rigid object, rather than as an individual who is involved in constant movement and change, called life! Allopaths would do well not to accept that sleep is a mere turning "off," from "on" while awake, technique—a mere parting from consciousness—but rather, is a switch to a "second" consciousness, another realm, of dreams rich in adventure and wisdom. The famed writer Edgar Allan Poe explained that the Self (in my opinion he meant the conscious) has a double that is mysterious, half-hidden, yet somehow exerts an influence over behavior and feelings (referring to the second conscious, the unconscious).

Twenty-five percent of our sleep is REM sleep during which we dream; this should not be dismissed, as it is the opportunity to learn more about ourselves. It may be recommended for sleep problems to see a sleep specialist, who may study the levels of brain deactivation with their different stages. Here, too, opinions will be different and quite opposite of each other. In an article in *National Geographic*, "Want to Fall Asleep? Read This Story," Michael Finkel wrote:

> "Many sleep experts aren't interested in the specific images and events in our dreams … and even if dreams are imbued with emotional resonance, they are devoid of significance." Then again, "Other sleep experts strongly disagree … where the content of dreams is part of an involved mechanism by looking at the larger significance of new memories and how they should be useful in the future." (July, 2018, pp. 72-73)

After all, allopathic (conventional) physicians are trained to overlook individuality, focusing on the presenting disease rather than discovering the patient's unique identity. Their first goal is recognizing the disease *in* a patient, called diagnosis, in order to be able to apply the corresponding protocol. But classifying the patient with a disease name is depriving him of his identity and individuality, and in order to understand a patient's dreams the physician must learn about him as an individual.

What about dream interpretation and alternative physicians? Chiropractors? Naturopaths? Can their art of healing explain dreams? No such luck! It is not part of their expertise. Maybe Traditional Chinese Medicine (TCM) physicians who have studied the ancient Chinese books have some insight; for example, the Yellow Emperor's *Spiritual Axis* says, "When the Gall Bladder is deficient one dreams of fights, trials and suicide," and an imbalance in the Heart causes "dreams of fire, volcanic eruptions and smoke" (Maciocia, 1989). Regardless of how much I love TCM and have studied and practiced it for decades, I wonder how many of its practitioners can adequately treat clients disturbed by their dreams, as dream analysis is not taught in acupuncture schools.

Well, at least we have the homeopaths! Their modality and science certainly should be able to penetrate deep into the mind-body connection, linking diseases to unbalanced emotions. Unlike allopathic medicine which groups patients into large categories, homeopathy recognizes and treats the *individual.* Homeopathy's founder, Samuel Hahnemann, was the first physician after Hippocrates known to approach each patient as if he were the only one in the world—with great wisdom and without jargon or presuppositions. (He was also the first to advocate the humane treatment of the insane and of epileptics, who were considered insane at that time!) While allopathic medicine treats the disease (by suppressing symptoms), homeopathy treats the individual *with* a disease (by going to the root of the problem). As TCM proclaims, the individual is a microcosm within a macrocosm.

But when one examines Hahnemann's masterful treatise, *Organon of Medicine*, very little can be found about dreams. Throughout the six editions from 1810 to 1843, only one phrase seems to have come up: *"Recurrent dreams are important."* No further explanation and no further investigation of dream interpretation have been proposed by any homeopath since then unless they have studied the works of Carl Jung. In his book, *The Symbolic Quest*, the late Edward C. Whitmont, M.D., was such an exception (Whitmont, 1969). Although Freud, back in 1899 in *The Interpretation of Dreams*, produced the first breakthrough work of what was called "soul craft" (Freud, 1998), dreams for Freud were always a disguised fulfillment of a wish, which was rather a narrow interpretation, and therefore I prefer the insight of Carl Jung.

Homeopaths could use this important "other" part of the human being in healing their patients—the unconscious and its messenger, dreams! Newly proved remedies contain all kinds of dreams, but I have never seen any symbolic subjective translation of these dreams in relationship to the prover's existing conscious situation. Dreams are just treated like the other proving symptoms—registered as facts without depth analysis and therefore, the homeopath misses the true meaning of these valuable messages. In order to be successful in practice, the excellent homeopath must strive to possess a sensitivity that furnishes him with psychological antennae that will discover the abundant dirt and secrets at the bottom of every individual. He needs to see the hidden and hear what is not said except at night by his patient's dreams. It is perplexing that looking for the truth often brings so much resistance. Is it because we live easier in a world created of fantasy, lies, and projections; a life cloaked in the folds of moral hypocrisy? Is it for this reason that dreams—revealing our other side—evoke such strong reactions as to be called nebulous philosophical distractions; because they undress us to full nakedness?

The subject of dream analysis is very difficult, not only for intellectual reasons, but even more on account of personal, subjective resistance, as it demands from the homeopath (or anyone else) ruthless self-knowledge and courage—two characteristics in short demand for most. The Delphic oracle "Know thyself" is an excellent precept but not a favorite or popular topic, as it disturbs, quite often, our seemingly peaceful abode. Yet one of the meanings of life is to find out how to meet and resolve our *own* difficulties! How many among us have the courage and humility to draw back the curtain to find the truth? Should we not aspire to that, in order to reach greater health and freedom, and rebel against the bonds of self-slavery?

Understanding urgent dream messages is a necessary help and a useful guide on the road to self-actualization. An attempt to reach self-awareness should become the main, if not the minimum, condition of human existence—a rope knotted to form a ladder leading from animal to Plato's philosopher king.

The road to self-actualization is not a passage that jumps from one seven-year period to the next, but rather from day to day, even from minute to minute, as one stumbles along, often sidetracked, feeling hopeful when a new milestone is reached on the treacherous journey, as the soul remains in apprenticeship, tested anew and anew, ultimately emerging as the eternal phoenix from periods of decline and setbacks. It is a life full of fits and starts, lacking for most the coherence and self-control much sought after. Only theater life is as such, as it is an area that connects one set of events to another. Real life is more like monologues directly from the heart, agitated and interrupted by the feelings of each moment as it passes, portraying real experience, the changeless truths of ordinary humans.

We can only hope that changes will come intentionally, from looking inward, exploring our dreams and trusting our soul to find footing again and again on this slippery road. At the end of life, we should be able to look back and digest how far we have come through a spirit of courage, determination, and creativity, rather than viewing life as a train that never left the station. A fully functioning existence is not distorted by most sycotic and all syphilitic miasmatic traits, but produces a person who *is* what he *can be* (the highest virtue of man)—not an individual who never takes a risk, who is afraid of failure and novelty, and who, in spite of calling himself a "spiritual" person, never investigated his dark or shadow side; in other words, what Jung and many other psychologists called, "a *complete* individual (*not* perfect), trying to reach self-realization"!

If you want to live undisturbed in your fantasyland, identifying with the wise old man, even God, or the expert teacher who only preaches because he or she considers himself above everyone else, then this book is not for you. Keep on making a lot of noise, in order to not hear the truth by which you could gain self-awareness. But when you are unprejudiced, then by all means devour this book. What awaits you is the discovery of a new Self, in which you must become a child again, ready and excited to embark on a new journey, to discover a country you never thought existed. You have to become the lion with a brave heart, the eagle with a sharp eye, breaking through old barriers and buildings—not a ruminating cow, who avoids stepping into what you fear the most in yourself, the exploration of the vast dark continent of the unconscious. If you want to create a new world, you must oppose the old one in which you had too much light that blinded you, while never illuminating the darkness for new guidance.

Make your curiosity greater than your pride. Don't shy away and shrink from examining anything false and fanciful that you hold dear. Discover that you are not the one and only, but one among many. After reading this book, you will wake up with new insights that not only will benefit all your patients, but foremost, you and your loved ones. We can state that there is progress in physics and biology, and allopathy claims the same, but the latter forgets far too often to apply the progress in dynamic social psychology. The existence of the irrational and unconscious sector of our nature, and its messenger-dreams, is still neglected by the masses, physicians and homeopaths included. Irrationalities in dreams can be understood rationally as they are responding to laws of homeostasis, reflecting reactions to external conscious events.

May this book stimulate the reader to devote his energies to the study of the unconscious, of which most lack even basic knowledge. And precisely because it is the beginning of its study for most, it will excite the real human being and physician to devote his interest to the topic. Don't fall into the common trap of longing to return to a never-ending state of inertia, fearing that you will lose the protection of the old familiar status quo! You must try to establish Tao, a very Eastern idea, to integrate your unconscious into your conscious in order to discover yourself, wherein hopefully you will find companions. Tao stands also for "The Way," a path or road, the way to a destination; a path to be followed in life to produce wisdom, harmony, and "right conduct."

I am out to reach lovers of the truth, inner-directed people, young and old, professionals and non-professionals, lovers of the ideas and insights of Plato's *Republic*, and lovers of progression even when discovery of the Self puts one at risk for pain and confusion as well as abuse from others who preach their own science. As Hahnemann showed us, the divinities you should worship are "Thought, Art, Genius, and Truth." May you find the willingness to fill the empty pages of your existence; may light come over you and your life be spared from falling apart, little by little, like fallen ashes. But if your life does fall apart, may you rise like the phoenix from its ashes, and begin a new life. As an ordinary fellow human being, I am so close behind you, that if you stretched out your hand I think you can reach me in what we call *life*, a mixture of good and bad, virtues and vices, light and darkness. Be spurred on by the difficulty of this enterprise! You have something definite to work for. End your apprenticeship and start your real existence. Enjoy this great collective enterprise which will release you from the bonds of boredom and loneliness. May your soul fly out the window for new adventures, as new life always starts with the death of the old one. Why would the phoenix not show disposition to rise from its ashes? Why would the phoenix be reluctant, dragging its talons, resisting all new goings? Putting your house in order at last is one of the most exciting activities you'll ever engage in, and the benefits for everyone around you, and for yourself in the first place, are incalculable. We now seem to live in a society that has almost forgotten the decency of what it means to be human. Progress and healing are always needed yet remain to be in short supply.

My intention is to stir thought, disturb your peaceful fantasyland and provide some introspection into the Self, hopefully helping you grow and move towards the person you are meant to be. Be an adventurer and discoverer filled with courage and curiosity. Reclaim your life by understanding the clear messages of the unconscious, and no longer be ruled by repetitious misfortunes—a collective task for humankind—and follow a path that you most likely have never trod before. I challenge you not so much to agree or disagree as to grow. To quote Aristotle in the opening sentence of his *Metaphysics*, "No desire is more natural than the desire for knowledge." Quotes from Jung in this book are not a substitute for studying all of Jung; my ambition is to lure others on to that undertaking! May you grow old and always continue to learn!

NOTES

There are many factors in the patient histories which I cannot, with respect to professional discretion and the economy of space, include in the case examples presented in this book.

The first section of the book is devoted to general aspects of dream psychology, the language of dreams with important dreams during man's life, the different themes in dreams, and the three different classes of dreams: recurrent, series of dreams, and archetypal dreams.

The second section will examine the elements of the conscious: the ego formation, the persona, its uses and malformation, and the four conscious functions of Jung with the two attitude types.

The third section elaborates on elements of the personal and collective unconscious with specific archetypes such as the shadow, anima, and animus, and their roles in human lives and dreams. Particularly of interest is the human love story, always the result of projection of the sygizi (anima and animus).

Finally, there will be a fourth section explaining the birth of the cyber delusion, its role, how to find it in the homeopathy practice and Repertory, and a chapter about following the direction of cure under the guidance of dream analysis.

A brief appendix of relative fixed symbols is found at the end, as well as references.

Terms unfamiliar to the non-homeopath are defined in the Index, as are all remedy names, listed in full.

Homeopathic remedy names and quotations from provings and from the Repertory are italicized.

"Delusion" was capitalized for rubrics under that large and important subsection of the Mind in the Repertory.

References Note

Aphorisms

Aphorisms referred to are from the *Organon of Medicine*, Sixth Edition, by Samuel Hahnemann, translated by Jost Künzli, Alain Naudé, and Peter Pendleton.

Quotations from Provings and the Repertory

Proving symptoms and rubrics are referenced from the *Essential Synthesis* by Frederik Schroyens.

Literature Citations

For older literature cited in this book, such as that written by S. Hahnemann and C.G. Jung, the dates given in the citations are the reprint dates or editions. Please see references cited for more information on the original publication dates.

SECTION ONE

General Aspects of Dream Psychology

1

DREAMS, THE KEY TO AN UNKNOWN WORLD

"The nature of the body can only be understood as a whole." — *Hippocrates*

Understanding the Conscious to Help Find the Simillimum

Objectivity and truthfulness, the driving forces of all strivings for freedom, are always the first victims. The thinking intellectual, especially, uses his conscious function to confirm and rationalize predetermined irrational ideas and fixed delusions, which at first always seem logical, compelling, and truthful. As we will discover in Chapter 8 ("The Four Conscious Functions"), when we neglect our feeling function, protected by ingrained subjective convictions, we are unable to see the harmfulness of our actions as we can find all kinds of superficial "logical" arguments to validate our thinking and consequent irrational decisions. It is especially the cyber delusion (see Chap. 15) that is the dark force in a person, for it governs all behavior, no matter how honest personal intentions seem to be. A perfect example is a deceived woman, immersed in the *Nat-m* jungle of hatred and revenge, who wants at all cost sole custody of her child "as it is in the best interest of the child," while the real motive is a sadistic and revengeful punishment of the father. This should also be a warning to those people who descend into a *Nat-m* state when martyrdom is sought for a cause, with uttermost disregard for their own basic needs. For such *Nat-m* persons, life itself does not progress and seems to circle around one center of pain; suffering becomes one long moment, creating a paralyzing immobility of life. An aphorism from Lou Salome, Nietzsche's platonic love and admirer, describes it very well: "Women do not die of love, but waste away without it" (Hayman, 1980, p. 252).

Homeopathic provings/rubrics that express this notion are well known: *Delusion (Del), wretched when looking in the mirror; aversion to company, fond of solitude; face, wrinkled; dwells over past disagreeable occurrences and recalls them; thoughts, haunted by unpleasant thoughts.*

A *Nat-m* person should learn not to remember past wrongs. When deceived by her lover, she regards the other woman, who she wants revenge on, as poisonous vermin that must be exterminated at any price. She withdraws in solitude, but solitude is conducive to whatever she takes into it: hate, revenge, sad thoughts, persistent grief—all of which she wants to recall—and suppressed anger. The latter, as Mark Twain said, "is an acid that can do more harm to the vessel in which it is stored than to anything on which it is poured." She even makes a great business out of her "crusader's plans," expressing her views and suffering on websites and blogs, which is ideal now that she lives only for that purpose, neglecting her personal needs and often those close to her. It is amazing that such a person can fit infinite grief and hatred into such short of a life. Although this person is active in her mind, it is just another form of inertia, hindering growth and full potential. In her revenge, she focuses on the other person's vulnerability; she wants to hurt *especially those who have offended her!* It is an act of restoration of her honor (*Ailments from wounded honor*). And many encountering such a *Nat-m* person will quote the acerbic but always insightful Oscar Wilde, "Some cause happiness wherever they go; others *whenever* they go!"

Every homeopath in practice has been confronted with the difficulty of discovering the patient's critical information from this vast continent of terra incognita, this unknown, hidden land containing the shameful, painful, and private parts. "Private" comes from the Latin *privare* or "to deprive," which is to say, this is "property," the use of which everybody is deprived of, except the owner! But is this the right course? When will the patient let his guard down to tell us what he is otherwise so busy suppressing, repressing, or projecting onto others? How can we loosen the man's character-armor of the affects from his concealments? There is a way! He will relax when you ask him, "Tell me about your dreams." He might laugh and say, "Listen to this crazy dream I had! I had this ugly woman chasing me!" He will do so without reservation, not knowing that dreams—the messengers of the unconscious—will reveal much more of his personality than the homeopath ever can obtain from the patient's divulged limited conscious. Dreams fill all the gaps of the limited, well-guarded self-knowledge, the patient's blind spots, guiding us with more precision to the simillimum and hence to the patient's greater well-being and growth.

The homeopath needs to pay attention not only to *what* the patient recounts in dreams, but also to *how* he communicates them: coherently or inarticulately, politely or aggressively, with sneers or a mask-like face, with gestures or zombie-like behavior, as all can be valuable clues as to how candid the patient is in the narration of his history in general. Does the patient remain silent (e.g., *Nat-m*), become angry at your probing (*Nit-acid*), shut down (*Silicea*), try to overpower you with "superior" knowledge and language (*Lycopodium, Lachesis, Sulphur*), or change into an overanxious person repeating himself just to convince you of the seriousness of his disease (*Arsenicum*)?

All too often in the homeopathic practice, not only the patient but also the homeopath is focusing on trivial problems. For the homeopath, "trifles" are *only* important when his patient *despairs* over trifles, pays too much attention to them (*conscientious about trifles*), or is *overanxious* about trifles. Usually "trivial" refers to the discussion of superficial things, banalities, or glorified gossip, rather than distinguishing between what is essential and what is nonessential in a conversation. However, when it comes to having a talk with our unconscious, triviality is out of the question. A dialogue between our Self and our unknown world requires honesty and hard work, making us come alive. Such dialogue is found in dreams where deep insights, not silenced by the noise of daily life, can be formulated and discovered, leading to greater well-being. Increasing consciousness—from the Latin *cum* or "with" and *scio/scire* or "knowledge" or awareness: to know with and by myself—can only be achieved when we become aware of what is hidden. This can only be accomplished through an active, and above all, honest and courageous effort, by integrating unconscious elements into consciousness, elements that were for such a long time repressed and suppressed. Only then can the unconscious possess a creative, positive, and healing force! What are some of those aspects of dreams we need to be aware of?

Important Aspects of Dream Analysis for Use in the Homeopathic Practice

Hahnemann cannot be faulted for not having incorporated dream analysis into the homeopathic practice, as the publishing and constant evolution of his six editions of the *Organon* and *Chronic Diseases* required a lifetime effort amidst constant opposition to the practice of his art. It is left to us, his disciples, to expand the homeopathic investigation to the unknown element of the human being—his unconscious and its messenger, dreams. The ubiquitous and baffling ASD epidemic has made the understanding of dreams even more important. Too many such children seem to be caught between the conscious and unconscious, or are withdrawn completely in the unconscious, as the normal selective conscious filter has been closed to elements from the outside world, making increased communication and exchange impossible if not undesirable to them. Children in general are caught in their own dreamworld (*fancies* and *Delusions of fancy illusions*, syphilitic characteristics if deemed reality), and understanding their dreams can help us navigate the maze of their world. Moreover, in-depth psychology—especially dream interpretation—enables the crossover to biology and medicine, with great benefit to the medical and homeopathic community. As the homeopath studies the contents of this book, besides receiving a new and expanded view of the patient's suffering, dream analysis will contribute important information to assist him in expanding many aspects of the homeopathic art.

Dream interpretation can be used to:

- find the simillimum (expanded by the elusive cyber delusion, hidden in the unconscious—see my book, *Advanced Guide for Professional Homeopaths*).
- discover the shadow of the patient.
- know when to change the remedy or not during the homeopathic treatment as the conflict becomes resolved (*lysis*) in the dream (another aid to using Hering's Observations, with connection to the Six

Levels in TCM—see *Advanced Guide for Professional Homeopaths*).

- explain why a remedy does not work, even when there is no miasmatic block and the remedy seemed to be well-chosen, as the inner conflict is not acknowledged or remains obscure and the patient was not able to free himself from a strong high-feeling toned complex.
- tell the homeopath about the management: is he on the right track or not? Is he going too fast or too slow? Can he go full steam ahead (as the VF is strong enough) or is the dream indicating a hidden serious disease that should warn the homeopath to use low potencies and infrequent *small* doses of the remedy (the latter is *always* advisable).
- show the patient where he is straying from the direction of cure, creating an impasse, and whether certain aspects of his life remain unconscious—for instance, interests outside of the family business, or unused libido for any new vocation. (When people live blindly, with no self-reflection, the dream will be like a mirror, taking over the function of the intellect. No matter how much the patient will try to hide the truth, a dream, often *recurrent* at that point, will always remind him of the real situation until he is willing to correct it).
- warn the homeopath about dangerous aspects in his patient's life (latent serious disease or imminent death) to be remedied by the suitable medicine, or to obtain information through the compensatory dream when the patient's conscious mind cannot see the reality of his dangerous lifestyle and ambition. (A corrective dream, beyond the control of the patient's conscious mind, will warn the dreamer to

slow down, talking directly to the dreamer—or the dream will end in a catastrophe.)

- tell the homeopath how the patient is hiding unconsciously (in his shadow side) dormant *good* qualities, which when integrated into consciousness would provide the patient a greater meaning of life and vocation as well as furnishing a ground plan for future activities and potentialities for personal development.
- tell the homeopath about the prognosis (direction of cure, and prophetic dreams) and about the psychological, mental, or physical causality of his neurosis (NWS) as well as errors of lifestyle (Aphorisms 77, 5, and 7), so that the patient does not become an obstruction to his own cure by repeating the same mistakes over and over again. (Dreams are helpful in differentiating between organic and psychogenic diseases.)
- add elements, unknown to the patient and physician, to the subjective and objective symptoms, on which the homeopath can rely for the diagnosis, including knowledge of the patient's true temperament and constitution as he *really is*, not as he *wants to be perceived*—in other words, the Emperor without clothes. (Dreams are indeed the homeopath's number one ally, by ruthlessly puncturing the patient's illusions and delusions of grandeur, by telling him to take command of his life and pull himself out of inertia and blind alleys that stop his individuation and create a deadlock in his life, showing him that he is traveling an undesirable road—the "road most traveled"—motored by unrealistic inflations.)
- provide the patient with an urgent message and

warning that he is making a wrong decision in life —a decision contrary to generally accepted moral standards—which will lead to many missteps. (For instance, when someone is thinking about leaving his spouse and children for a woman many years his junior, a dream may possibly confront him with a point of view opposed to his own desires and convictions, making him look at his conduct from the standpoint of his moral nature.)
- give a wider view about the true causalities or what derailed the patient from his life course, by examining his formation of anima and animus, or possibly, by revealing that he has unconsciously been forced to function in his archaic conscious function.
- shorten the length of any analysis and homeopathic treatment.

Further considerations of dream analysis are as follows:

- Judiciously applied doses of the simillimum help the patient to bear the pain and conflict when faced with analytical dream work and he discovers the hidden truths in his unconscious, avoiding a psychotic break.
- Spiritual questions (meaning of life) are often answered by the unconscious, guiding the patient in midlife crisis, retirement, and approaching death.
- The psoric need of the patient is reflected in the dream with a total opposite compensation: if there was lack of love, the dream often creates intimate and loving behavior. If there was too much protection, rather called "domination," anxious dreams are created in which the dreamer is pursued

by someone that wants to kill him (see Chap. 2, under "Rule of Compensation and General Purpose of Dreams").

- Dream analysis encourages the healer to investigate his own dreams: not only will he understand what the real crux of the patient's suffering is, but the contents that normally would stay latent in the patient, due to the process of contagion, could lead to pathology in the physician. By analyzing his own dreams, not only does the homeopath have opportunity to gain deeper understanding about the patient's suffering, but equally finds the key to his own simillimum. Just as we have concomitants (accompanying symptoms) with the chief complaint of a patient, psychic contaminations must be considered a concomitant of the physician's work.
- Last, but not least, if the patient understands the urgent message of the dream, and he acts upon this message, a remedy may not even be needed!

Looking at these many advantages, which will be all clarified in the next chapters, as with the absolute need of taking his own simillimum, the homeopath must see the necessity and find the courage to apply the same perseverance to investigate his unconscious as he does his patient's, rather than remaining in the dark while claiming to enlighten others! And, lo and behold, doing so may remain very unpopular, as he might discover that he himself is not able to live up to the standards he demands and expects from his patients! Even Jung found those benefits of analyzing his dreams, as it warned him of his improper attitude towards one of his patients. In *Memories, Dreams, Reflection*, he writes how he was admonished by his dream that he looked down on his patient rather than feeling empathy and compassion; this interpretation, once communicated to the patient, was immediately followed by a change in the patient's situation and a release from her impasse, annihilating the *counter-transference* problem (Jung, 1963, p. 133). Because of the process known as *transference* and *countertransference*, the homeopath, through a dream, receives not only information about his patient's simillimum but also about his own. Unconscious contents are always projected upon others, and because this is true also of the homeopath, transference always affects both parties. No therapist involved is ever a "blank piece of paper."

There is also a possibility of latent negative transference to the homeopath: a patient's hostile emotions towards one of the parents can easily be projected towards the therapist with failed therapeutic result if this negative transference is not drawn out of concealment by confronting the patient with it. When the patient seems too polite at all cost, too nice, and seems to be all too willing to be an open book, we can be sure that this "perfect" patient's positive attitude is masking distrust, deceit, and anger. The mask of politeness is just a means of protection, as the patient does not want to start on the wrong foot. So the homeopath and therapist must understand that every case coming to him starts with an attitude of distrust; it does not mean this patient will outright lie, but he wants to conceal aspects of his life he deems "unimportant," *even when they are the trigger to his illness*, and more importantly, *part of his genetic structure.* But, as we will discover, not obeying the unconscious leads to a process of self-immolation.

After reading this book, the homeopath will understand that the possessor of the dream story that started the introduction should have investigated her unconscious to discover the skeletons in her closet before divorcing her husband. Also, she should have been made aware that her threatening dream was nothing more than a projection of her own archaic animus and the result of lack of true love, the kernel of all jealousy. Jealousy never waits for reason!

Moreover, the reader will discover in this book that all of us need to start the Herculean task of cleaning our own Augeas's stable where masses of deposited manure threaten to overtake our conscious life. Where Hercules was ordered to clean King Augeas's vast stables in one day, we mortals can at least use the rest of our life to take on this immense venture and try to find the hero archetype in ourselves, where each step forward rewards the owner with becoming a more enlightened and complete person. Such a shift from ego to Self is truly a healing of the soul. Our first goal in life: to cultivate our own garden!

Note

The interpretation of some dreams could have been more expansive, if it were not for my desire to protect intimacies of private life which should not be published. Occasionally, in addition to the interpretation of some of my own dreams, I share dreams of personal acquaintances, and divulge the conscious life of the person with his or her consent.

2

THE LANGUAGE OF DREAMS

"There have been times in my life when I have fallen asleep in tears; but in my dreams the most charming forms have come to console and cheer me, and I have risen the next morning fresh and joyful."
—Johann Wolfgang von Goethe

While the sages of Ancient Greece advised one to "Know thyself," to become more spiritual and whole, the encouragement is largely neglected, even shunned, consciously or unconsciously by present society. In addition, surprisingly, the more erudite the person, the quicker any thought of delving into the unconscious and listening "wide-awake" to its messenger, dreams, is discarded. Leave it to the primates and children, guided by the unconscious to believe in fairy tales (myths, and folklore) because such tales resonate with their dreams. In fact, in primitive tribes, people planned their lives and futures around the "big" dreams of the chief or medicine man, which were used as a guideline for the welfare of the tribe. As Jungian psychologist and scholar Marie-Louise von Franz wrote in her book *Dreams*:

> Primitives believe in two kinds of dreams; the big meaningful and the ordinary small dreams ... Great and important dreams are very rare and only a very big man has big dreams —chiefs, medicine men, people with mana. (1985, p. 66)

Modern man has not yet learned to use dreams as a source of continuous self-diagnosis: to see where he stands psychologically, to evaluate his degree of modesty or grandiosity, or to check the many other aspects of his psyche he is usually unaware of—or refuses to visit. Rather, he wants to shut down the voice of this continuous dialogue, helped by the rationality of the ego, and so misses the opportunity to look in the mirror and see himself how he really *is*; not who he *wants to be* or wants others to perceive him to be. In the mirror we see the image of our soul: it is an allegory of self-reflection. Examining the structure and physiology of the brain with MRIs and PET scans will never furnish an explanation of our psyche!

The "great dreams" of the chief or medicine man—so valued by primitives—had no relation to the conscious life of the tribe, but were like an oracle or vision, direct and autonomous products of the unconscious taken seriously because they prophesied the outcome of an urgent situation like famine, war, or other dangers. Such archetypal dreams also occur in modern times on a personal level, at the threat of a severe mental illness—a psychosis like schizophrenia—where an unconscious content overwhelms the ego with risk of fracturing it. But for the Native American Indians, dreams were the guiding light given by the Great Spirit to the souls that wander in the darkness.

Native American Indians, intimately connected to a balanced life with Nature, knew that animals served a great purpose in their spiritual development. Nature and humanity were inseparable; animals and humans were living in unity. The Native American Indians' myths and tales are filled with animal-people who guide and teach. When going to war, protection was sought in magic, contained in small bags filled with special herbs or animal parts, and drawings or animal parts on their shields represented symbolic power to the bearer—like eagle feathers or bear claws, believed to convey the power and ferocity of those animals. The way the Native American Indian painted himself and his horse was also believed to protect a man going into battle, except when this power had been defeated by some infraction of sacred rules: e.g., dreaming of the wrong animal, eating the wrong food, failing to carry the special grass or stone, or ruining this magical power in many other possible ways. Power was also believed to come to them from the "unseen world" or unconscious, which they visited in dreams. The question, then, arises: were the Ancient Greeks and subsequent cultures, even the primitive tribes, the real "modern" people when it comes to integrating and accepting dreams as part of their lives, consulting them as a psychopomp,[1] while modern man should be considered "primitive," as too many among us consider dreams "nonsense"? What about those "senseless" dreams? Should we listen to them with open ears?

Are Dreams Senseless?

Few are the mortals among us who have not exclaimed, upon being disturbed in their dreams by catastrophic and weird tales, "Thank God, this is just a dream! Just go on with the day and pay no attention to these absurdities, they have no importance to waking life." And maybe, the only dreams we feel are worth listening to are the series of "daydreams" our illusionary world is constantly creating, not understanding that they can be dangerous, as they smolder on like a fire, sometimes consuming us completely as they connect us with our complexes. Daydreams, which are akin to fantasy, wishful thinking, and overestimation of our capacities, often receive a better reception by our conscious mind than ordinary dreams. We could not be more wrong! Dreams are using a more intelligent language than our actual consciousness. Often, a dream may appear senseless, like the scene of a crazy Mardi Gras, but it will become obvious that it is we who lack the common sense and critical thinking needed to read its enigmatical message from the nocturnal realm of our psyche, where the unconscious has relatively free play and displays for our minds what true democracy is. While daytime is often used to create a persona of a king riding in his car in regal pomp and splendor, nighttime allows the shunned and outcast to come out from the nooks of the unconscious mind, compensating this one-sided, exaggerated attitude. It is as if at night there is someone else talking to us, in a frank and uncensored manner, bluntly stating how he sees us, which is quite different from our perceived reality. Dreams shake our fixed belief that it is only our conscious will that makes the choices for our life journey, and perceptions of ourselves and others. Sometimes only later, even years later, after much study and contemplation, are we confronted with our own blindness and experience that discovering the truth has a liberating effect.

We are astounded at the kind of elaborate mysteries we can write in our sleeping state, especially if in conscious life we cannot produce even the simplest letter. There seems to be a night muse at work, a poet and raconteur, who is capable of inspiring even the simplest soul and of elevating him to a "man of letters." However, upon awaking, we may also think that either a trickster or demon must have been at work for weaving such an alien, flimsy tale that produced nothing but confusion and perplexity—if not irritation. How to explain the contradictions, disconnections, and impossibilities in the created mystery, which surely draw nothing but disbelief and laughter in our daytime life? Few among us are willing to share with others this nocturnal "insanity," this "freak of Nature," primarily for fear of being laughed at and considered feeble-minded. "How can you believe in this nonsense?" is the usual remark made in response to dreams. While during the day we consider ourselves reasonable and intelligent, the night seems to be able to transform us into weak-minded, deranged fools. So, somewhat sheepishly, we withdraw and convince ourselves to pay no further attention to the literary product of our unconscious mind.

Alas, by doing so—by neglecting this direct expression of the nocturnal psychic activity—we miss the best chance to get to know ourselves and be guided safely on our way to becoming a better individual. By ignoring dreams, we lose out on instructions for our future, and lessons from our past. Of course, it is much easier to justify our neurotic character traits when reminded of them through the dream message, and say, "That's simply the way I am," rather than have a serious look at the message—a look at why our character has become what it is and not something else, for what specific reasons, or due to what incidents, that needs to be helped through analysis and remedies. (Character traits *can* be changed!) Frequently, we keep an uneasy feeling about some dreams, haunting us for several days precisely because they possess incredible psychic energy.

Even the trusted physician with whom we might share our nightly tales just smiles and waves away our concerns with a laugh, and asks us instead to "Focus on what is really important, what ails you, and how any anomaly can be measured through the trusted, medical, 'proven, evidence-based' science." That, of course, is called "real science" according to conventional medicine; the rest we can leave to story tellers who entertain and mesmerize our youngest children with fantastic tales when we put them to bed. While parents happily tell fairy tales to their children, they have no idea that they talk to them in a language close to the collective unconscious. Not just medical doctors, but adults generally put this same language—dreams and fairy tales—on a primitive and childish level, therefore indulging more and more in the conscious (the only kind of life that they believe has value, and is under control of their will), losing any chance at wholeness. No wonder neither physician nor patient make any attempt to relate the dream content to the present or past life of the patient. I wish physicians would understand that fantasies are the source of creation for many artists, writers, and sculptors who have worked with and investigated their unconscious. Alas, the physician finds these stories of the unconscious completely against his scientific values of the conscious, and therefore their contents will never be acknowledged and assimilated into the conscious.

This is, of course, a very seductive way of thinking, as it casts those incomprehensible stories to the realm of forgotten territory so that we can keep on believing that we can control our environment and destiny and face obstacles in life with deliberation, thought, and a mind that is not intruded upon by continuous, insensible nocturnal thoughts. This attitude is the result of the present unbearable dominance of intellectualism that neglects research into the soul and unconscious, despite the "psychosomatic and holistic" terminology used in health practices that hardly bother with investigating the other world, the unconscious. The unconscious is constantly forced into the background by the proclaimed scientific progress made by dissecting man, piece by piece, obliterating our wholeness. Such one-sidedness is not scientific, but rather a mark of barbarism, as it reduces man to a mere machine. As much as physicians claim, when their tools fail to resolve the physical dis-ease (whatever its name), "You might outgrow it," such "outgrowing" of psychic suppressed complexes—which are repressed emotional themes such as an inferiority complex, power complex, authority complex, Oedipus complex, father-complex, etc.—never will occur, but the possessor will instead be tortured by them at inopportune and unexpected moments, due to their autonomous character. The unconscious has a life of its own.

Along with doctors, both the average and the highly

educated person seem to be convinced that the unconscious should be left alone, and should only be used in fairy tales to amuse our children or, as in the past, before technology took over, as the chief form of wintertime entertainment or at the campfire in the summer to chase the ghosts away! This often reflects a repulsive fear of something that is unknown, and best be left alone! But what we do not know is that if we keep on talking about our dreams, we reveal more about ourselves than we ever want to share with others, even with our trusted physician! Just like in investigations and interrogations into crime, the more the suspect talks, the more he betrays himself and becomes the Emperor without clothes, producing signs of an uneasy conscience. However, if we become more introspective, it will be easier to see that the unconscious is the real existence, while the conscious is a contrived Shangri-La, a paradise where we only think we are out of the turmoil and torment of life!

One of the reasons that we react so adversely to dreams is not only because they are so mysterious and disjointed—expressed in a foreign symbolic language speaking in images—but often, because they are ruthlessly honest and declare something about us or close loved ones that seems completely opposite our reality in life, at least as *we want to see it*, but obviously not as it *is*. They reveal harsh psychological and spiritual facts regarding our reality, and the ego must be strong enough to assimilate its content, hence the necessity of our insight; otherwise rejection and disbelief result. Take the example, for instance, of a woman who dreams about her "husband," who appears in her dream as a domineering, know-it-all opinioned being. In reality her spouse is an easy-going personality, admired by all who know him, quite the opposite of the person who appeared in her dream. It is, of course, normal that this woman easily casts aside the dream as pure nonsense, but what she fails to see is that the unconscious tried to convey something hidden to her regarding the real husband: that she puts him too high on a pedestal, and might become too dependent on him, inhibiting her personal path to individuation, her goals and desires. Or this dream might reveal something about *her*, by its apparent discrepancy. Indeed, as discussed further (see Chap. 12, "Animus"), every woman "carries a man inside her"; the masculine in her hides its existence in the animus, her "recessive maleness." This dream, following the rule of compensation (discussed later), is purposeful, stating something about her abnormal "maleness" or animus—that it is a dogmatic, steamrolling opinion maker, known to all her friends, and of course her husband, who are the direct subjects of its exerted power—but easily denied and set aside by the dreamer. This "firmness" suits her well in the life she desires—to live selfishly, according to her standards and opinions but without real love. Unbeknownst to her, the dream told her that her animus was in a deplorable state, creating obstructions and difficulties not only in her life, but especially in the life of others. So, do dreams offer the possessor a way to better health and quality of life?

A World in Service of Health and the Individuation Process, Belonging to the Dreamer Alone

The Greek philosopher Heraclitus of Ephesus (500 BC) declared that, "The waking have one world in common, but the sleeping turn aside each into a world of his own." While dream language is the universal language common to all people, apart from the collective part of dreams most are an *individual compensation* to a somewhat *distorted conscious situation*. Some people might complain, "I always have bad dreams, while my wife always dreams of vacation and pleasure." As much as we sometimes declare, "I had a bad dream," there is no such distinction between good and bad dreams, for if, and when, our dreams' messages can be assimilated, dreams will always be in service of health and wholeness. It is our non-acceptance and non-understanding of them, without a correct change in our conscious attitude, that will lead to recurrent nightmares (see Chap. 5, under "Recurrent Dreams"), as the Inner Therapist or the Guiding Self—the knower beyond his knowing—will never cease to work, holding an ever-fertile dialogue with the conscious, providing guidance throughout life without ever asking for payment. However, a person does pay a price when he refuses to listen to this free and often urgent advice of the inner workings of this being, as ignoring it is punishable with illness, accidents, bad relationships, neurosis, and even psychosis. Indeed, in dreams we can part from shame and common sense, as our dreams can be "infected" with the most vile, unnatural, irrational, and indecent things—even incest, or killing a beloved child.

More than one *Sepia* woman, often suffering from post-partum depression, has had such shocking dreams when she becomes separated from her feminine feelings while being over-whelmed by a sense of *too much duty and responsibility*, and stress or ailments from *emotional excitement* and *sexual excesses* (too many pregnancies). Even in the most noble and respectable person there seems to be a lawless wild beast peering out in sleep, as good never exists without evil. We should never forget that a dream speaks primarily to the dreamer, to his own inner psychic life, and *each of the figures in the dream represent some part of his being.* It was Jung's genius who introduced those different aspects with the names of persona, anima, animus, and shadow, some of the most occurring archetypes in dreams. The dreamer must ask himself about whomever appears in his dream, known family members or unknown figures: "What part of me is like this person?" (The term for this is *projection*, to be explained further.) And, "What does this figure represent in my life?" Only when these images are assimilated in term of their relevance to the patient's psychological conscious life situation, will they become more helpful to the dreamer in his life journey. Important to remember, is that if no part of the dream's action applied to actual events or to the actual person in the dream, for instance a husband, friend, family member, etc., the dream is an *allegoric description* of the image qualities that actually belong to the dreamer. They were only projected onto the husband, friend, or family members, creating "ordinary" personal allegoric dreams, which are more frequent than archetypal ones, although interplay of archetypal and personal material is not uncommon.

Obviously, we live in a world where listening to our unconscious is not a favorite topic, as it might portray us as an antisocial and self-absorbed person, the opposite of what we project to the outside world. If we dare to follow the voice of the unconscious, listening to our dreams will eventually bear fruit. But often, in the process, we will discover that we need to do something we do not like at all. Seemingly worse, we will have to follow advice making us do things *others* don't like! Yet in every case, listening to the unconscious message will reveal not only how to improve ourselves, but also how to improve our relationships with others! Provided that we realize we are not projecting the image of the other person for a quality we possess but instead lack, the dream gives us the opportunity to improve ourselves. Or, the image may tell us genuinely something about the real character of that other person—objective information that would have eluded us was it not for the dream. Both interpretations, projection of an inner aspect of the dreamer himself, or true information about another person, are valid. We should take the unconscious seriously, something that requires honesty and courage of the dreamer—not the most common virtues of humanity!

Besides personal benefit, heeding our unconscious has another great effect: every single individual who dedicates his life to following his individuation path—*the search for wholeness and developing human awareness*, a process of continuous death and rebirth—unconsciously influences those around him. Such a person is on the road to a divine capacity for love and creation, to developing his reason and critical thinking, to having a sense of Self without feeling the need for artificial relatedness in status, race, or profession. This causes sparks to fly, as deeds always speak louder than words! As a Chinese Master expressed: "When the enlightened man is alone and thinks rightly, it can be heard a thousand miles away." Anything else leads to stagnation and regression! As much as we are exposed to catastrophes of fires, earthquakes, and hurricanes, the greatest danger comes from exposure to the elemental and primitive forces of our own psyche. But how to understand these dreams using a new language, the language of relative fixed symbols?

Relative Fixed Symbols

Dreams are the most accessible and honest way of investigating the contents of the unconscious. As Sigmund Freud said, "The interpretation of dreams is the *via regal*, or royal road, to knowledge of the unconscious activities of the mind." Dreams are the messenger/psychopomp and spontaneous product of the unconscious, and therefore, not unexpectedly, say things beyond our conscious comprehension. They are pure Nature, not a freak of Nature, not falsified by any conscious purpose, not controlled by a censor to conceal the real meaning of the dream from the ego (as Freud once claimed). Therefore, a dream always *means what it says* in the most genuine way. We must assume that a dream is just what it should be, no more, no less. If a dream presents a negative aspect about the dreamer, there is no reason to suppose that a positive aspect is intended, no matter how much one tries to distort its content towards a favorable light. A dream expresses facts about how we envision ourselves, others, and the world unconsciously, although obviously it does not *restate* exactly what happens in the reality of our life (except for parallel dreams, explained later). This is called *subjective* reality, as dreams restate what is "forgotten" in conscious life. As we will discover in the dream principles, the unconscious, through dreams, *presents a point of view which enlarges, completes, or compensates the conscious attitude*, offering us a wider lens by which to see our life differently. The dream supplies the missing elements that the ego is unaware of; its images are carriers of messages trying to enlighten us about facts we are unable to grasp with our rational mind. To be in contact with dreams offers the hope of altering our deformed ego-standpoint, in the light of a larger reality unknown to us.

A dream shines light on our *blind spots*, the forgotten elements of a conscious situation, revealing dormant qualities in our personality while putting the mirror in front of us and asking us to look at "the man in the glass," the real person as *we are*, not what we *desire to be* or what other people *want us to be*, so that we can become more complete as a true individual. However, the difficulty we encounter is that dreams do not have a *general* meaning and we cannot translate them as we would translate a text from one language to another—for instance, from English to Spanish. Dreams which are identical in content can have two different meanings for two different persons. Dreams speak in the language of *images, or symbols, archetypal images and allegory*, and the creation of symbols is the most important function of the unconscious. The unconscious forces humankind to learn a new language, not taught in regular schools but produced spontaneously in dreams, using the tricky and baffling language of symbols that appear over and over again in myths, fairy tales, religious stories, and works of art of every kind of people throughout history. According to a book of root words, "symbol" comes from the Greek *sym*, meaning "together," and *bolo*, literally "to throw or strike," and *bolus*, or "lump": "throwing or lumping things together."

It is the things thrown together that are *not fully understood* —unconscious elements, only partly conceivable—which can only be gleaned through the union or marriage of the conscious and unconscious, at which point the symbol ceases to exist as it becomes part of the consciousness. Symbols are primitive expressions of the unconscious, manifestations of the archetypes in this world, building blocks in the psychic structure of every human being and guidelines for the process of individuation. Indeed, as we will see in the *compensation rule* of dreams (explained later), these symbols can only be helpful and relevant when assimilated to the specific psychological and life situation of the dreamer. For one person, the same object, the moon for example, represents just that, the moon, a known entity or a sign, while for others it represents a feminine symbol, yin, feeling and receptivity-toned (even when it occurs in men), or it is the first place souls go after death—the place of departed souls. The moon can also bring up associations to lunacy and lunar rhythms. The main thing in interpretation is to try to find out what the symbol *means to the patient*. We can immediately understand that especially the intellectuals or the dominant conscious thinking types, cut off from the figurative language of their psyche and from the rest of their conscious functions (especially feeling first, and intuition second), have the most difficulties in deciphering their dreams, while the primitive man puts less distance between his conscious and unconscious life, using almost equally his four conscious functions (see Chap. 8). The more civilized man is less inclined to follow his instincts and the message of his dreams.

What most of us underestimate is that whenever we share a dream, we are revealing more about ourselves than we ever imagine, and that the unconscious is a constant guide and wise adviser to our conscious life. We should realize that we will achieve a serene and happy life only when we learn to live with a world that is united, made whole, by our conscious and unconscious. To the homeopath or physician who studied this universal language, the real person behind the mirror appears—the one that freely and without hesitation divulges everything, especially the dark side the healer wants to know in order to attain a true cure on every level. In dreams we can commit the worst crimes, violence, and murder—even against our loved ones, with complete indifference and without remorse. Dreams do not use any of the disguises we usually wear in the conscious world, and they can reveal to us and our therapist something about our inner Self. So rather than considering dreams fantasy or superstition, this unique universal language—common to all races since the start of time—divulges the deepest genuine psychological and physiological facts, dressed in the cryptic language of symbols.

The only problem is that these symbols are *not* universal, because a dream in most cases is an unconscious reaction to a conscious *individual* situation. Individuality is and should be a sacred word in any medical science: in homeopathy, it is a hallmark feature and principle, and therefore interpretation of dreams, deeply tied to individuality, must be and is easily integrated into the homeopathic science and art. It is plain foolishness to believe in the ready-made, systematic guides of dream interpretation found in bookstores, *as no dream symbol can be separated from the individual who dreams it.* Dreams cannot be decoded by a glossary found in "dream dictionaries." The latter are worthless, as the physician must always inquire about the patient's present conscious situation so as not to violate the individuality principle well-known to homeopaths. Symbols are called "relatively fixed" because their meaning in a dream is *not absolute*: the meaning of the same dream symbol is not necessarily the same for different people, not even for the same person at different stages in his life. Indeed, this enigmatic language, which has great diagnostic and prognostic value, can take on a totally different meaning in the same person if, for instance, it speaks through dreams before puberty, during puberty, or in middle age. No dream-symbol has a fixed meaning in every detail, but it is possible to have frequently occurring symbols with a *general* meaning. The specific meaning of symbols will always be determined by the dreamer's associations, explanations, and amplifications (explained later).

There can also be more than one meaning for the same image appearing in a person's dream. For instance, "flying" in a dream might be related to gaining freedom in a prisoner-like *Staphysagria* marriage, or might reflect a person who tried to fly on his own "wings" or power—an act of foolishness when he overestimates his capacities and ambitions in life, often leading to injuries, mishaps, and even death. It is evident that no interpretation of dreams can take place without knowledge of the dreamer's conscious situation, just as we cannot give a homeopathic remedy for a symptom without knowing the patient's life story and mental/emotional/physical state (Aphorisms 5 and 7). There is a continuous exchange between our unconscious and conscious, in which the unconscious, through dream symbols, carries important messages with sage advice from the instinctive, natural part of our mind to the rational part, in order to illuminate the unknown and dark spots of our consciousness.

There are a great many relatively fixed symbols, and understanding them requires common sense and intelligence—it is not a mechanical system, and depends also on the erudition of the dreamer; on how much he is interested in philosophy (from the Greek *phileo*, or "to love," and *sophia*, or "wisdom"), as well as psychology, folklore, mythology, archeology, religion, alchemy, philology (the study of language), and history. It can happen that dream symbols can be too complicated to initially understand. All we can do then is wait for a further unveiling in the next dream to get more clarification as is shown in series of dreams. Above all, dream symbolism always has a personal, individual character and needs to be clarified by the dreamer's association to the image, to *what the image makes him think of* (discussed further in this chapter, see "Association and Amplification"). The dreamer's collaboration (following our homeopathic law of individuality) is essential if we want to give a decent and more scientific explanation of the dream, otherwise it is just sophisticated guesswork! And if this was not challenging enough already, there always seems to be a positive as well as a negative meaning of these relative fixed symbols. How to navigate this?

Positive and Negative Meaning (Duality) of Relative Fixed Symbols

Opposites cannot be put in separate watertight compartments: as it is above, so it is below; as man can be filled with virtues, there is always the companion component of vices, the latter ones more contagious than the former ones as they infect by contact. Almost all the symbols are capable of a positive as well as a negative meaning, and more than one meaning, and hence are called *relative* fixed symbols. Let us consider some relative fixed symbols.

Take the example of the *Mother* symbol. Positively, it is connected to nourishment and fertility—the nourishing Mother Earth, protection, reciprocated love, trust, and the womb that creates life, the Great Goddess. Also gardens, still waters, a country, the universe, and any circle (the most perfect geometric figure, the protection when children draw a magic circle in which they feel safe) are examples of this nourishing Mother archetype, the Divine Mother or Mother of Compassion and the counterpart of the "wise old man," the image of the animus and the Father (see Chap. 13). Mother refers also to the place of origin, and to Nature, the womb, the unconscious, our instinctive life, and the vessel that carries and nourishes.

But all archetypes are ambivalent! As much as they can be

white magic, they can also be black magic; they can work as both good and bad. There is the nourishing *Calcarea* mother (white magic), as opposed to the rigid, rules-oriented mother, the Terrible Mother or *Kali carbonicum* mother who has the *Delusion, an abyss is behind her*, reflecting her great anticipation anxiety. In dream language, "abyss" refers to the hidden, the darkness, and the world of the dead. This negative devouring Mother archetype or sarcophagus (representing a negative anima symbol which means "carnivore"), *Kali-c* becomes a witch, a dragon, or an ogress clipping the wings of her children, holding her children in utero, smothering the life out of her family, and preventing them from building their own ego (black magic). There is also the Kali god in India, the "all" god, as it has positive and negative aspects, loving *and* destructive. Archetypal figures always contain a duality—two sides of the same coin so to speak: a side pointing upwards (favorable), and a side that points downwards (unfavorable). The dreamer needs to decide if the archetypal image in his dream carries a positive or negative sign in order to know the role it plays in his life.

There is also the Black Virgin Mary, symbol of power, passion, and majesty, the opposite aspect to the traditional Madonna's motherhood or tender maternity. While ploughing in the fields, the infamous Rasputin saw the vision of the Black Virgin Mary, which sent him away on his journey, a wandering pilgrim trying to find his soul. As history has shown, this was with mixed results: after being initiated into the Khlysty, Rasputin had exceptional religious qualities that were offset by his demonic sexual appetites. These opposite aspects, embodied by Rasputin, were reflected within the Khlysty doctrine that each person was the reincarnation of God and therefore they should love and worship each other. These images are symbolic of different psychological situations (the individuality law in homeopathy).

Dreaming of a *snake* may have different meanings from one

person to another. Among the archetypal and recurrent animal figures, the serpent occupies a unique and ambivalent place and can be found in hundreds of dreams. In some regards, it is the symbol for supreme wisdom and the great healer or redeemer. On the other hand, it is the tempter of evil, to poison—the devil himself. Devil comes from the Greek *Diabolo*, or *Di*, meaning "across," and *bolo*, meaning "to throw" (throwing something like an obstacle across our path and creating problems). The snake is possibly also the symbol of healing/spiritual awakening, resurrection and self-renewal, or the shedding of old skin or persona. It can stand for femaleness, the darkness, night, yin, death, sexuality, and the instinctual knowledge of irrational nature and fear—an anxiety-provoking symbol. Whenever a snake appears in dreams, it symbolizes a piece of the instinctive psychology in us, something of tremendous and fiery power. It represents the vital and the instinctual stirring in us, our unconscious dark side. The serpent in Oriental psychology symbolizes the treasure of wisdom. It can also be a symbol of danger, of being caught in its coils, swallowed, or poisoned, representing the demonic-evil. A snake is also an anxiety symbol; monkeys and horses, for instance, are instinctively afraid of snakes. When a snake appears at the sickbed in dreams it can indicate foreboding of death. The snake's duality is also seen in the caduceus of MDs,[2] the Hermes psychopomp, where the two natures unite—*Sol* and *Luna*, symbols for man and woman. Analoguous to this, the greatest poisons in homeopathy are the greatest healers (*Arsenicum* and *Lachesis* being just two examples).

Animals in general, representing the instinctive life, are often helpers in dreams, and it pays off to listen to what they do or say, but the dark side is also present, as they can be tricksters, leading us astray.

When a *child/baby* appears in a dream, the same duality can be perceived (good/bad), and the physician needs to see what role this archetype plays in the patient's dream. It can refer to the inner child of the dreamer, to everything that is unfinished, just started or in need of growth, a symbol par excellence of the reborn psyche, evolving to independence, reflecting the death of the infantile personality and the rising of the adult personality. It can point to the process of becoming a new person, a renewal and rebirth; something new has been born, a new value, new attitudes—paving the way for a future change of personality, which is the meaning of the eternal child or the Savior. As the alchemists say, "No new life can arise without the death of the old one." Positively, this points to potentialities and possibilities in the dreamer's developing personality, to whatever has great possibility to grow and be fulfilled in the dreamer's life. A work in progress! Negatively, it points to *immaturity or infantilism*. The "land of childhood" can remain an enduring source of childish inclinations and impulses, often common to the *Calc-c* type. Such a person can behave in life as though everything will always remain the same, to which exasperated friends and family might ask, "When will he/she grow up?" Again, whichever of the two possibilities it is, depends on the patient's associations and amplifications.

A *young* person appearing in a dream refers to a person who has not lived, an unlived life, one who has not developed enough yet or is inexperienced. Always ask the *approximate age* of the child in the dream. A 3-year-old child in a dream may relate to some experience of the dreamer at age 3, or it may reflect something that started three years before the dream appeared. Ask also the sex of the child: a little girl appearing in a dream of a man might indicate a new aspect of the anima (see Chap. 11), and similarly a little boy in a woman's dream, a new aspect of the animus. *Death* of a child in a dream suggests that developmental possibilities have already been destroyed and little personal growth can be expected.

Not all symbols are of a personal nature; some seem to be

present in the collectivity of humanity. What are some common examples of this, and how to use them?

Symbols of a Collective Nature

Dream images or symbols that are not of an individual but of a *collective* nature, a universal element, can be translated *without* associations and amplifications, through symbolism only, without having to increase the content of the dream. When we say about a woman, "She is a snake," or "a witch," we all know what it means. As mentioned before, a serpent is the source of healing, wisdom, and power of transformation ("shedding the old skin") and immortality in many cultures, but is also a dangerous, devilish tempter in the Old Testament. As the sayings go, "I am surrounded by snakes," and "She speaks with a forked tongue," expressing the dual personality we often find in such a person (*will, two wills, feels as he had*). If we say about a person, "He is a fox," we all know we refer to a cunning trickster and false guide in many fairy tales, but also to an imposter in real life. When we state, "He fights like a lion," a symbol for power, courage, and ferocity is meant. Here again, we use symbolic language that does not need further amplification to understand its meaning, as the lion is the king of the jungle, feared by all. Following the rule of compensation, such interpretation will give us some opinion of the dreamer's momentary psychic situation. ("Compensation" is derived from the Latin verb *compensare*, or "to offset or counterbalance, to stabilize or weigh" one thing against the other.)

Another collective symbol is the owl, which stands for the bird of Minerva, the goddess of wisdom. It is interesting to note that in other cultures, "wisdom" is associated with different animals. For the native Africans and Hindus, the elephant is considered the wisest being, ahead of humans. For the Native American Indians, an eagle (the chief had a single feather in his hair), or a bear were symbolic for wisdom. The appearance of animals in dreams always refers to instinctual drives that want to reach consciousness, bringing with it an important message for the dreamer.

Such general images in a dream are very important for children's dreams where we have few or no associations. Even adults can have dreams without associations, dreams that are very difficult to understand since (almost always) the information might lie in a piece of mythology or alchemy. It is here that interpretation of relative fixed symbols is necessary. It is important not to get to an interpretation through speculation and guessing; *knowledge of the dreamer's* ***conscious content*** *is a must.* After all, the dreamer does not manipulate his dreams as he sleeps; the dream is just presented to him, and nothing in his dream is forged or incorrect. Even as every individual is different from any other, the scientific thinker will always find some general principles and laws in the manifoldness of individuals. In order to understand the homeostasis,[3] or psychological equilibrium, the revolving door between conscious and unconscious, we need to clarify the *rule of compensation*, which is the basis of a psychic self-regulating system. What is the rule of compensation which produces the general purpose of dreams and makes them more intelligible?

Rule of Compensation and General Purpose of Dreams

TCM already depicted humans 5,000 years ago as a picture of yin and yang duality: not only in their character but in every aspect of their life. There is also day and night, white and black, rationalism versus empiricism, intellectualism versus sensationalism, idealism versus materialism, optimism versus pessimism, and the persona versus the shadow (see Chap. 10). We see this same duality in homeopathic portraits, like the fastidious and messy *Sulphur*, or the religious fanatic and agnostic *Lachesis*. Therefore, we should not be surprised that the language of day and night is not only entirely different, but that both are of equal importance in our life. The rational thought of conscious life (Logos) contrasts with the autistic thinking of the unconscious or the dream language. All of us are at least bilingual: we shift necessarily from one language to another when we put our heads on our pillow. And no doubt, without shifting over to the enigmatic language of dreams, our emotional and physical well-being can be disturbed. This interchange of language safeguards us from descending into the hell of psychosis, and moreover, makes life a revolving door so homeostasis can be achieved. Remember, *the main dream purpose is an unconscious compensatory act towards an individual conscious situation*. Dreams are windows to allow us to look in, to see what is going on continuously in the unconscious.

While most dreams are compensatory, other dreams function in a different way, such as *prospective* dreams, those that anticipate a psychological development, extra-sensorially, and predict future events. But as a rule, as an act of psychic self-regulation, every one-sidedness, challenge, and maladjustment or delusion in conscious life is compensated in dreams. Anxieties, worries, and fears of the day often find appeasement in dreams, a self-healing force that plays the role of the inner hidden physician, one that always is on duty to resolve the conflict situation between the unconscious and consciousness! When an individual is suppressed and dominated in his/her conscious life (e.g., *Staphysagria*), her world built on a back flayed by whips, dreams often turn to a healing compensatory act. Such dreams might reflect being able to run away, to fight a battle, to jump, to climb, and even to fly with wings that seem to provide unexpected ways of escaping her life as a serf. Her actions in dreams are spurred by the daily bully or oppressor in real life and are the first sign that she longs to become an independent person instead of the unjustly accused slave she presently is.

A sense of relief can be produced when symbols are understood, bringing hints of advice and help to many problems in our life ("sleeping on the problem" as we say). By turning towards dreams and the unconscious, we can find out more about our life in order to make fewer mistakes. Even if that genius carpet weaver is at work within us every night, his patterns are so fantastically subtle that we struggle to find the meaning of it all. However, the purpose becomes somewhat clearer when we take into account the homeostatic action of the dream world. As Jung wrote in *Dreams*:

> The more one-sighted the conscious attitude and the more it deviates from the optimum possibilities of life, the greater becomes the possibility that vivid dreams with a strongly contrasting but purposefully compensating content will appear as an expression of the self-regulation of the psyche, establishing a psychological balance. (1974, p. 39)

The dream is an urgent message from the unconscious telling the dreamer to change his conscious attitude, as the unconscious is in complete rebellion against the values of the conscious. If the conscious attitude is excessively distorted in one direction, as seen in an over-valuation or inflation of ego-consciousness (delusions of grandeur)—often because the dominant conscious function forms the essence of the ego (see Chap. 9)—the unconscious may express in dreams an equally exaggerated, but opposite compensatory tendency.

The secret to psychological health is to use the unconscious as a helper. If we put ourselves consciously too low (the positive side of the shadow, see Chap. 10), the unconscious will lift us. Whenever we put ourselves too high—as observed in delusions of grandeur and psychic inflation—the unconscious will pull us down. This pair of opposites, the conscious and unconscious, need to come to a fruitful cooperation and a happy marriage, a continuous infinite dialogue, as the dictatorship of either one will lead inevitably to a revolution, resulting in many neuroses and psychoses. Compensation through dreams shows the corrective, healing, and directive expressions provided by the unconscious and its messenger, dreams, that show their purposeful nature in service of health and life itself.

I can assure you that once people know you have wandered onto the slippery road of dream interpretation, the next question will be, "I wonder if you can explain to me this dream I had yesterday?" The wise homeopath should not fall into the pit of haughtiness and inflation, ready to demonstrate his newly discovered, immature knowledge, by jumping on such an occasion, especially if it is a single dream, and worse, not knowing anything regarding that person's individual conscious history. Only those blinded by delusions of grandeur could not resist such a request, as the danger of deception and suggestion is too great!

Compensation and *complementation* are overlapping concepts. Both provide the elements that make up the dream content, the story of the dream. As mentioned above, compensation refers to the balancing correction of the extreme one-sidedness of the conscious position and viewpoints: all the excluded, often ugly parts in the conscious will show up in the unconscious, providing material to come back as a return-to-sender through dreams. Time to open those cast away letters, to let them guide our life in a different direction! Less compensation is needed by the dream if the conscious attitude has a position near the middle of the life situation or expresses a correct attitude. Complementation, on the other hand, adds different missing pieces, *not necessarily the polar-opposites* of the conscious attitude, but as a goal to complete or widen our view of the problem posed by the dream. The functions of both compensation and complementation (association and amplification) serve to correct our blind spots, the parts that our conscious wants to forget. When the conscious attitude of the dreamer is appropriate to his outer adaptation, to the degree of realization of his personality development, the dream will usually appear more gently compensatory, offering *slight* corrections to his conscious position. If his conscious attitude is ill-adapted to his objective situation or to his subjective needs, or both (we all at some point have illusions going to delusions), then his dreams appear to have a *guiding prospective function.* If the conscious attitude is correct, the dream may further emphasize the conscious attitude, or help the individual in his individuation process, or, most often, no dream is necessary as the situation is stated correctly.

Besides compensation in dreams as an expression of psychic activity seeking equilibrium, most people try (albeit with varying success) to live out their compensation. In order to stay in the distorted, one-sided, exaggerated conscious state, we must be able to find the opportunity in which we can live out our cyber delusion of grandiosity. If we or our family can maintain the high financial standards and privileges attached to our desired high position, we may be lucky enough to live out our life in complete ignorant bliss, having survived a rather frail balance of which we were totally ignorant of. Here we think of *Platina* with the *Delusion, others are small entering the room while she is great.* Any admiring glance fails to stir *Platina's* heart or cause her to drop her eyes. What's one more admiring look? It does not mean much to her, except for the pleasing thought, "I was outstanding today, as usual." *Platina* is not alone in such an attitude, as she has company in other characters seen in homeopathic portraits.

What is another example of an outspoken, one-sided conscious situation?

Example of a One-Sided Attitude of the Conscious

It should come as no surprise that most people refuse to listen to their dreams when it comes to guiding their life. The result will be a *recurrence* of these dreams (see Chap. 5), and unfortunately, as no change is made in the lifestyle and psyche of the dreamer, illness is always apt to call his attention to the fact that a change in his life *is* needed. For an illustration of the compensatory action of dreams aimed at a need of change towards an exaggerated individual conscious situation, *Lycopodium* is a perfect example, contrasting his outspoken one-sided conscious attitude (persona) with his correcting opposite irrational unconscious or shadow side. A *Lycopodium* guy may look to his working world as a marvel, but his wife, children, and servants see nothing marvelous about him, suffering under his dictatorship of blunt talk, full of contempt and void of true love and empathy, all tumult and baseness within (*contemptuous and hard for subordinates and agreeable, pleasant to superiors or people he has to fear*). He usually treats his wife with the unthinking chauvinism of a man totally unaware of an alternative. He looks like an emotional guy: when being thanked for a certain "benevolent" deed (one most likely beneficial for him), he is sometimes so overcome by a rush of tender affection that his eyes well up with tears (*weeping when thanked*). Yet his outward show does not correspond to his inward disposition, as he sits on the lofty throne he desires. *Lycopodium* always overcompensates, as he seeks power (*love of power*), wealth (*desires to be considered rich*), or a form of sovereignty over others (*dictatorial, speaks with a voice of command*). What he lacks within (*self-confidence, lack of character*), he seeks in the outer world.

Although many might consider him a powerful person, himself included, the reality is that he has no power over himself. From the ill-governed intensity of his opinions and convictions (*speaking with a voice of command*), he makes certain that he will not be called into question (*intolerant of contradiction*). He can be irascible when contradicted, often leading to a violent quarrel (*anger from contradiction and about former vexations; mania in rage*), as this, to him, is a mortal injury (*offended easily; takes everything in bad part*). He speaks to most people with great contempt, his nose in the air, as he harangues loudly and unsparingly—assuming an air of command and imposing his arrogance—so that anyone who obeys him wants to hit him. He can be firm and determined, even if led astray by a smoldering long-lasting emotion, and therefore, blindly and obstinately, holds to his opinions (*obstinate*) even when they are sustained by illogical reasons, convinced he is immutably right, the axiom for which he lives (*intolerant to contradiction*). Although considered an intelligent person, his is more like a "Swiss-cheese intelligence," characterized by a multitude of holes when it comes to the ability to integrate his auxiliary conscious functions, while conducting his life solely by his dominant thinking conscious function. This might serve him well in his profession to some extent, usually through power, conviction, and leadership, but he utterly fails outside of that environment—with his family and other social relationships. He is not conscious of the needs and feelings of others who he considers his subordinates, and worse, unimportant entities (*contemptuous, hard for subordinates and agreeable, pleasant to superiors or people he has to fear*). He tends to forget if not outright abandon his children (*forsakes his own children*), not from malice but simply because his agenda does not include them, as it is only filled with inward ambition and *love of power.*

For Nietzsche, the three worst curses or vices of humankind were *voluptuousness, passion for power,* and *selfishness.* He spoke unconsciously of *Lycopodium*, the prototype of those vices! To some degree everyone needs a healthy dose of the three vices to survive in this world, but *Lycopodium identifies* with them. In *Lycopodium's* case, unconscious inferiority tallies with conscious megalomania, a cocky ego hypertrophy and an appearance to be bold. Everything that is lacking in his conscious is present in excess in his unconscious mind—a fatal mistake preventing true changes in his character—but a dream will remind him of what he is ignoring in his conscious. His love for power and dominance sweeps him away on a four-horse chariot beyond the ends of the earth, a risky voyage to unknown shores, doomed to failure at some point—although he hopes to live a joyous life, in the manner of Turkish fashion, reclining on downy cushions. *Lycopodium* does not seek the epicurean pursuit of pleasure, restrained and responsible, but rather grotesque self-indulgence based on power and sexual conquests (*libertinism*), part of his fabric of everyday life. But for most *Lycopodium* persons such an attitude brings nothing but a sense of hidden insecurity, performance anxieties, and stressful situations (*irresolution in action; undertakes many things, perseveres in nothing*), while hiding a face of *low self-confidence* under the veneer of harshness and contempt (*contemptuous, hard for subordinates and agreeable to superiors or people he has to fear*). For *Lycopodium*, pleasure seeking is a code name for vice.

This lack of insight into *Lycopodium's* sickness points to a neurotic character trait rather than a simple neurotic trait. *His conscious megalomania and desire for power is balanced by an unconscious compensatory inferiority. Lycopodium* wants power so much (*love of power*) simply because he knows he lacks internal strength (*lack of character*), and so, he needs power to be the person he purports to be. The lower his self-esteem and confidence, the more he desires and insists on being a leader; instead of acknowledging his weakness, he reacts with *defiance,* which is nothing but childish obstinacy. Such a person forgets that where power rules, there is no love, and where love rules, power is not needed. Sadly, the moment a situation demands responsibility, commitment, forming a permanent relationship in marriage (*the idea of marriage seems unendurable*), starting a new job, or taking care of his children, his true colors come through. He has a *fear of undertaking something* and *he flees from his children; forsakes his own children* and has *aversion to domestic duty* and *to being kept in his house.* Clearly, *Lycopodium*, lacking patience and insight because of his strong protective armor and mask, is unconscious of what he is doing, of the real human values he is destroying through his irresponsibility, leading to an inability to achieve a corresponding fulfillment of life. When he comes home to his family, *Lycopodium* drops the mask and his role as actor ends.

Let's examine further *Lycopodium's* conscious attitude contrasting with his unconscious, which eventually will lead to *reductive* dreams, a needed guideline and compensation for his megalomaniac nature. "Reductive" comes from the Latin *Reductio at primum figuram,* meaning "Reduce to the first figure," or going to the root of the problem, often going back to childhood where an abnormal link or complex with one of the parents can be established (*un fils-à-papa*, or "a mama's boy," linked to a domineering father or mother). *Lycopodium* has *dreams of his boat foundering,* expressing failure to reach his port of call, aptly found in the rubric *fear, of being unable to reach his destination.* Such a dream comes as a shock to this person's system, as in his created conscious world he has built up only an image of success and confidence, having rarely not succeeded in what he has proposed to himself: becoming CEO of a company, a successful business man, or a professional man such as a lawyer, physician, or politician. But "not reaching his destination," expressed by his dream of his boat foundering as well as recurrent dreams of *failures in exams,* refers to not reaching the intention to become a more complete human. He is not someone who has never stopped trying to become more enlightened to move towards what everyone should aim for: self-realization as a result of listening to his inner voice, setting aside conventionalism and conformism (soulless mechanisms with their collective seductions and necessities). *Lycopodium* might have a hard skin in business and relationships, but in order to not get injured by the unconscious, he should be reminded that humility creates the most protective skin.

If there is one outstanding common characteristic among *Lycopodium* children and adults, it is the great *fear of failure*. Such a person does not like what he is not good at, and he attempts to control his fear by avoiding any field of activity in which he does not believe he has a reasonable chance of success. He sticks to topics with which he feels safe, and in the case of a *Lycopodium* child with ASD, to his preferred activities. This *fear of doing wrong*, and *everything will vanish* (fear of failure), and of being "unmasked" also produces some degree of competitiveness (*he employs every possible means to achieve his ambition*) and *suspicion* in *Lycopodium* (*Lyc.* is the strongest black type remedy for suspicion in *Synthesis*), since he is driven by a love of power. Of course, his reductive dreams, which mean "to reduce" his persona or lift the mask to expose himself, are the best possible gift that he can receive. This person needs to be shocked to even find the courage to change (with the homeopathic remedy assisting him in the process). If he is willing to listen, and when he is finally unstuck and can make strides on his individuation path, such dreams can become a life changer. I said, "If he is willing to listen," not an easy task for such a thinking person. Indeed, what induces man to choose his own way is "vocation," from the Latin *vocare*, or "to call upon or summon," and *vox*, or "voice," "to be called upon by an inner voice," a voice that transcends materialism, avarice, and egotism, a difficult project for someone who has *love of power.* But *Lycopodium* is intelligent, *deceitful*, and has *a disposition to contradict*, ignoring "nonsensical" dreams unless a visible physical ailment appears. In the first place, he will consult a physician for sexual problems, part of his power image or persona.

His CD, *everything will vanish*, takes on special meaning in his sexual relationships, where he is king of one-night stands and uncommitted sex due to his expectation of immediate pleasure and gratification. Because of sexual desires and thoughts, the married *Lycopodium* is the most prone to unfaithfulness in his relationship, being a sort of hunter like *Medorrhinum*. For both remedies, the expression of this Don Juanism is nothing but a mother-complex in which they seek their mother in every woman they meet. *Lycopodium's* rather debauched sexual lifestyle eventually leads to sexual insecurity. *Lycopodium* is so self-absorbed and his powers of self-observation so acute ("Did I perform like a great conqueror? Was I the great lover?"), that he starts any conquest with the fear of not being able to succeed (*fear he will not reach his destination*). Eventually this anticipation anxiety leads to the sexual performance failure for which *Lycopodium* is so well-known: *impotence, penis small and cold and relaxed; feeble erection, strong desire without being able to have an erection in old people; erections wanting after sexual excesses; erections wanting with his wife* (only remedy).

The *character* of compensation or the *necessary amount* of compensation is connected to the whole nature of the individual—his predominant miasmatic state or inborn fixed response pattern, constitution, temperament, and core delusion or cyber delusion (CD)! *Lycopodium* is mainly a sycotic/syphilitic remedy, choleric in nature, and has as a CD: *fear of doing wrong* and *everything will vanish*. It is always helpful when we set out to interpret a dream to ask: *"What conscious attitude does the dream compensate?"* But which attitude to choose when different possibilities of interpretation present themselves, as there are several possible explanations for one symbol appearing in a dream? Following the rule of compensation, the one to be chosen is the one that is *most opposed to the dreamer's conscious position*. It is clear in the case of *Lycopodium* that, although saddled with an inflated persona, he will be pestered by recurrent dreams of failure: failure in exams, or trying to fly, or to reach heights which he cannot conquer.

To bring further understanding of dreams, numbers appearing in dreams have specific relative symbolic interpretations. It is worth our time to examine this topic closely.

Numbers Appearing in Dreams

The number in a dream always has a special meaning. When numbers appear in a dream (with no mythological meaning) we may ask if they stand for years or months. When a precise age of the dreamer or a person in the dream is mentioned (e.g., 7 months old), we do well to ask the dreamer to look back seven months to see what happened in his conscious life. For another example, if a dreamer dreams of a 2-year-old child, the analysand/dreamer needs to investigate the ever-important subjective associations he might have, and think what happened two years ago: did he start something new in life, was there an important event in his life? If the dream puts the analysand at age 5, what happened at age 5 that now needs working through in the dream therapy. For instance, if someone dreams of the number 10, we can ask what happened 10 years ago, or what incident, event, or therapy started at that time. Our unconscious has an uncanny ability and relationship to time. When I need to go on a trip and take a plane at a certain time, I am amazed that I do not need to set my alarm (although I do, as a precaution), but never fail, I wake up minutes before the alarm goes off.

What does it mean to dream of *birth*? When we were born, one world of experience ended for us (the womb existence or unconscious life) and another began (the outside world, or conscious), going from paradise to reality. Birth in the dream has the same meaning: it is the beginning of a new life, a new attitude, a new project, leaving the old behind (the death of the old). It is a new step in the individuation process, and expression of huge changes in our life. When we dream of birth, we could also count back nine months and sometimes uncover a very important event that happened at that time. There is also a special meaning attached to specific numbers appearing in dreams. Let us examine each closely.

Special Numbers and Their Symbol

These numbers refer to the number of persons and/or animals appearing in dreams:

- **Number 1: One** stands for the unconscious, as everything is still unseparated.
- **Number 2:** A double image can mean two sides to the matter, good and bad, positive and negative, white and black, active and passive, a unification or reconciliation of the pairs of opposites or *Coniunctio*, a joining together of the male and female. **Two** is the number symbolizing the emergence of previously unconscious parts of the personality into consciousness. It is a marriage of conscious and unconscious; such a "marriage" is sometimes represented by a *hermaphrodite, a union of the strongest and most striking opposites.* **Two** is the absolute number of linear in general, and the experience of *linear time* particularly. Two points generate a straight line; a symbol of linear events moving steadily from the past into the future or from birth till death (two ends of a rope). The appearance of **two** in myth and dreams is often a reliable clue to the concern for the passage of time and its impact in the form of aging and the

inexorable approach of death. **Two** is also called the number of symmetry and balance.

- **Number 3:** Pythagoras called **three** the perfect number; it is the number of synthesis, the union of body, mind, and spirit. Also: the masculine *Holy Trinity*, the Christian deity or the active creative force made manifest by the three in Heaven (Father, Son, and Holy Ghost), a sacred number for western people (father, mother, and son). The fourth person in the spiritual realm is undoubtedly somewhere in the dark or unconscious, or as in TCM, in the yin, representing either the devil or merely the inferior conscious function (see Chap. 8). **Three** also stands for connection with *time*: the past, present, and future. **Three** is generally connected with the flow of movement, and with time, as there is no time without movement. The appearance of a clock in a dream represents the man's memento of the flow of all time. The number **three** also means that some fateful point has been reached and something unavoidable will happen. Doing the same thing three times is a magical trick to make something effective, and in many fairy tales it leads to a solution: there are often three steps and then a finale. **Three** leads to four, which leads to a result!

One of my patients, a very intellectual person who considered dream analysis and psychology worthless, had the following dream after a consultation.

Dream

I am standing on a pier and I am going to board a ship. On the narrow plank leading from the pier to the ship, I have to repeat the same thing three times, which I do. I wake up in a relaxed way.

Analysis

This is a clear message from the unconscious to board a ship (the Self) and go explore the unknown unconscious, leaving the conscious world (the pier) by walking on a plank (connection from the conscious with the unconscious). Repeating the same thing **three** times indeed led to a "solution," as he woke up more relaxed, and consequently, was then far more interested in telling me his dreams to see a relationship to his rigid conscious life.

- **Number 4 or the quaternarian symbol: Four** is the number of individuation; something is added to the Trinity. It is an ancient symbol of *completeness* or *wholeness*, the emergence of human consciousness or bringing order to chaos and representing individuation (four corners of the earth, the four cardinal points of the horizon, the four winds, the four directions of the compass, the four seasons, the four elements (Fire, Earth, Wood, Water), the four humors and temperaments (*melancholy* or sadness; *choleric* or anger/irritability; *sanguine*, the excitable optimistic person; and the *phlegmatic* or slow passive person), the four arms of the cross (the empirical basis that conquers the powers of darkness), the four phases of the moon, the four-petalled flower, and four-lobed leaf (also representing wholeness)). The number **four** also stands for the mystery of birth, life, death, and rebirth, and the four main colors of the rainbow: red, yellow, blue, and green. **Four** also stands for the **four conscious functions**: when four people appear in a dream, they refer to these functions. If during a dream initially three persons are present, and then a fourth comes out from nowhere (=unconscious), it indicates the appearance or integration of the primitive or archaic function of that person, since it was delegated to the unconscious—also known as the taboo function, the dangerous one to visit (see Chap. 8). The number **four** represents also the four gates of consciousness, in the East. The number **four** always expresses the coming into being of what is essentially human, the emergence of *human consciousness, transformation to the Self.* A mandala (a Sanskrit word for "magic circle") represents the Self and Perfection. In Buddhism, a mandala is part of its religious ritualistic paintings, always containing the square, the so-called courtyard of the monastery, with the four gates of consciousness portrayed by the colors red (feeling), blue (thinking), yellow (intuition), and green (sensation). A mandala is regarded as a symbol of the basic order of the psyche as a whole; based on a quaternary system and a general designation of the circle motif. When people draw a mandala that only has three corners it would mean that one function is lacking and could be called a "disturbed" mandala. Other symbols of the Self, a sign of wholeness, are a ball, a globe, a clock, a wheel, a coin, or a horoscope (all circular). Additionally, a garden with a fountain, the inner court of a castle, a square table, a four-petalled blue flower, a cross, and any quadripartite structure like a square house, all express the centering aspect of the Self from which comes strength and protection. Sometimes, instead of the number **four**, multiples of **four** appear: 8, 16, 32, etc. There is also the foursquare stone or the crystal, the philosophers' stone, and lapis lazuli, symbolizing the treasure at the center of the psyche. Symbols of the Self are also gold and a fortified city, among others. In the Apache Indian tribe, a boy had to accompany the warriors four times on the warpath before he could be admitted to the council. They believed firmly in the magic of the number **four**.

- **Number 5:** The number denoting relationship is **five** (whole of one person + someone else!). Sometimes **five** is called the number of marriage because it unites all the previous numbers: 1+4 and 2+3. It stands also for the five senses! **Five** represents the pentagram, or five-pointed star, that represents mankind, the link between heaven and earth, man with feet on the ground, arms reaching towards the horizon, and head in the skies. It is also an eternal symbol of supra-personal love.
- **Number 7: Seven** corresponds to the highest stage of illumination, the stage longed for and coveted, the highest stage of the process of integration before the enlightenment from the collective unconscious can start. It symbolizes the process of individual transformation and the complete realization of oneself (*self-actualization*), a process reached by very few people. It signifies completeness and mystic unity and fulfillment. A second meaning for the number **seven** is *time for a change*: "the seven-year itch"! The relevance of **seven** to time also goes back to the seven lunar days, lunar time being natural time, used in primitive cultures.
- **Number 9: Nine** is the number of Mothers, the world of mothers, or the collective unconscious, on

account of the nine months of pregnancy. It is also a magic number representing the perfect form of Trinity in its threefold elevation.

- **Multiplicity:** When in dreams a great number of animals or people appear, this is characteristic of unconscious life processes, and the more unconscious a process takes place in a person, the stronger it is dissolved and fragmented into a mass, often indicating a dissolution or organic problem in the person. Of course, it can also indicate the infection and contagion we can experience when we are swept up by the emotion of the masses, like at a sport event, where one is dissolved as an individual and becomes easily part of the mass "hysteria." It also may convey a *collective* dream, a message and problem common to humanity, reflecting a universal problem linked to humankind, not just to the dreamer but belonging to the collective unconscious, what Freud called the super-ego.

While we have mainly contemplated dreams based on the compensation rule, there are also dreams where *no compensation* takes place. They are called parallel dreams. How do they present?

Parallel Dreams

While most dreams take a compensatory stand towards the conscious attitude, parallel dreams seem to be a mere repetition of preceding events of the day or days before. These account for most children's dreams. But they can certainly occur in adults too, especially in response to a shock or event that causes psychic trauma such as the 9/11 event. These dreams, obviously, are not compensations but are essentially a *reproduction* of traumatic experiences. Unfortunately, as is the case in the 9/11 event, these dreams can roam in the unconscious for quite some time as news media bring back the traumatic stimulus every year, which is horrific and harmful for *Calc-carb* personalities and others who are sensitive to *hearing bad news* (*Staphysagria, Lachesis, Ignatia,* and *Phosphorus* to name a few).

To study dream analysis in further depth, beyond relative fixed symbols one must understand the terms **association** and **amplification**, indispensable tools to better understand the carpet weaver of the night.

Association and Amplification: More Understanding of Dreams

Contrary to Freud, who was more an obsessive rationalist, Jung did not use *free association*: starting with object X and then letting the topic go to Y-Z-A-B, etc., thereby being far removed from the starting topic, X, at the end—in other words gliding from one association to another, without regard for the initial idea or concept, leading to the discovery of some complex not usually represented in the dream and leading the therapist too far away to tell accurately what the dream conveys. More than once, Jung had to tell his patients, and even his students, "stick to the dream image," do not fall into the mass of free association (which points to emotional thoughts unconsciously captivated in the mind), excluding the irrelevant ideas that the dream image might bring forth. Otherwise, at the end we are stuck with a heap of free associations that have nothing to do with the original dream theme.

Although Jung still refers to the dreamer's associations *only* (not his or whoever does the analysis!), these meaningful associations and connections are the easiest to obtain, are of paramount importance, and refer to anything that can come to the dreamer's mind—notions, memories, or reactions (rational or irrational) he might have when thinking of the dream image. This is analogous to what the homeopath investigates to find the essential background of his patient and the real psychological significance (the essential rubric) on a thought, emotion, or reaction, by continually asking, "Why?" and "For what purpose?" Similarly, the dream therapist must continue to ask: "And what else does this image make you think of? How do you see this? What makes you think of this person, and what is noteworthy and peculiar about him or her? What ideas do you associate with this image? What emotions does it evoke in you? Where have you seen or heard this? What occurs to you in connection with this image, what comes to mind?"

If this line of questioning does not immediately ring a bell, the therapist can ask the dreamer to keep the dream image in his mind for the next few days, to see if possible revealing associations to this image appear. It is of utmost importance to know what an image or symbol really means for the patient. When parents appear in the dream, the dreamer's conscious consideration must be given to these images, and the way they appeared to the dreamer, what role they played in his life, and their positive and negative qualities influencing his conscious life. This list of questions should continue until there are no further patient's associations found, and then at that point, these associations reveal their psychological background and their possible origin in certain memories of the past. When the patient suddenly claims that he has no associations at all, or no further associations to that one single image, the possibility is that the therapist touched on the nucleus of the patient's suffering, on the constellation of his cyber delusion, which sometimes provokes mental inhibition so that no further associations can be found from the dreamer.

Make sure that if the dream image is a "cow," then "What else makes you think of this?"—the next association always has to refer to "cow," *not straying* from it, always coming back to the image of the cow! When the dream's investigation continues, the resurrection of *all the associated memories pertaining to each element* in the dream is required to get a "full translation" of the dream, in order to be able to explain the main points of the dream. Personal associations of the dreamer also help to shine light on his blind spots, even when the dream content has a paucity of information—in other words, is a dream of which only a few fragments are remembered. The therapist should not dismiss out-of-hand such a "trivial" dream, but rather should continue to ask questions probing for a deeper meaning: *"Why and for what reason?"* (Again, those two key questions we always ask in the homeopathic process to find the exact rubric for a case, are also helpful in dream analysis.) These snippets lead to further discovery, as they always reveal more of the dreamer's character and situation.

Further understanding of the dream can be obtained by first putting the dreamer's *amplifications* into the context for each of the images appearing in the dream. Amplification is derived from the Latin *amplus*, or "spacious, increase," and *facere*, or "to make," so amplification is "making more space" or enlarging/completing/expanding the dream content through the collection of a quantity of parallels. This process of elaboration is amplifying an existing image until it becomes more visible, by bringing the patient back repeatedly to the *actual* image. It is an expansion, a conscious enrichment when looking at archetypal parallels for a deeper understanding of the dream symbols. It is enlarging the dream's personal context with parallel and corresponding motifs from myths, fairy tales, folklore, alchemy, mythology, history, philology, philosophy, art and literature. Consequently, *first* in dream analysis the dreamer's amplifications and associations are evoked. It speaks by itself that the patient's contribution to amplification is not an intuitive process but depends much on his degree of intelligence, erudition, and willingness to investigate his personal unconscious.

The *first source* of amplification takes place and produces material from the personal unconscious of the analysand, from his own memories and feelings which are evoked in response to it. These are called *accidental symbols,* as they are *personal* and certainly not relative fixed symbols or *universal* symbols, which are part of the second and third level. The second level contains cultural material assimilated to the image. For instance, a Spaniard accustomed to bull fights would react quite differently to the image of a bull than someone from India where bulls are revered and wander unharmed in the streets. The third and most abstract level consists of archetypal images (see diagram on p. 57). There is a clear hierarchy in this amplification: the personal material *always* takes precedence over the other two levels. If the dream becomes clear within the range of the personal amplification, there is no need to proceed further to these universal and archetypal clarifications. If the dreamer's associations and amplifications are not enough, only then the *therapist's* amplifications (but *not* his associations) are added to the process of dream analysis. So the therapist's amplifications and explanations are always subordinated to the dreamer's, as personal elements need first to be worked through, and the therapist must pay close attention and conduct a proper investigation while paying attention to *his* emotional responses to the patient's dream material, as not to contaminate any dream interpretation.

Here again, analogous to homeopathy where the homeopath should take his own simillimum: if he acts as the dream therapist, he must make sure he has investigated his own shadow side, otherwise his own complexes will be added to the patient. All these associations and amplifications are elicited to ground the symbolic and allegoric images of the dream, and this process needs to be done with every singular element of the dream. We must know what it means for the dreamer when he dreams about an animal, object, person ... not what the analyst thinks about that animal or object, but what connection it has for the person who had the dream. It is important that the dream material will be understood allegorically and symbolically in terms of the dreamer's current psychological situation—his *conscious existential situation.* This analytical process furnishes an excellent opportunity for therapist and patient alike to discover character tendencies (good, in the case of a positive shadow—see Chap. 10—or bad) that are overlooked, inaccessible, or avoided, an important step to becoming a more complete person.

PHASES OF AMPLIFICATION

From the Latin *amplus*, or "increase, spacious" and *facere*, or "making"

PERSONAL MEANING TO DREAM IMAGE

Accidental symbols: non fixed (1)

CULTURAL MEANING

Universal symbols: relative fixed (2)

ARCHETYPAL CONNECTIONS

Universal symbols: relative fixed (3)

(2 & 3 depend on erudition and intelligence)

While compensation creates a vastly opposite reaction or image in the dream, putting the accent on the blind spots of the dreamer as if holding a mirror in front of him, this is not the same as complementation. From the different sources of complementation available, they *add* information to the meaning of the dream, but not necessarily the opposite of the conscious situation. These universal symbols widen the patient's view of what meaning is offered, a technique done by the patient and therapist, and often find assent of the dreamer. I think it is an exciting aspect of dream analysis as both parties, therapist and patient, are stimulated to investigate and study so many other branches of education, opening many doors to further erudition.

In homeopathic seminars, I saw that some teachers applied only an objective dream analysis, therefore missing important information obtained by subjective analysis that would guide them to the simillimum, and to the patient's real-life situation. What is the difference?

Subjective/Symbolic vs. Objective/Symptomatic Dream Analysis

Dreams always must be analyzed in two ways. Dreams are looked at first objectively, on the concrete personal object level, but always need to be taken one step further, at the subject level, the patient himself—what the dream says about the dreamer him/herself. In other words, the dream figure reflects the inner (subjective) or outer (objective) person. How to discriminate? If we meet a crippled person or a beggar in our dreams (nothing in common with our real life), they demonstrate that we are harboring them, that we are just like them and among them, and an urgent investigation of the unconscious is necessary to improve our life. Let us presume that an affluent patient comes to you and tells you that she had a frightening dream of being poor, of living on the street with a critical and cruel husband, hungry and cold. Can this be a foreboding dream of a catastrophe in the patient's life? If this dream has nothing to do with reality and there is no foundation in fact to be found in her actual life for this message, we must ask the associations to her husband. If the husband is a decent person, warm and affectionate, and her relationship to her husband is positive, the dream has to be analyzed subjectively, in which case the husband in her dream refers to her animus, her "husband within" (see Chap. 12), which is possibly cold and critical, unable to contribute to a warm relationship with her real husband, a situation she is unable to see as her own real individuality, a lack of Eros, or art of relations.

Let's take another example, where the dreamer receives the picture of his father as an evil person, a person who pursues him with a gun and tries to kill him. This shocks the dreamer, as in reality (consciously) he feels nothing but deep love and admiration for his father who seems to be the good example (objective interpretation). Why then this threatening image or subjective meaning? In this case it can well be that strong fatherly guidance has clipped the son's wings, as he depends too much on his father's advice, stifling his own initiatives and causing low self-confidence. This dream, through its compensating nature, warns the son about this suffocating relationship and tells him not to put the father on a pedestal, while encouraging the dreamer to take more personal initiative so that the road to Self will indeed be built from personal experiences, successes and failures, so important in life!

To take yet another example, in which you dream of your mother-in-law, where you want to kill her because she is excessively arrogant and controlling. If the dream image corresponded with reality you would not dream about this situation, as a dream *will not restate what you have already seen correctly and adequately* (objective dream analysis). But if your mother-in-law is a nourishing, loving and supportive person, and your objective view is less than truthful, then your mother-in-law has to do with the "inner woman figure"—your anima (in the case of a man, the female within)—and these characteristics you have projected onto her are owned by you, the dreamer (see Chap. 11). Only when you see part of the true picture, but are blinded by your own prejudice, will you then dream of your mother-in-law, since dreams try to correct your one-sided incorrect opinion (law of compensation). Also, in this case, the dream could be used to discover things about your mother-in-law that might have alluded you, that were unknown to you, amplifying your viewpoint to show that she really is controlling (dream analysis on the objective level).

Especially when the dream is about somebody with many dark and evil traits—a person who is despised and hated by everyone, someone who you never would have anything to do with—it is obvious that almost everyone will deny being that person him or herself. It is no surprise that such a dream seems to refer to "someone else." Only by analyzing subjectively such a dream, by opening the secret door to ourselves, can we shine the light on the dark spot in which we are identical to this despised figure. It takes much courage to do so, as such discovery is a shock to the system, ripping the mask off our face. I would always suggest consulting your spouse, also, who hopefully will be helpful and honest enough to confirm your inadequacies, as we all have them. And lo and behold, then we must admit: "I am that immoral person, even the devil at times." Then a new and exciting land will be discovered by you! In a dream we see the world entirely from within; it loses its objective meaning and is transformed into a symbol of our own, purely individual experience.

I remember a patient with a morbidly hypochondriac disposition, who in spite of numerous tests giving him a clean bill of health, always insisted on repeating the same tests or doing progressively more invasive diagnostic procedures (*anxiety, hypochondriacal; Del, time has come to die; Del, being doomed; Del, is about to receive an injury;* and *Del, being sick*). One night he had a nightmarish dream that a new doctor diagnosed him with cancer, which of course brought the person in an alarmed state to my office. If I first would analyze this dream on the object level, I might conclude that this is possibly a warning dream of an incurable illness that I might have overlooked. But in view of his habitual, one-sided hypochondriacal attitude, I would most likely view this situation on the subject level, as he might indeed suffer from an "incurable illness," that of a serious imbalance on the psychological inner level. Indeed, *Arsenicum* in LM potency, in watery judicial doses, brought this patient out of his impasse and endless repetition of anxiety attacks about his health, to the great joy of his family.

Now that we have looked at different tools and aspects to understand a dream, the question comes to mind, "Who is this great director/creator of such variety of dreams?"

The Creator of Dreams

When we look at the mysterious content of dreams, the question arises: who is this being or entity that creates such outlandish tales at night, sometimes disturbing our sleep with morally objectionable things about ourselves, while other times bringing us stories of love, feasts, and pleasures? Sometimes we are relieved and exclaim, "It was just a dream"; other times we wished we never woke up from this fanciful, alien world. It looks like at the time when our soul is the least disturbed (during sleep), there is most perturbation in its imagination! Is there a trickster at work, maybe a magician or a wizard who at will brings us from pleasure to despair? In French we say *faire un rêve*—"to make a dream"—as if it is up to our conscious mind to make up a dream. But we are only instrumental in this creative process, and through the law of compensation we will advance towards self-realization if we find the dream's meaning. The ideas conveyed in dreams come without us and despite us: we play no active creative role in them. Accurate observation shows that we never can influence our own dreams consciously, they are not under our control. This symbolic experience simply happens to us and speaks to a situation as it is; dreams indeed are autonomous and meaningful products of psychic activity of the unconscious, not controlled by free will. If this was not the case, humans would resort to and wish for the corniest dreams of riches, festivities, banalities and yes, excesses. However, the conscious mind has nothing to do with the creation of dreams except for creating a counter position to an abnormal, excessive conscious situation (rule of compensation). The unconscious retains its strict autonomy. Even *lucid dreaming*, to be able to realize in the dream that we are dreaming, does not allow us to change its meaning, direction, and nature. The only thing we can do, although it is presented in a foreign language, is to try to understand what message is offered and how it can be used in a beneficial way in our conscious life, to alter and adjust our ego response to the dream's message. Mastering lucid dreaming can lead to seeking answers or insight about specific problems, and to the reveal of cathartic encounters.

Why does a dream possess this cruel nature of not telling us its meaning directly? A dream, being a product of Nature, carries the duality of Nature—the reconciliation of a pair of opposites. Nature knows nothing about right and wrong, good and evil, pleasure and pain: she simply acts. She creates a beautiful child and kills it with a germ. She creates a fine mind and imprisons it in a non-functioning body in Alzheimer's disease. She may destroy a beautiful piece of art, just when it was finished, through a ravaging fire. There is no purpose and plan in all of this, no justice or injustice, no charity or cruelty. As we all know so well, Nature can be cruel (hurricanes, floods, fires, etc.) and can be benevolent (the nourishing aspect), but the choice is not ours! "Nature has good intentions," as Aristotle once said, "but she cannot always carry them out!" Nature can be tyrannically inconsiderate, relentlessly enforcing its mighty powers, but also provides for our needs, including for healing. An example of the duality of Nature is easily seen when we consider the effects of a burning rash after contact with poison ivy or stinging nettle, while the homeopathic preparations *Rhus-*

tox and *Urtica Urens* show the remedial character of those same plants for acute shingles and acute gout, respectively.

Dreams are neither deliberate nor arbitrary. This product of the unconscious, after all, keeps man sane in many insane situations, even without his consent. Sure, we are in the dream, this created drama, this fantastic film, but only to find ourselves in a certain predicament, a certain problematic scenario, without any apparent conclusion most of the time. So, let us not waste our time to wait for a dream to tell us what we ought *to do*—it just tells us: "Here is where you are, figure it out how to go from here!" We are the object of the dream, put in the middle of a Greek drama, not its maker. If fatal destiny awaits us, we are often seized with a prophetic dream where the unconscious lets contents ascend into our consciousness that are still unknown yet. If we are on the wrong course in life, we often get an early warning, sometimes through symbolic dreams, like fire or lightning destroying a house (the Self), before illness sets in.

Every part of the dream and all its actors refer to the dreamer himself. A dream therefore *is always a projection of what the dreamer unconsciously thinks about himself, about other people, and about the world.* Therefore, nothing appears in the dream which the dreamer does not put there himself. And the dream should always be treated as one whole piece; we should not lift one piece of the dream and translate it as a chapter of a book, as this would not be the whole book, just as neither is "the foot the whole man," as Hahnemann pointed out (A7, *footnote*). A dream is not an accurate picture of the objective reality and should never be treated as such. *It is however an accurate picture of reality as it appears to the dreamer, his own perceived reality.* This kind of reality is called ***subjective*** reality. To put the content of this chapter in a practical way, let us now attempt to translate a short fictitious dream.

Translation (Analysis) Exercise of a Made-Up Dream

Normally, each part of the dream will be investigated for its close association and the dreamer can usually find more than one association. Bringing a correct interpretation to the dreamer of his nocturnal tale is analogous to the lead detective of a crime bringing enough elements to the prosecutor to bring an indictment. If we have not fully investigated the case, the prosecutor will say, "I have not enough facts to bring an indictment. Go back and bring me more." In the same way, we must "translate" every image of the dream before we will obtain the assent of the unconscious to release its important message. We must try to understand such a dream as an *answer for the conscious situation* of the dreamer.

How to find the "translation" of the dream? As mentioned before, we try to enlarge each important image of our dream with *personal* associations and amplifications enriched with possible relative fixed symbols related to these dream images. Once we have replaced each dream image with its clarification, then we can reformulate this dream just like we would translate a text to another language. This is like translating the language of the patient into the language of the Materia Medica and Repertory, when we replace the patient's expressions by rubrics that amplify and explain these expressions. Following, I present an exercise involving a made-up dream. Try to insert what we have found, as a possible explanation, as if into an equation:

> I am watching a lake and see a black knight on a black horse standing in the lake, when the night has fallen. I also see an owl in the light of the moon.

This personal amplification and association must be done with **every** element in the dream. The dreamer who sees this vision stands for his ego-consciousness who watches a lake at night—in other words, he is investigating his unconscious. In a real dream case, of course, I would ask about personal associations and amplifications. In this made-up example, we will only use relative fixed symbols and my own amplifications. **Water** is the most common symbol for the unconscious. A **lake** is associated with the relative fixed symbol of the *personal* unconscious, and I put "personal unconscious" instead of lake (the **sea** represents the *collective* unconsciousness where all psychic life originates, the mother of all that lives). A **knight:** the white knight stands for protection! It is a human type superior to all others. In the past, the education of a knight was directed to strengthen him: physically (so he can protect), but moreover, to develop his spirit and soul (the noble knight on the white shining horse), his morals and his reason, in order to prepare him adequately for his tasks in the world. The **horse** is the symbol of the bodily vehicle, and the "rider" is the spirit. It reflects the survival drive, all that has powerful energy to move us, but also the subhuman animal side or unconscious, the animal life. A **black horse:** his unconscious libido looking for his natural master, the shadow; it reflects the unruliness of the passions, unacceptable passions; threat of death; threatening changes. This knight is in black, and medieval tales and legends most frequently refer to a black knight, reflecting relative shortcomings while carrying out his duties. Maybe the dreamer is evoking a protective person in his dream! The **color black** stands for sin, the hidden, rebirth in seclusion, or withdrawal and sorrow. Thus, the black knight stands for withdrawal, penitence (contrition, regret), and sacrifice. The black horse and the black knight are half-evil elements that correspond to the descent into darkness or unconscious. The white knight is the chosen one, the natural conqueror, and stands for innocence and purity. Alchemy presents us with a rising scale of colors (an evolutive, progressive scale): black, white, red, and then gold as the final stage. The descending color scale goes from blue to green, from heaven to earth.

Moon(light): represents the feminine, love, romance; also represents the woman's strange, sensual, and overpowering attraction, as well as the unconscious. **Owl** may symbolize wisdom in general, or the wisdom belonging to the unconscious (night=unconscious), or intuition (associated with woman, who is associated with the moon, or knowledge of the collective unconscious as owls see best in the dark). Some mythologies connect the owl with death, and an owl might act as a messenger regarding the death of a family member.

In the end, when the patient adds personal associations and amplifications, we can see what the whole dream means. For this analysis to be effective as a tool in the healing of the dreamer, the question can then be asked: who needs to understand *first* the meaning of the dream, the patient or the therapist (homeopath)? And how to communicate with the patient?

The Process of Communication of Dream Interpretation

Any professional has the tendency to think he needs to be the one enlightening the patient, but when it comes to understanding dreams, the patient comes first! The only hard and fast rule Jung made about dream interpretation, is to listen very carefully to the unconscious, and *say, first to oneself,* "I have no idea what this dream means" (Jung, 1974, p. 69). With the help of associations and amplifications (in the first place the patient's, and then the physician's amplifications *only*), the physician only puts forth *proposals*—more than one explanation, till one explanation finds the *patient's assent,* as only the patient can agree with the translation (and it is *his* decision only) and thus with the meaning of his individual dream.

It is of the utmost importance that the patient understands the dream first—that the interpretation "clicks" for him and that the therapist will not be overcome with arrogance and a sense of superiority and an inflated ego, as it might lead to an act of transference to the therapist who seems "to always know the answer," but in reality will only slow down the healing process. Any suggestion by the therapist too early in the process of analysis will be met with the most intense resistance and indignation, especially if this explanation touches on a high feeling-toned constellation (the CD for the homeopath). Whenever the patient puts up strong resistance to our analysis, the more energy he will put into protesting the validity, not only of the interpretation but also of the dream itself, which he will then call meaningless.

The truth, when not understood and told too early, is always offensive and never investigated further or accepted, and only leads to fruitless battles and discussions with the analyst. It is wise and imperative not to force our interpretation on the dreamer if he is not willing to go to the content and message that has been revealed. We must proceed cautiously with the patient's associations and amplifications to his dream, which is a slow, individual, and necessary work process, and will avoid moral indignation and repugnance in the patient. Such caution will result in calm and accepted verification when the clarification brings an emotional conviction to the patient. Besides using his intellect, the therapist must consult his feeling and intuitive functions to understand a dream, a product of the unconscious, putting himself in the right atmosphere for understanding the dream and supporting the patient.

How to communicate the dream interpretation must be tailored to the individual—to the kind of patient we have in front of us—who is often struggling with his complexes. Take the example of a *Verat-a* patient I saw in my office. He was dressed in the persona of a bishop, with a big cross hanging over his chest. He brought up names of famous people he met (not in reality), and oracles he had from the almighty God in his dreams (*Del, he is a prince; Del, he is distinguished; Del, he is in communication with God; Del, he is in heaven, talking with God*).

His wife told me in private that he was violent (*destructiveness while drunk; dictatorial*), disrupting religious services in the city (*Del, himself to be Christ*). He had inherited a big sum from his parents, and now was dealing with his inferiority complex with irrational, childish deeds. While preaching to the homeless and prostitutes, he *squandered the money*, adding to his grandiosity. Not only were the dreams compensating for his exaggerated inferiority complex, but his actual behavior, without any doubt, indicated *Verat-a.* If I explained to this patient bluntly what his dreams meant and how childish his behavior was, it would have made him only "smaller," which would be counter-productive, even cruel. I instead took the opportunity to be "interested" in his "encounters and adventures," tactfully and patiently, not confronting him with the brutality of the truth. In this way, further dreams, and above all his simillimum, could expedite the direction of cure. I gave him one dose of *Verat-a* 10M (there was no sense in giving him LM potencies as he would have abused the remedy). When I saw him back the next month, he was totally transformed into a calm, even meek person who could now start realizing that by not seeing the tragedy of his behavior, he was destroying his life. This was a case where anyone could see the speed in which the simillimum can work, rather than having to strip the patient's excessive persona off piece by piece, over many years.

For Jung, there was no such thing as a correct interpretation of a dream. A dream was successfully interpreted when the analysis made sense to the dreamer and could be used constructively by him or her. Only the dreamer can say with certainty what his dreams mean. The certainty usually comes in the form of a *wordless* "Aha" of recognition, a kind of gut-level "yes" or intuitive deep-down feeling response; a "touché!" Despite dreams being a universal language, other people can come up with possible different meanings of a dream, and when suggesting them to the dreamer, are very likely to evoke more exclamations of recognition in the dreamer as well. By taking every possible meaning into serious consideration, the dreamer can usually find that there is one special meaning of a symbol that "rings a bell for him," something that clicks for him. *The dreamer's own "Aha!" feeling is always the best guide, as it carries an emotional conviction for him.* Something clicked, and if not, it is either because the interpretation was wrong, or the dreamer has not reached the point where he can understand this dream.

There is also value in a negative "Aha." Take for instance, in a dream group a certain meaning is suggested, but the dreamer will respond with a negative "Aha" that says in effect, "No, that is totally wrong," as it is so far from the mark that it makes the dreamer realize *what is really true!* This also means that we don't have to analyze and make associations for every person, topic, or word in a dream—only that much of the dream text needs to be "translated," until the "Aha" comes to the dreamer in a satisfactory way. Much like translating a foreign language: you don't have to translate every word to find out what the whole text means. And chances of touching upon more meanings is greater if several people are involved in the process, so no interpretation is "dumb" or off the mark. It is always helpful to see others' dreams with "fresh eyes."

In this chapter, I discussed useful elements and guidelines of the dream language, such as relative fixed symbols, symbols of a collective nature, the rule of compensation, meanings of numbers in dreams, association and amplification, and subjective/symbolic versus objective/symptomatic dream analysis, as well as the importance of how to communicate dreams to the patient.

I will now proceed in the next chapter to investigate the most important kinds of dreams in man's life.

3

IMPORTANT DREAMS DURING A HUMAN'S LIFETIME

Dreams are not disturbers of sleep,
but rather its guardians against disturbances.

While dreams are always important for humankind for self-healing and progression, the interpretation takes different meanings in the different phases of a human's life. Let us investigate some of them, starting with early life.

Early Childhood Dreams

Until age 5, before outgrowing the helplessness of a baby (the weak infantile consciousness), a child has a consciousness that is still very close to the collective unconscious with its archetypal dreamlike images. Therefore, fairy tales, "Once upon a time"—pure expressions of the collective unconscious, the prenatal imaginary world—are welcomed, as they reflect the child's language. They speak about a world familiar to him and are often used by parents to educate their child about life in general. As such invasion of archetypal contents far exceeds the comprehension of the immature child's ego, we cannot expect personal associations or amplifications from such a young child. Archetypal images such as appearances of snakes, monsters, pyramids, or castles can be perceived as frightening, or charming and alluring. Animals as well as the parents often figure into children's dreams.

Alas! Dreams about parents can have untoward effects. No doubt the child remains close to the Mother type of the collective unconscious, and the child's prenatal psyche and early psyche is open to the psychic influences from the parents. Parents should not be regarded as being a separate entity but as part of the child's universe. Lévy-Brühl[1] called it the *participation mystique,* or mystical participation, in which the child feels any unrest and psychic trauma stemming from the parents, to the point that children dream about the unresolved conflicts of their parents, an awful heritage and transference that few parents are aware of. Such childhood trauma often has a wave effect throughout the rest of their life.

No matter what we think, the secrets of parents always have an extraordinary influence upon the young lives of children. In any neurosis of a child we need first to examine the relationship between the parents to know the whole individual psychic situation of the child. Parents may insist that they never fight in front of their children, but children sense unrest, and the more they are loved the more they are influenced by the hostility between parents. The invasion of unconscious contents into the conscious always carries the danger of dissociation and shattering of the weak, still developing child's consciousness, leading to infantile schizophrenia, which often occurs before the prenatal psyche needs to separate from the parents' unconscious (especially the mother's) at ages 4-5, when the child ventures out in the foreign world of school and organized society, away from the security and nourishing aspect of the home environment. The child instinctually senses the responsibilities and challenges ahead now that she leaves the comfort of the early childhood paradise. She must adapt to a new world, and all depends on if this child is ready for this adaptational work: *Pulsatilla* and *Calc-c* children will have difficulties, while *Sulphur* and *Phosphorus* personalities will welcome the challenges, enjoying their expansion of freedom!

At age 6, a normal child is beyond early infantile consciousness, but of course much work lies ahead to develop the core personality of an adult. At this early age, dreams of a child of his mother (or anyone who has a vital relation to him) represent in the first place *that person* in the dream. Around age 8, being somewhat beyond the carefree and sheltered world of the collective unconscious, a time of transition to ego consciousness, challenges and psychic traumas such as bullying by other children or a too strict, harsh, or stern teacher or parent, or incest, might throw the child into fear and confusion, leading to withdrawal, timidity, and lack of grit, often repeating a theme of terror in the child's dreams. Such early dreams (often archetypal in nature, see further) are important, as they frequently express the child's future destiny and his later personality; the child will carry these characteristics over to adult life, changing their character and initiatives. The occurrence of recurrent dreams from childhood on—often remembered and told when they are adults—continue to play a role in daily life for the adult, until finally, through psychotherapy or the simillimum, the adult is released from these infantile shackles. Discovering why an adult has had these sinister dreams since childhood will be important, even if the situation in which they arose has long been erased from memory. By looking at what happened in the patient's life when these dreams recur, discovering the trigger of a painful feeling-toned complex still roaming in his unconscious, will be a key to his simillimum. Childhood dreams still remembered as an adult are very important, for they have been preserved in the unconscious because of their impactful and shocking nature;

they are dreams that have made a deep impression on the dreamer.

Besides the collective unconscious and the mystical participation, a third source of children's dreams are the daily occurrences, called *parallel* dreams. It is always important to ask the parents what happened the day before the dream occurred. Was there any trouble at school, an upsetting event, disagreement with a friend, any change in her familiar environment like a best friend moving away, or the child herself moving? Was there any important event like the child hearing bad news, such as the death of a family member? *Hearing bad news* has many different origins, and especially a *Calcarea* or *Phosphorus* child is very sensitive to what *they* perceive as bad news.

That such recurrent unresolved dreams can have a negative impact on the individual even as an adult is easily seen in the conscious situation of the following patient. Note, this is a parallel dream occurring at a young age, repeating itself as a parallel dream later. There is no rule of compensation in this dream, as her dreams reflect the terror and isolation taking place in her conscious life.

As a 6-year-old child, a time in a child's life when separation from the parents starts, especially from the mother, she was caught in a country where war and its cruelties were daily horrors with constant threats from bombing. Often at night alarm signals could be heard, announcing the threat of bombs. On those occasions she hurried to her parents' bed but was told to go back to her own bed—that she was a big girl now. For the rest of the night she would be curled up in bed, terrified, feeling completely alone. From then on, severe separation and anticipation anxieties recurred, into adulthood. For such a small child, the mother is the figure who appears at the right moment, from whom protection and love is expected. At that age, still living mainly in the collective conscious, the most important and only archetype is that of the mother. In a fairy-tale world, the fairy (mother) is all powerful, superior and with many magical qualities, a wise, guiding figure and helpful spirit that brings solutions in the most complicated and dangerous situations. The "crime" unconsciously committed by her parents (especially the mother) was *Ailments from being forsaken*, causing a state in which she felt *forsaken with a sense of isolation.*

This situation can also be called a Post-traumatic Stress Disorder event (PTSD), translated in the rubrics as *fear of the fright remains,* a syphilitic entry point to her case for which we have two remedies: *Aconite* (2) and *Opium* (3). The CD of *Aconite* is *she is about to die,* reflecting an immense fear of imminent death. We see *Aconite* also in the *Delusion, she is away from home*—home being a relative fixed symbol for security and protection (mother!), as expressed in the proving symptom *long lasting fear, ideas haunt her, cannot get rid of them.* When someone wants to return to the womb, it means also returning to the unconscious, even the collective unconscious, to be near the archetype of the Divine Mother (symbol of love, tenderness, nourishment, and security). The "return to the unconscious" in this patient was reflected by *chronic insomnia*, and a feeling of lightheadedness (*faintness after a frightful event*). Clearly, a person in an *Aconite* state, consumed by the idea that she will die, wants to remain hypervigilant. At night, when sleep should set in, all inhibitory processes fall away; then an *Aconite* person is at the mercy of all the suppressed emotions that have been hiding in her unconscious. This patient would say, "I am awake but I am not" (*Delusion, insists she was sleeping while awake*), would become easily angry (*anger with fright; anger with silent grief*), and became asocial and withdrawn (*aversion to people, has no affection for anybody with almost indifference towards her friends*). Despite her actual situation (*she cannot banish anxious apprehensive thoughts even in gay company; intolerant to contradiction*), the CD *is about to die* has become a fixed idea that can resist even the most eloquent, rational argument, inflating her fears to immense proportions.

The remedy needed is obvious: *Aconite* in its chronic state, resulting in psychic and physical inertia. Her dream, recurring from an early age, predicted her present state. She is caught in a state of being detached from the earth. She is living in a cave, the most original place to live, slipping into the maternal womb, which was so much denied at age 6. This hiding is also an isolation that effectively severs the patient from her environment, and can thus be called isolation from consciousness, "being there but not being there," not able to participate in the normal activities of life, resulting in a vicious cycle where the endpoint is "permanent isolation." This remedy was never given (she was not my patient, but I received her dreams later from her therapist), so her dreams have a recurrent theme. Let us find out what messages her adult dreams were projecting before any remedy was given, and how an event as a young child has made such a lasting impression in her life.

Dream

The first dream I remember is with trains. Trains everywhere. For some reason I am living in a really noisy place surrounded by train tracks and trains coming and going. Sometimes one has to cross the tracks, but you cannot tell if a train is coming or going. It is always night. Then I am on a train, at night, in the middle of these snowy mountains and the train is going way too fast down the mountain. I cannot do anything about it, so I just close my eyes and let the noise and G-forces take over.

That's all I remember. It was a stressful dream.

Analysis

Trains, like airplanes and buses, are *collective* means of transportation (not like a car—more personal). Here we see how this patient is diving and traveling in the unconscious (night), going too fast down the mountain (hurling into the unconscious), looking for the protective Mother type, totally out of control and not under her willpower at all, so all she can do is let herself go, governed by these forces of Nature—these deep instincts and forces of the unconscious—immersed in the unconscious (closing her eyes). Of course it is stressful, as she feels she is swept up by the force of an invisible entity (G-force), the unconscious, where she is entangled in all the old frightening memories of her childhood, when she was in her bed, scared and curled up by herself, when all she could do was close her eyes, overtaken by her fears, just like in this dream.

Next dream

There is a play I went to (in real life) and for some reason in my dream I am seeing it again. They want me to sing a number I have not rehearsed or known about so I will have to improvise on stage. I decline. I know it is a once-in-a-lifetime chance to sing on stage, but I don't know what I will be singing! And I am very aware that when I get nervous, I sing off key. Then for some reason two composers come to give autographs outside the play, and I leave the play (even though I like it a lot) to see who these people are. The one that everyone wants signatures from I have never heard of, but the other one that no one is lining up to is actually someone who had written a song I really liked, so I end up talking to him. When I return to the play it is already over and I am disappointed.

I don't remember anything from this dream except that I woke up screaming, "Help me!"

Analysis

This is the play of her life in general, her Greek drama so to speak. She has a chance to sing (which is expressing her inner feelings, her real Self, and thus reflecting more of her creative potential), a chance of a lifetime, understandable in view of her history, but she does not know the content of the song or hasn't had a chance to rehearse it (because in her dream it is the first time that the unconscious prompted her to express her deepest feelings—something she never felt she could do) and she was afraid she would sing off key (expressing herself wrongly). Then **two** composers appear (duality of the opposites—one known, one unknown) and she is attracted to the unknown one (the unconscious), who had written a song that she really liked; she resonated with the message of this song, the message of the unconscious, so she talked to him. He was probably the wise old man (see Chap. 12, "Animus") giving her advice. When she returned to the play (becoming conscious, going towards the light) the play was over, which upset her greatly. She is still isolated, and had not the opportunity to express her feelings, which would have created much satisfaction as she could be more herself. Hence her cry: "Help me!"

Another of her dreams

For some reason I am working at the large mall not far from where I live. However, that day my former male boss is there, asking for a meeting late at night. He says, "After work I'd like to speak to you." I know this was about why I had left (in real life), and I really don't want to talk to him. Still, I have to go do something in the bowels of the mall, and when I return to the area of my office, my purse is in the meeting room and the room is locked. I am getting very anxious because it is very late (in the dream) and I will be stuck without my purse, and I know there were still people inside, and they will be locked in too. No one wants to or is willing to help me solve this.

Analysis

This is very much the same message as the previous dream. The mall (referring to the Self) is where she is asked by her boss (her animus) to speak at night (unconscious), referring to investigating her unconscious, something she did not want to do (too scary). When she returned from the bowels of the mall (= the personal unconscious, part of the Self), she found out that the way to the meeting room (integration to the conscious) was blocked and her purse (containing money and identification) was in there. She of course wants her purse, as money is the symbol of psychic libido and psychic energy to move forward. When we put or have money in the bank, we have psychic energy in the storehouse of the Self, the unconscious. Here in this dream the money is out of reach in her purse—a loss and disorientation of psychic energy to move forward. Money means power to change things, to do things. Her identification papers in her purse—to confirm her identity (Self)—were out of her reach too. Other people would be locked in also, showing again this is an archetypal message, as this message (lack of ego and identification) does not belong only to the dreamer but also to mankind. It seems like she is still unable to move forward, to integrate the dark contents of the unconscious.

It is often helpful for the homeopath to let children *draw* what they have dreamed about. Images of the unconscious may appear in dreams and visions and may seek representation in drawings and paintings. Drawings often picture the trauma which has already appeared in the dreams—either monsters taking them away from their parents, or a family with one of the family members omitted (who is absent in their life). I had a child in my practice that was so often shifted from one family member to another (because of work and illness of family members) that he drew a big bird carrying him away in his dream, a frightful expression of the actual family situation in which he roamed around in the world as an orphan, not belonging to anyone. This child, taken care of by so many people, had not felt safety in anything or anyone. He first drew an angry threatening monster from his dream that changed into a winged creature after application of the simillimum. "Wings" are a symbol of liberation, of being able to rise and be freed from an oppressive situation, a symbol of transcendence. When a child can draw the horror of a dream, it liberates him to some extent from the psychic burden and stabilizes his or her consciousness. The picture softens the sting of the terrifying experience, so that the power of the fantasies is lessened. Here are his drawings:

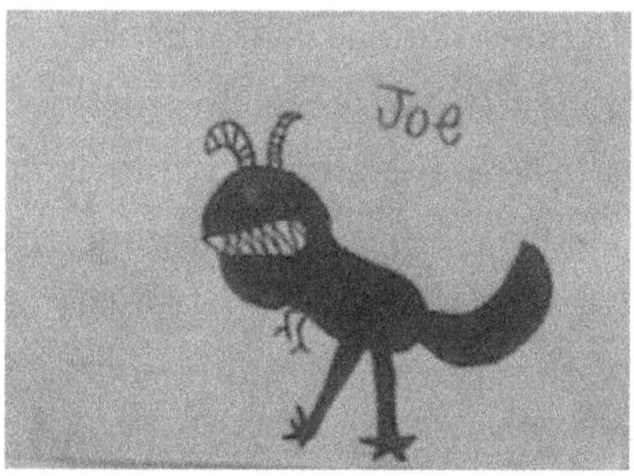

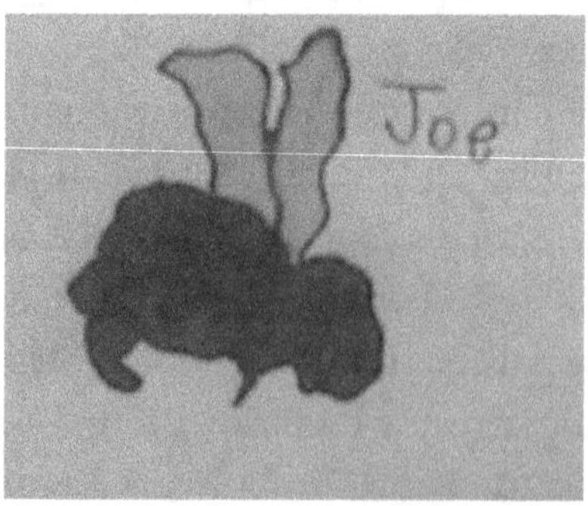

Drawing or painting what was seen in a dream should also be extended as a tool for adults, even for those who do not possess a grain of artistic talent. We are drawing what we see inside us, not what is presented outside of us! Anyone and everyone can be a modern artist when he gives form to the inexpressible. This brings us to another important stage of life in any human being: puberty. What kind of important dreams present themselves?

Dreams in Puberty

Every parent has witnessed the natural process of transformation in their child during pre-puberty and puberty. They are puzzled by the "new" child that has come to live with them, as the old child is dead and a new child, one in a high state of excitation, has been delivered to their doorstep. But all transitional periods follow the path of "death" of the old and "birth" of the new, and at this point in life the early, main infantile manifestation of vital activity or libido that found expression in sucking and being fed is converting itself into sexual libido. It is blind youth, just emerging from childhood, thrown into disorder in accordance with a poorly understood instinct. There is newfound excitation, a giddy, amped-up energy with the jangling dopamine of awakening adolescence. It is the recklessness of a bubbling and indestructible spirit flowing from the joy of burgeoning youth. When young, eternity is too big to grasp. The years are elongated, shaky, and seem countless. The ego has undergone a dramatic growth spurt, with the resurgence of increased self-awareness, but this can lead to impulsive behavior and dangerous situations, especially for those in whom the sycotic and syphilitic miasm are awakened.

Besides being an age of confusion, it is also the time of conquest for its own sake and for the sake of sexual investigation. It is the age of making fun of the moral values parents talk about (but may seldom practice), a wild and brazen growth episode. It is the fight to be their "own," not wanting to be followed and controlled by the shadow of their parents. There isn't anything that such a teenager would not do to procure five minutes of entertainment. Nothing seems serious in life for such a fellow. Even St. Augustine described the turmoil of his adolescence:

> For a time during adolescence I burned to find satisfaction in hellish pleasures and I dared to run wild amid all kinds of shady passions ... The eruptions of puberty like mists rising up from muddy swamps of my carnal desire, clouded my heart and made it dark. (Lincoln & White, 2001)

Why is this act of Nature so constant in the young, although in different degrees according to the predominant miasmatic state?

The sexual awakening—the passion of sex frequently becoming a tyrant—creates upheaval and disaster in its path. The arrival of the sexual tsunami has created havoc in more than one such child. Especially in young men, a *Kali-bromatum* state can be created with the *Delusion, his mother's house has been invaded by lewd women*, expressing the confusion created in young people as they are overwhelmed by these primitive urges that well up from the depth of their being. The less expressed at home about sex, the more they fill their thoughts with it. New extended rules are implemented by parents out of precaution and fear—much because of what they remember doing at the same age—filled with melodramatic and exaggerated ideas. Unfortunately, these prohibitions triple and quadruple the value of the "forbidden fruit," and it becomes more sought after than anything else. Most parents are not professional reformers and guards, only spasmodic ones, filled with memories of their own youthful guilty pleasures. So, reform breaks out now and then, with considerable intervals in between. Entering college, the adolescent often has the birth of lust, alcoholism, and madness combined, not a solid base on which to build a future life. And for those ensnared by the syphilitic miasm, there will be nothing he will shrink from—no taboo, no crime, no horrible activity—propelled by greed, passion, a sense of misplaced entitlement, and pure selfishness.

Another danger at this point is the possible appearance of the initial phases of *paranoid schizophrenia* characterized by bizarre ideas, ideas of persecution, and the loss of the power of rational associations, as if a wire had been tripped in their brain. With the social and spiritual separation around puberty, "great" dreams appear as this child begins to grow into a specific human world, freeing himself from the collective unconscious. The separation from the parents is an archetypal situation that has been repeated, many times over, over billions of years. The young person must give up his childish desire to cling to his parents and grow up (leaving the "eternal child" to some extent). Otherwise his developing life energy will be disturbed, if he cannot cut the psychological umbilical cord from parents and childhood. The more the child grows, the more he develops a quest for freedom and independence. But at the same time, it creates a feeling of powerlessness and anxiety. Separation might be difficult, but if this separation is not achieved it leads to more difficulties! The struggle for freedom and independence can cause neurosis in the struggling child who keeps returning to the magic helper, the parent, when making decisions about how to deal with life. And discipline, from the Latin *discere,* or "to learn," must come from the parents, who should teach by imposing order that can ultimately be internalized. The parents must find an appropriate response to the child's growing independence. It is indeed hard for the parent to close the open hand out of love ("tough love"), and to keep modest as a giver.

Unfortunately, in our society, parental education often

results in the elimination of spontaneity, and a substitution of original psychic acts and thoughts by superimposed parental feelings and wishes. All kind of complexes are created by this, hindering the journey of individuation. It is at this moment (puberty) too, that the emphasis in dreams lies in instinct and sexuality, as the anima for males has been separated from the mother (Oedipus complex), and now is transferred to the other sex in the outside world (and vice versa for females). Premature puberty detonates the sexual complexes lying dormant till then. Parents appear confused as they offer long speeches and lectures about what is forbidden and dangerous, but at the same time, sometimes wonder why their boy is not interested in girls. It becomes a game of incitement and prohibitions: "Don't do this, don't do that," and then creating confusion, "Why are you not interested in going to this party?" Mom wants him to be more independent but expresses on the other hand her fears about all the harm out there (*fear, something will happen*).

Besides the sexual tsunami, two other issues arise in the adolescent's life. First there is the flaring up of any latent miasmatic state. Even when there is some forewarning of the havoc ahead by certain unspecified symptoms like occasional violence, aggressiveness, clinginess, or other symptoms, puberty (like menopause) will rouse the full strength of the sleeping dominant family miasm and personal miasmatic state, often changing the child into an uncontrollable person. It is here that homeopaths can achieve excellent work, by subduing and exterminating as much as possible the parental heritage, or dominant family miasmatic influences.

As if this turmoil was not enough, every parent has witnessed their child's natural struggle to find a balance between basking in the childish security of the home (safety issue), and the desire to find increased freedom and adult independence (growth issue) with acceptance of adult responsibility. Many teenagers struggle with the issue of finding their life path, overcome with this alternating state of confusion and assertiveness (e.g., *Silicea*), never knowing when the need for security will overtake the desire for freedom, a process that can continue into adulthood. Newfound powers are easily beset by fears, anxieties, and a lack of confidence when life throws obstructions in the path of the individual. Divorce, financial problems, or sudden illness in the family can cause loss of personal independence and necessity for the security and emotional and financial help from home. Such conflict surging in young people is the source of telltale dreams, especially in characters like *Pulsatilla*, *Calcarea*, *Silicea*, and *Phosphorus*. While the first two constitutions always try to remain close to home even into adulthood, it is especially *Phosphorus* with her tubercular character that struggles with the choice between home and freedom. Love and empathy for family are outspoken, but as "the world is her other home," so is the desire to connect to the rest of the population.

All the aforementioned existential situations find an expression in "great dreams." Here are two of such pubescent dreams that are analyzed, with the accent on separation issues.

Dream

A 13-year-old girl, not yet in puberty, dreamt when her parents planned to go on a trip a couple of months later that she was walking on a bridge with her parents and a tidal wave came over the bridge. She became separated from her parents who were washed away by this wave.

Analysis

Tidal wave: Like rising waters, this represents the unconscious, its devouring aspect, threatening to engulf the conscious ego and distorted emotions, preventing the emergence of true independence. It may also symbolize the surge of sexuality or the sweeping strength of some emotion (in this case fear of abandonment). At this point the ego feels carried along by the experience rather than being in control. The dreamer must learn how to ride the waves like surfers do, but this requires confidence, daring, and balance. For this *Calc-p* girl, it was still too much to bear—the thought that her parents for the first time were going on a trip without her (although a family friend would take care of her). Anxiety is an "enormous wave" that may threaten to engulf its victim; it is one of the tidal waves representing human conditions. It all had to do with strong anticipation anxiety about being separated for the first time from her parents at pre-puberty, a difficulty that is universal, not only belonging to this girl—it is an archaic image derived from ancient human experience. The anxiety stems from not yet having a firm foundation of consciousness, still insecure and childlike. Here the wave of the unconscious sweeps over the bridge separating her from her closely needed support of the immediate family.

The old, still-infantile position must die in this girl, so that the tension represented in this dream between her still insecure, precarious ego and the threatening danger of the unconscious (the tidal wave) can be dissolved. Other settings of such dreams, besides a tidal wave, can be a stormy sea, a rocky coast, ships struggling among the waves, a sailboat not being able to sail due to lack of wind, and a train station where many trains depart but the dreamer is unable to board one, and so forth, reflecting the struggle in puberty.

A bridge: Some of the different relative fixed symbols possible are the following:

1. A place of danger, precariously positioned over an abyss. Psychologically this represents the weak spot of consciousness, the place where it might cave in.

2. Crossing a bridge is an elegant symbol of transition between two periods in our life: a passage from youth or childhood to adulthood, to a new phase in life, namely puberty (as in this case). We also need to build a bridge in order to cross the gap between the conscious mind and the unconscious —"bridging the gap." It symbolizes a critical juncture in the dreamer's life, a situation that calls for a definitive decision, a way of passing over obstacles and difficult situations, a frequent symbol for a fundamental change of attitude. Consider the sayings, "I have a bridge (or a river) to cross before I get there," or, "I will cross that bridge when I come to it." If the bridge is in danger of collapsing, this may reflect the anxiety of the dreamer about a transition in life—like leaving home to go to college or going from one job to another. A similar symbol in dreams reflecting a situation of transition can be "going through a mountain pass."

The question in the case presented needs to be posed: "Is this bridge long enough to carry the girl from one developmental stage to the other; in other words, has she been adequately prepared to master this next difficulty in life?" This youthful dreamer is still afraid; her unconscious senses the danger and the inability to cope with the new problem she is confronted with. Apparently, she needs reinforcement through the indicated remedy (*Calc-p*), along with parental reassurance, otherwise she can fall into infantile regression. Although she is not devoured by a giant monster in her dream, she falls prey to another element that scares her: the tidal wave. Water also symbolizes a place of transformation (and a healing power, represented in the Christian baptismal water that washes away all sins), which now for her has a frightening and destructive character. Contrary to the primitives, we do not have puberty rites in our society that would facilitate and prepare the young person for the separation from innocent ignorance to adult responsibility.

3. Life is also the bridge between the cradle and the grave, the bridge between the past and the future.

A difference between the image of a bridge or a *pier* in a dream may be obvious. A bridge is a continuity of consciousness, connecting land to land. A pier is an abrupt halt between land (consciousness) and water (unconscious); it is approaching a border between consciousness and unconsciousness, coming to the edge of consciousness, a place of danger from something alien and possibly devouring, where we can fall in the water. It also has a dual symbol, however: of danger where one can drown, or of healing and purifying, an element of rebirth when exploring the water (unconscious). Standing on a pier versus a bridge could also be called standing on shaky rather than firm ground, so there is always an element of hesitation and anxiety present.

This dream reflects a merging of the personal problems of this youngster and the collective aspects of her puberty problem —in other words, portraying archetypal images derived from common ancient human experiences. An elegant solution besides acknowledging her separation anxiety and not mocking it, and reassuring her she is protected (her parents will stay in contact, easy to do in this electronic world), is to give her constitutional remedy, *Calc-p* in a 10M potency once, 1 tsp. from a 4-oz. dilution cup.[2]

As further dreams and physical symptoms appeared it became clear that *Pulsatilla* was next needed by this girl. Here is her next dream, with first the description of her conscious situation.

Conscious situation: Her symptoms are wandering joint pains, bedwetting, bland leucorrhea, and constantly cracking her knuckles, twisting her back to crack it, and has stopped running because it seems to cause her knee and hip pain.

When asked about any dreams she remembered recently, the last was as follows.

Dream

I dreamt that my brother is getting married and I am asked to be the MC and am asked to talk about his life and why I think it was a good match etc. I feel it is my responsibility to be nice and fill that role, but I don't really want him to get married so young and feel that he needs more experience before making such a big decision.

She also said that this dream about her brother getting married was a sad dream because she felt he had made a big decision rashly, and she didn't think he should have done it as it would change his life forever. Sad also because he wouldn't be able to date "50 other girls" to decide who he was going to get married to, and he was only 16. She felt she didn't know the girl well enough to really represent her at the wedding. It was a very serious, solemn, and sad thing.

Analysis

Looking at the regressive infantile behavior and the wandering joint pains and the discharge (leucorrhea), *Pulsatilla* comes to mind, especially since she is entering puberty! Her dream also points to *Pulsatilla*, depicting the lack of animus she has developed so far. There is still a strong bond to the family, and in reality, her brother represents her animus in need of more growth before she can separate herself from the family and explore the world without their support (subjective dream interpretation). The need to meet "50 other girls" tells us how much more she needs to experience the meeting of the animus and anima to feel more secure to make the next independent steps in her life. Presently she still needs the shelter of the home; there is no desire to travel (*Calc-p*), and no desire to meet many other people.

A second puberty dream, of an older girl (age 17)

I am in a car with my mother on my way to the train station to go to college. She leaves me, while I am crying, at an intersection just before a bridge under which my train is to stop. There are many people and many cars at the intersection, and I am trying to be polite and let others go before me, but as a result, when I heard the whistle of the train, I knew I missed my connection. As it is the last train, I know that I cannot get to college that day. I want to cry but cannot do so.

I wake up relieved.

Analysis

Car and train: Buses, trains, airplanes, and cars are all vehicles which she must take to further her path of individuation, to become psychologically more complete, and independent. They all have horsepower, representing libido or Vital Force in which one can go from one place to another, indicating a transition to something new. Cars appear, by far, most frequently in dreams, and play a major role in dream content at many stages of life. They often represent the amount of energy available to the ego to use when confronted with tasks in life. A *scooter* is even more particular, as it requires even more individual handling when taking turns and stops, indicating a self-steering, highly individual form of transport. *Moving* in a dream (be it walking, or running, or traveling in one of these vehicles) is always progression in life as it shows an active process of psychologically becoming an individual! Traveling is moving forward on a path of individuation, not only to become more whole but also to attain personal goals and take control of one's life. Movement also represents notions such as ambition, progress, and achievements, as well as breaking family ties or fleeing from something, for instance a stifling and controlling relationship.

Cars, trains, and airplanes are also *vehicles of power* and as such stand for the vital energy of one's impulses, particularly the instinctual sex life. For adolescents, cars can express the greatly expanded freedom of movement that comes with becoming old enough to have a driver's license (age 16 in the United States). For adults, cars are multifaceted images of one's individual Self, with the color, type, age, and condition of the car a metaphoric mapping of corresponding aspects of the dreamer's personality. For instance, driving in a stretch limousine (like at graduation day in the United States) could express a desire for more public attention; a dream of malfunctioning brakes could reflect life being out of control; a dream of being stuck in a crowded minivan could relate to problems with one's family. Life is a journey involving constant movement and progress, and we are in trouble if we are stopped too long by the side of the road or in a parking lot. Driving a truck is linked to work, to our efforts to get something done, to get things moving. Driving a convertible car, open to the sky, the air, the wind, and the elements, often represents the sense of adventure and liberation associated with youth, vigor, and speed (*Phosphorus*, *Lycopodium*, and *Sulphur*). When there is no driver in the car it might reflect terrible fears about the passage from life to death (*Ars, Plat, Phos, Calc*). Trains, buses, and airplanes are public ways of traveling, unlike a car, showing that the dreamer is controlled by the collective as opposed to the individual. *Ships* have a more numinous, or spiritual, character as they carry us through life. *Bicycling* is, of course, individual and a positive way to travel; as with *walking* or *running*, bicycling utilizes one's own power.

Do you like to be the driver, or be driven, as is the case in the preceding dream? It is better to be the driver than the passenger of the car, for when we are at the wheel, we direct the course of our life. When someone else is the driver and we are a passenger, someone else is controlling our life, with or without our permission, and often the dream ends badly as we don't take charge of our destiny. In this specific dream, the girl's mother is the driver, reflecting the daughter's hesitation to separate, her dependency and search for motherly protection and nourishment, still at age 17. It reflects the fear of transition in her life, of leaving the shelter of home to attend college.

Bridge: See the explanation of a bridge symbol above (p. 86). In this dream, the car is stopped before crossing this bridge.

College or classrooms: These represent learning of lifelong importance to achieve new steps on the way to individuation, to learn something to assist us in our development. It is a succession of many different schools to go through, a "lifelong lesson."

Intersection: An intersection reflects a crossroads with many different options. What road should I take? "We are at the crossroads to make a decision—which way do I go, freedom or dependency?" In this dream, many people and many cars are at the intersection, pointing to the fact that the choice between independence and freedom is a collective problem, belonging to mankind throughout the ages, not just a personal one.

What does this dream tell us? It is obvious that this dreamer was ambivalent and not ready to leave the protection of her mother and home. Just before the bridge to cross (the transition to be made) she steps out in tears, reflecting her fears and despair. By not taking this train though, she misses the next opportunity to grow, to advance on her individuation path, as she has a sense of inadequacy and is held back by her mixed emotions. In real life she was not ready, not mature enough to leave home, hence her "politeness" to let everyone else go in front of her. She can't cry as she realizes that the failure to catch the train was on purpose; she is still too much tied to the motherly security and love. In fact, she wakes up relieved, not in terror! This was the dream of a *Pulsatilla* girl.

Animals figure often into children's dreams. One boy, age

10, had till then a recurrent dream: "I was terrified when being chased by a big bear. I always woke up screaming from this nightmare." Being attacked by wild animals such as a bear—a feeling of a threat—represents deep instinctive urges trying to break through the conscious from the unconscious. When he entered puberty the next year these dreams disappeared, as the sexual primitive urges were successfully integrated in a balanced way.

Why does dream interpretation go back centuries, and why is it that some people are convinced they never dream? What does modern medicine tell us about this?

Why are Dreams Forgotten?

We try to recall dreams—whether they are happy or sad, or more frequently weird and apparently nonsensical—but the more we struggle to find more details, the more they seem to be buried in forgetfulness. "We often forget our dreams so speedily: if we cannot catch them as they are passing out the door, we never set eyes on them again" (W. Hazlitt).[3]

This sentiment is often unrecognized. There are many, way too many, people who claim and are utterly convinced that they never dream, but the reality is they simply do not remember. Through modern sleep studies where dream activity is shown during a unique condition of nervous excitation, called REM (Rapid Eye Movement) activity, it has been proven that all people dream and that this should not even be a point of discussion. Except for infants under the age of 6 months and the very drunk (as alcohol is a dream depressant, as are sedatives and psychotropic drugs), all of us dream as much as five times a night, and the state of dreaming takes up nearly 25% of our sleeping time! By the decreased state of conscious attention, the unconscious and its messenger dreams are activated. But the voice of the "carpet weaver" is not always heard, or if it is, it may be that the sleeper does not want to hear it! Many people stubbornly hold to their opinion that dreams never occur, believing this because their consciousness obliterates the voice of their dreams with overbearing noise when awake. The voice that gets blotted out (dreams) is a direct intervention of the Self, and therefore the opportunity for dreams to be a guiding light in life is missed. Let's have a closer look at why so many people have this stubborn opinion, and still can be wrong.

Do we always remember everything that happened during the previous day, or days? No! Our filter of ego consciousness immediately disposes of things that are not crucial or worthy to remember, and their content finds a reasonable destination in the garbage can called the unconscious. There is only so much that we can remember on a given day; we constantly need to make room in our consciousness for other impressions. Perceptions are often too weak in our waking state to create memories; we remember long and vivid events due to their intensity. This is the same with dreams. Singular occurring dreams, with a content that is neither very pleasant nor shocking, are easily discarded as the "nonsense" they are deemed to be. If an event during the day repeats several times, or even twice, no doubt it will stick and find a place in our memory. So is it with dreams! *Recurrent* dreams—especially from childhood to adulthood, plaguing the dreamer like an insistent tax collector—will finally get the attention of the dreamer, reminding him that something will have to be done to end this incessant torture. So recurrent dreams, or dreams with shocking events or very joyous themes, will more easily be recollected than single, mundane, everyday dreams! *Series of dreams* are another opportunity for our psyche to start paying attention to our dreams. Such series of dreams, those harping further on the same theme yet somewhat evolved and changed, might tempt our curiosity to explore their content to make sense of these fairy-tale-like constructions.

Why some recall all dreams, in detail, while others

remember none, is a phenomenon I wish to comment further about from a homeopathic standpoint. I think, firstly, that the dominant conscious function plays a role. Extraverts are less inclined to dive into the unconscious, while introverts listen more to their dream's voice. The constitution therefore can play a role: the extravert intuitive *Phosphorus* and introvert thinking *Sulphur* might be more inclined to want to remember and investigate their dreams. *Calc-c* and Earth personalities like *Pulsatilla* might be fearful of delving into the unconscious message, aware of this or not, even though *Calc-c* types are interested in being counselors and astrologers and connecting people with dead relatives and pets (*likes to be mesmerized*).

There are also sensitive, introvert types who do not recall their dreams. But looking at those patients, we see they were able to find positive compensations to their present, somewhat turbulent conscious life. Perhaps they achieved psychic equilibrium, a similar role dreams play, through adequate compensations. Consequently, the dream message may be tempered if not silenced, as a certain psychic homeostasis has been attained, so no warnings are necessary. Or rather, the patient easily sets aside those unconscious messages.

Then there are children, even adolescents, who pretend they never dream or simply remember no dreams. In that case, especially when their indicated remedy corresponds to an in utero event, it is wise to ask about the mother's recurrent dreams, as the mystical participation for a young child and even the fetus will reflect in the mother's dream too. If the patient's remedy picture, e.g. *Mag-p*, has "no dreams"—at least none in our proving symptoms—we need to look at the conscious picture: *Mag-p* has *difficulties concentrating*, *aversion to thinking*, and *study aggravates*. Not good tools to get involved in the unconscious process of dream recall.

There might be many more reasons that an individual does not remember dreams, which is not equal to *does not dream*. We can only hope that besides encouraging patients to become actively involved in remembering their dreams, the simillimum will liberate their dream messages.

As already mentioned, most dreams seem to be composed of fragments of a story, shattered pieces of a puzzle that require a closer look in order to make sense of it all. The dreamer is not usually presented with a clear image. Dreams speak in a subliminal way, vague and less rational, and are often utterly chaotic, like small fragments of a broken mirror, difficult to put together and unable to cross the threshold of consciousness. No one in his common sense would tell such a disjointed story, or demand from us to "piece together a broken mirror" so that we could write a decent, comprehensible story told by the unconscious. These unconscious phenomena mostly present themselves in a chaotic and unsystematic form, a flood of thoughts that seems crazy—not rational. It is easy to dismiss the dream as incomprehensible, seemingly dictated by an unknown lunatic, pieces that do not form a worthwhile story to remember! And the danger always remains that if the analyst insists on more details, the dreamer, to please his physician, gladly makes up lapses in the story, making it inaccurate and falsified.

As the stars of the night suddenly disappear when daylight sets in, so the consciousness has an obliterating effect on the unconsciousness. Dreams flutter away with the nocturnal darkness. Just a small delay in trying to put dreams on paper is enough for immediate recollection to begin to fade. Recall of any dream drops sharply after waking from a REM period, the period when the dream state reaches its highest intensity. This is why, when I personally want to remember a dream, I dare not fully wake up but keep my eyes half-closed until I find paper and pen, and write (or rather, scribble) everything down before the dream content disappears into thin air. No doubt, for most of us, the more time elapses between the dream and waking state, the easier it is to forget its content. Sudden awakening results in more recall than a gradual one. Usually the last dream remembered was created when it was the last thing still in the unconscious but already mixing with consciousness.

Some people—for example, a *Phosphorus-Carcinosin* personality like my wife—can recall dreams in the greatest detail, even a day or days later. She can tell me the amount of people that appear, how they looked, the color of their eyes and hair, what they were doing, if they go on a road that bends first to the left and then to the right, whether they come into a certain structure and how the rooms look—with many more details than I bother to catch even in my waking state. I, like most, must use other "tricks of the book" to help my faulty dream memory, as previously mentioned!

It is also interesting that when I start asking my patients to remember dreams, they suddenly begin to recall them though they did not before! It is as if the unconscious rewards us when we start paying attention by attempting to recollect our dreams. At the end, we will have to conclude that it is not always possible to interpret *every* dream. As dreams follow the rule of compensation, there may always be enough psychic internal resistance in us to keep our dreams guarding their secrets with greater jealousy than the Sphinx. Unless we have the capacity, drive, and curiosity for psychological knowledge, along with intelligence, self-discipline, and courage, our dreams will remain a mystery.

Remembering dreams also demands a certain amount of psychological stamina and equilibrium: dreams tend to shock, as they can release deeply buried secrets that normally would never become conscious, throwing their message in the face of the unsuspecting dreamer. Knowing that dreams are mostly compensatory, trying to wake us up from our well-guarded self-satisfaction and illusion, we must be very careful not to suffer (or cause) a mental breakdown when undergoing the process of analysis. Especially for patients with the unfortunate syphilitic heritage, artificial compensation for their created latent psychosis can break with disastrous results: suicide, depression, destructive tendencies, and schizophrenia. The latter is a world that is a mixture of distorted visions of God and the devil, of insanity and the highest degree of genius, all welded into a single horrible experience.

Of course, as much as there is some mental resistance to dreams, during sleep many inhibitory mechanisms at work during our waking time are inactive and therefore give us a chance to glimpse the dark continent of the unconscious—a territory that, while dark, is more enlightening for those who want to see than light itself! When evening falls, the threshold of the unconscious is lowered, and the images of the unconscious can pass across it.

The previous subchapters have been devoted to an analysis of the different elements occurring in a dream. How to put them all together, and is there another component that helps us do this? This leads us to the structure of every dream, which shows the way to start the analysis.

The Structure or Schema of Dreams

We first structure the dream as a story, a course of events. Most conscious stories have a beginning, a middle, and an end, but this is not the case with dreams. A dream is a short drama taking place on our inner stage. Most dreams have the structure of a classic Greek drama, formulated in four stages. To understand the dream, we must break it down into sentences or elements of a Greek play, and thus work on the problem posed by the unconscious. What are these four stages that we will use to analyze each dream? In order, they are as follows.

Locale or setting: The setting is the place, time, and *dramatis personae* (the participant(s) or actors involved; known and unknown persons, animals, or monsters), usually already found in the first sentence of the dream recall. It is the opening scene which introduces the setting and characters. We need to count the number of people at the beginning and at the end of the dream and notice the number symbolism and the part that it plays (see Chap. 2, under "Numbers Appearing in Dreams"). By counting the amount of people belonging to the conscious and unconscious, we can see what portion of life (existence) in the patient has the upper hand—the conscious or the unconscious. For instance, say that in a man's dream, besides the dreamer himself (the "I" in the dream), there appears an unknown woman and two unknown males. These **three** persons all belong to the dreamer's unconscious, so the patient's conscious mind is completely absorbed in the one, fully dominant integrated function: in this case, the unconscious has an advantage of 3:1 (the dreamer is person number **one**) over the conscious. In further dreams, this ratio can change, say to 1:3 (only one, unknown female appearing, and two known males), indicating the effectiveness of therapy when suddenly the conscious gets the advantage, showing successful integration of unconscious contents. When *many* people are present with the dreamer, it means the problem posed in the dream is a *collective* one—not just belonging to the individual dreamer but to the whole of mankind. Also, the dreamer should describe the place where the beginning of the dream takes place and the dreamer's associations to this place. If the person the dreamer meets is unknown to him, let the dreamer describe or visualize this figure, how he/she looks and what is striking about that person (attitude, moods, temperament, persona, etc.).

Exposition, or naming the theme: The next component is the exposition or naming the theme, which is the illustration of the problem of the dream, a statement of things. "Here is the problem (or issue) I am struggling with." *It states or names the theme or problem.* A conflict or crisis begins to form. It contains the theme, or the question posed by the unconscious. What question does the unconscious pose? It is a demonstration of the situation from which things start.

Peripateia: The third component is called peripateia (from the Greek *peri*, or "around," and/or *patos*, or "path," or "the public pathway"). It is the development or culmination: the illustration of the event that takes place, the developing story, the ups and downs of the event, moving out of the fixation and showing trends and possibilities. It involves a thickening of the plot, an uncomfortable situation, what is happening (a certain escalation that may become truly dramatic), how the dreamer deals with the situation, etc. This can go on for quite some time until we get to the climax, a crisis being the high point of the drama. Either something good or bad is going to happen to resolve the deadlock in the action. The dream action leads to increased complexity of the dream, until it reaches the climax and changes, sometimes in the form of a catastrophe, or a decision to be acted upon, or something occurs that throws a completely different light on the problem, leading to the fourth part, called the lysis.

Lysis (resolution), or catastrophe: The lysis, or its opposite, the catastrophe (a Greek word for tragedy, e.g. falling from a mountain), is the response to the conflict. This element of the dream brings a solution or result of the dream, a work in progress. Is there closure or no closure? The latter, called *unresolved crisis,* is a situation that indicates no salvation and no solution, which often (but not always) points to an unfavorable prognosis in which the dreamer is in a dangerous position, especially when the dream's content is meager, as a vital problem has found no resolution. Lysis portrays possible strategies that the dreamer might employ to cope with the issue presented in the opening scene, or a helpful image might appear at that time. Sometimes the dreamer gets "nearly" killed, or "nearly" falls off a mountain; at that point a backdoor to escape the situation has been left open to avoid the final catastrophe. Of course, there is *no standard* lysis! A catastrophe attempts to shock the dreamer's consciousness with an *urgent warning* (change your life style; whatever you are doing now is not working, or there will be a fall off a mountain, another accident or a fire, etc., or you are taking on more than you are capable of handling), or less likely, the catastrophe acquaints him with a fixed situation. If there is neither crisis nor lysis, it is a situation that leaves open the way in which the response and development might go. Naturally, we would like dreams to always be like a crystal ball—to tell us about the immediate future and give us advice on what to do to avoid life challenges—but rarely is that the purpose and goal of a dream. The lysis and "solution" that is offered often baffles us, as if a cruel tease of the unconscious. But in fact, it is a lesson from the unconscious to take its content seriously, to work hard and be honest when investigating it, or the content will forever escape us.

In very rare cases, the unconscious (or its messenger, the dream) does tell us what we *ought* to do, except when it is obvious. Several solutions are usually possible; the dream simply presents a choice of possible solutions, rather than actualities, if there is a lysis. Lysis or catastrophe always points to the future, to what is in the making, what is possible or even likely. The dream seems to say, "This is where you are now! This is how it is with you!" Dreams can even be prophetic, as we know. The dream may show where we are amiss and what possibilities are open to us, but unless we attempt to change and go those ways and wrestle with their difficulties, the dream message is in vain. On the other hand, in a vision (see further) there is no lysis, as the dreamer is passive and only watches a scene.

Trying to explain a dream is to descend into the unconscious, always a dangerous journey to some extent. We go there to get something: men usually "go fishing," women prefer to "go shopping." Contrary to our beliefs and expectations, it is a valuable treasure we may find there on our fishing trip, or in the marvelous store. We do not know exactly what fish we caught on this excursion, but when we come up again into the world of light or consciousness, this surprising catch mixes with the content of the conscious. This might lead to a frightening insight—that we were not as good as we thought—or on the contrary, it might bring a positive message when pondered.

Finally, the lysis leads us back to the point from which we started. We began with a conscious problem that burdened us. We then slipped into the unconscious, hoping to bring back a treasure to enlighten us. The dream will give us the message, the treasure, but don't rush it. "Sleep on it," we should tell ourselves! Even if we do not have a dream, or do not recall one, something may become clear during our sleep and an answer come to mind in the morning, or in the next few days.

To help you find these structures and phases of a dream, following are some examples. No attempt otherwise is made here to explain the dream with its relative fixed symbols (subjective dream analysis).

Examples of Dream Structure

Dream example one, male patient

I'm away from home to attend some event. I have to spend the night in a hotel where I have to share the room, and the bed, with a woman. She's a beautiful woman, about my age. In the evening, I'm lying on the bed while she is standing on the bed, doing her fingernails. She wears a long, thin, white night dress. One moment she comes to stand over my face; I look under the dress, up her legs—she's not naked—and I start massaging her legs. I realize she's trying to seduce me, but I'm determined I won't get into that (although I feel very much sexually aroused); I know I have a lovely wife at home who I don't want to betray.

I massage her legs being careful not to give any "sexual signals." Later we lie down, sleeping; she has wrapped her legs around mine and I enjoy the feeling but at the same time I have fun with the thought that she's making such an effort to seduce me.

Locale: Two people; the dreamer and a strange woman (1:1). Drama takes place in a hotel.

Exposition: The dreamer has to spend the night in a hotel where he must share the bed with a woman. She is a beautiful woman, doing her fingernails.

Peripateia: The developing story goes from**,** "She wears a long thin dress," to "I don't want to betray (my wife)."

Lysis: Good lysis; he enjoys the feeling and has fun at the thought that the woman is making such an effort.

Dream example two, male patient

I am invited to go play tennis by a male friend who I do not particularly like because he has a tendency to be overfriendly towards everyone, but it is clear that this is just a persona. This takes place in a hotel, in the underground garage of a hotel. I have my tennis racquet packed in my doctor's bag, but when I arrive in the garage, I hear music upstairs. I put my bag down and go upstairs and look for a good female dancer as I enjoy dancing. I meet an attractive lady and spend hours dancing away. When the orchestra stops, I go downstairs to meet my friend but now I cannot find my bag with my racquet. I keep on searching in different rooms and finally on a last attempt I find a cleaning lady who asks my name and proceeds to tell me she found my bag.

I wake up with relief.

Locale: Two males and two females: 2:2. The dream takes place in the underground garage of a hotel.

Exposition: The dreamer is invited to play tennis with someone who has a created, friendly persona.

Peripateia: He hears music, and later meets an attractive lady. When the orchestra stops, he goes downstairs and can't find his tennis bag, then meets a cleaning lady.

Lysis: A good lysis; a relief when the tennis bag is found.

With these examples, it should be clear to the reader how to proceed with the analysis of a dream, and how to put some order to it. I would be remiss not to elaborate more about visions, so that discussion now follows.

Visions

Who among us has ever had a vision? What does it stand for? My wife told me about the following vision she had while traveling in the Middle East. The intensity of emotions she felt during this vision never left her, and the vision held some of the most remarkable pictures etched in her memory. It helps that she is an extraverted, intuitive *Phosphorus*, so she has a very pure relationship to the inside and the unconscious. Therefore, a vision for her is taken in completely, as it was presented by the unconscious, not distorted by the shadow side. Following is her vision, beginning with the circumstance in which it took place.

Vision example

I went on a shopping trip to Damascus to look around for household furnishings. Among them were antique frames, inlaid with mother of pearl, that I found in a shop I have been to before on past visits to the Christian Quarter. After having the customary tea with the familiar owner of the shop, I decided it was time to return to my hotel room with my frames that were carefully wrapped up in brown paper and string. The owner had a helper in the shop that I had never seen before. He was in his early 20s, lean and tall, a very willing helper, of good disposition, and of African descent. The owner treated him terribly in my presence, treated him with scorn and orders, but the young man maintained his friendly disposition in spite of the abuse from the "master." The owner insisted that the young man help me with my package and hail a taxi for me. I reassured him that I could do this on my own. This went back and forth three times, then I finally gave up and said, "OK, he can do it for me." So, the young man walked with me to the street to hail a taxi, and when one stopped, I got in with my package. The young man leaned in on the passenger side to talk to the cabbie about what hotel he was to take me to.

While watching the young man in conversation, I had a vision: looking at him with open eyes, I saw in a flash that I was standing on a cobblestone street, very similar to the one I was just on, and I was covered from head to toe with an abaya (a loose over-garment, a robe-like dress, draped from the head, covering the whole body except face, feet, and hands, and can be worn with a veil to not be seen by other men). The color of my abaya was blue, my face was covered with a semi-transparent white veil. I could see my physical self as being short, meaty, with medium-brown eyes and very white skin. I felt aghast, a bit shocked to see the sight of myself as I was white, short, and plump. But next to me was my own black slave who was holding many packages for me in his arms as though I had just finished shopping. Next to us was my carriage with one horse and my driver, waiting for me to enter the carriage. I saw myself as a married, well-to-do woman with my own slave, carriage, and driver. This seemed to me to be in Ottoman times, either in Damascus itself or possibly in Istanbul, but being that I was physically in Damascus, I then concluded that this past life was also in Damascus. And the catalyst or trigger to this vision was the young black man that I saw in the shop being treated like a slave.

Analysis

What has happened? The inner unconscious material is so intensified that it becomes visible in waking hours in states of diminished consciousness. It is a direct invasion of unconscious contents into the world of consciousness, when the threshold of consciousness is somewhat lowered. We cannot say, "I would like to have a vision"—it is an autonomous creation of the unconscious, not under the command of our will. And if by any chance we have a pleasant vision, we cannot will it to last longer. It really is a vivid experience of the direct invasion of consciousness by an element from the collective unconscious, an archetype, while the person (my wife in this case) is still in contact with the conscious world (she knows where she is at that moment), and is not swallowed up by the whole experience. Therefore, having a vision is not at all synonymous with mental illness, where the unconscious has overwhelmed the conscious and there is only one world evoking hallucinations and other states of psychosis like schizophrenia.

A vision is a conscious, temporary contact with the images of the unconscious while not losing contact with the objective reality. Visions are in the same class of psychological interpretation as dreams and need to be studied and understood in the same fashion, except that they have no lysis like in a dream. In a vision, no action takes place; the dreamer is a passive observer, as the content consists only of an image (vision) presented to the dreamer. Visions may come from mischievous spirits as well as from the Great Spirit (American Indians). Well-known in history are the visions of Black Elk, the medicine man of the Oglala Sioux, who wrote in his autobiography *Black Elk Speaks* about his vision at 9 years old, when he suffered an acute febrile illness. Initially he kept the vision to himself, but an old medicine man told him that he must share it with his tribe. As a result, men and horses who participated in the reenactment of the vision became much happier, and some cures of diseases were even achieved!

Another vision was had by Sitting Bull, who restrained his 8,000 young impatient warriors from attacking Custer and his 650 soldiers at the battle of Little Big Horn, until he saw in another vision that he would defeat him. Crazy Horse, a famous Lakota chief, had a vision which was a premonition of the way he would die (a vision close to a prophetic dream). Crazy Horse was one of the bravest American Indians, involved in more than 80 battles, but his vision told him that he would not die in battle at the hands of an enemy. Rather, a man who appeared in his vision on horseback, coming out of the lake (the personal unconscious talking), was a soldier who killed him by stabbing him while he was held by a friend. This indeed happened, while he was held on the reservation where he had surrendered. Crazy Horse was a plain man who avoided personal display, and his introverted thinking character was expressed by the time he spent alone seeking visions and guidance, and simply to think.

Not everyone has, nor needs to have visions, they are just another way to have contact with the unconscious. But anyone who has a vision should pay as much attention to it as he should to his dreams. After all, these are natural products, not produced by the human will.

Before I end this chapter, which consisted of different stepping-stones to successful dream interpretation, I would like to share further hints about dream interpretation to make it easier for the reader to add "more meat to the bone."

Further Helpful Hints in Dream Interpretation

As dreams are individual expressions of patients' unconscious, we cannot force laws or even general considerations for dream interpretation on anyone. But at least there are some hints to help along the way that can be used to help the dreamer and therapist come to a satisfactory explanation.

- Always begin with the expectation that the dream will reveal something unique about the dreamer. Don't we say to an old acquaintance when we meet him, "What is new?" Also, in order to make the correct interpretation of the dream, it is essential to know and take into account what sort of person had the dream: what is his trade, position, age, intellectual character, and activities; in other words, all characteristics expressed by Aphorism 5 of the *Organon.*
- Ask, is this a favorable or unfavorable dream? What feelings does the dreamer experience after he wakes up? Was it a good feeling? Did it reflect joy, love, anxiety, or fear? Everyone experiences that this emotion upon awaking can color the mood of the dreamer the rest of the day
- What caused such a dream? What were the experiences of the previous day? Events of the preceding day or recent past are often woven into the dream plot. What happened? Was there an exceptional or strange situation?"
- It is always important in dreams to evaluate the dreamer's actions and responses: how does he respond to the message, to persons in the dreams, especially archetypal images? Does he ask further questions from the figures or does he run away from them (non-acceptance)? Or does the dreamer simply contemplate what is said to him?
- Is the dreamer conscious of anything about it, so he can amplify the dream? Has he come to the age that he can understand the objects in the dream: for

instance, a 3-year-old would not know the moon has craters, and a *Bar-c* person might not know what a wedding signifies.

- When analyzing dreams, we do well to start with a dose of humility and not think that we are a mana personality who has all the answers, which easily leads to vanity and arrogance. Whenever patient and physician try to unlock the mysterious message of the unconscious, they must never forget that this road of discovery is always a treacherous one, full of uncertainties and baffling questions. No matter how much we have studied and how erudite we are, there always will be dreams for which we cannot find the key to unlock the door to the unconscious
- Often the first dream after administering the simillimum brings to light the causality (trigger) and theme of the dream. Even more astonishing, some patients have an important dream the evening before the consult with the psychologist or the homeopath. It is as if the unconscious prepares the patient to rehearse important contents that were till then invisible to the patient.
- When the dreamer himself appears in a dream (the "I" in the dream), he usually represents only his conscious ego (*the dream-ego*), and the dream often foretells future activities of the dreamer; the other figures (people known and unknown, animals, objects) stand for the more or less unknown unconscious elements.
- If an unknown person (man or woman) appears in a dream, it represents an unknown aspect of the dreamer, an archetypal figure of the collective unconscious, a voice of the unconscious or the Self. Unknown persons represent a relentless "call"

from within that must be examined and answered. If an animal appears in a dream, it refers to the instincts of the dreamer, the entirely natural part of man, either still suppressed (if a wild animal, especially a black one; "blackness" means that this part of the person is still rooted in the unconscious), or partially integrated into consciousness (if a domestic animal, especially a white one; "white" is the color of innocence). Animals are also often helpers in the dream, as they are in fairy tales.

- When a voice is heard in a dream it can be an intervention of the Self, a voice with knowledge rooted in the collective unconscious, and therefore should be obeyed as the real truth; it acts as an absolutely authoritative character coming at decisive moments for the dreamer, often called an animus voice representing the wise old man (see Chap. 12, "Animus").
- With parallel dreams, ask: has there been an experience like the one in the dream? For instance, of near drowning, a car accident, of witnessing a disaster (even just on TV) like the 9/11 events in the United States? Has there been a PTSD event?
- In general, children dream more of animals than adults; women tend to report more nightmares, and remember colors in their dreams more than men; women tend to report a higher incidence of human interaction and speech than men; men have more physical battles with others in their dreams, and examination dreams. Such dream themes correlate with the theme of the CD of men and women, where women often carry a theme of love and speech in their delusions, while men's core delusions

tend to be more about action or performance, ambition, competition, and delusions of grandeur.

- Analyzing dreams can go on forever, as ending dream work is always arbitrary. To find "closure," ask yourself: Have I, and everyone else involved in the work (students, colleagues, etc., but especially the dreamer), found enough "Aha!" while we have been exploring the dream? If the next dreams agree with the interpretation, then we have interpreted the material enough. But if your psyche tells you, "You have not addressed the problem yet or answered it," then we must go further. And if these dreams do not reveal their messages, or are impenetrable despite plenty of amplification, they will usually repeat themselves in a slightly different form, bringing the same message (see Chap. 5, under "Recurrent Dreams").
- Anyone interested in dreams should keep a regular dream journal as even the most vivid dreams can escape when not written down. For most people, their majority of dreams are lost forever if not recorded within the first five minutes of waking. So, this should be done even in the dead of night. Use little penlight flashlights to write with so you don't wake anyone else up (your partner might not match your enthusiasm about your latest dream!). Nothing is flightier than a dream, which seems to elude even the best memory. Even if you remember only fragments, write them down, as something more of the dream may come to you. Dreams want to become conscious and reach the light of day. Leave interpretation of your dream until you are fully awake and avoid doing the interpretation as you are writing the dream down. Draw pictures of your

dreams; one picture is worth more than 1,000 words! Always record dreams in the *present* tense to make the dream record more vivid and compelling for the dreamer and to easily draw others into it when shared. Accuracy of reporting the dream is important: ask for as many details as possible. If the dreamer turns to enter a room, does he turn right or left? If there is a setting for the dream, ask whether it is indoors, outdoors, a city, a forest, etc.? If a woman is involved, "Is she old or young? Known or unknown? How does the woman look? What color are the walls of the building?" Nothing in the dream is arbitrary! There is no absurdity in asking any question at all that could lead to a more complete description of the dream images. The more details in a dream, the more it points to a purely *personal* problem. Sparse contents of a dream and simple images point more to *collective and impersonal* problems, problems belonging to the human species.

- The time of life of the dreamer is all-important. It makes a tremendous difference in the interpretation of a dream whether the dreamer is a child, adolescent, in midlife or old age. Always state the *age* of the dreamer.
- Simultaneous dreaming (same content) can occur between two people when their bond in the unconscious is deep (spouses, children and parents, lovers, etc.).
- When in the same dream the dreamer goes from one scene to another, and makes the dream somewhat complicated, each of the scenes gives us a different way to look at the dreamer's complex, and more information as to how to deal with it.

- When a *young* child dreams of her mother, the dream refers to the real mother, a person of vital importance to any young child.

This chapter has been devoted to an analysis of several different stepping-stones in the interpretation of dreams. It showed that great attention must be paid to details, that filling in gaps in the dream recall must be avoided, and that we should proceed, step by step, in a very disciplined way. In the next chapter I present some of the different *frequent dream themes* in the population.

4

COMMON THEMES IN DREAMS

"Dreams that are not understood are like letters that are not opened." — *Talmud*

Although dreams are individual unconscious peculiar expressions, requiring the dreamer's cooperation and insight for a correct and intelligent interpretation, humanity is plagued by certain frequently occurring themes, posing common archetypal collective problems. In other words, because they are archetypal in nature, it appears that such dreams have a general "common" message to whomever they occur. Themes of failing examinations, of falling, flying, being caught naked or inappropriately dressed, of pre-death and death. The latter two are just a couple of the most common motifs with prophetic capacity, encrypting an early awareness of a longtime situation or crisis before the conscious mind can grasp it. It is here that the dreamer should validate the preciousness of these unconscious messages when he tries to understand what they want to tell him about his conscious life situation following the compensation principle.

Let's investigate some of these common themes.

Prophetic Dreams

As much as dreams find their origin in conscious contents, some of them represent unconscious processes which have *no recognizable relation to consciousness*, alerting the dreamer about events that have not materialized yet, nor have any apparent cause. These are the prospective, or prophetic, dreams—those which anticipate future conscious events, like a voice of the Oracle of Delphi—warning or enlightening the dreamer. In the rubrics of the Repertory, among the remedies found under *prophetic dreams* we are not surprised to discover the nervous, anticipative *Aconite* as the main remedy, one who even *predicts the time of death.* We should also not be amazed to find *Phosphorus* with her close relationship to family members and the unconscious in general, and *Sulphur* with *cares about relatives,* to have prophetic dreams about an accident, or illness, befalling family members.

Pre-Death and Death Dreams

The unconscious looks at death in a very different manner than the conscious mind, portraying death in dreams in a very different language, often a symbolic one. Frequently in these dreams there are many allusions to destruction and/or restoration, suggesting impending disaster or rebirth. Some symbols found in dreams about death portray Nature: a tree felled by lightning, a symbol for death by apoplexy; a horse losing control and running itself to death, representing our physical energy abolished; a clock in which the hands have stopped, indicating time has ended for that person, or that the destruction of structures is more imminent than of the dreamer him/herself.

For example, I had as a patient a nun suffering from cancer, who dreamed of setting the city on fire. As in reality she was helping the poor, this shocked her very much, but two months later she died from the cancer. Her dream had presented her diseased body (the Self, symbolized by the city) in rather esoteric language—fire standing for disturbance in the unconscious. Cancer may be a metaphor for energy out of control, or of destructive, proliferative activity of a psychological complex, as seen in this dream. If a fire breaks out in the attic (upper conscious) or the cellar (collective unconscious) of your house (the Self), it means in those places there will be an emotional disturbance. Such a dream seems to come from nowhere, "out of the blue," without first giving a hint of its meaning and with no mention of death of the dreamer herself. It is often only after death has occurred that its meaning becomes clear.

Dreams of actual death (final death) can be taken prognostically, but more often they refer to a *symbolic death and rebirth process*, usually portending the need for a great psychological change. Rarely should they be taken literally, as they most likely refer to a psychological development or improvement: the dissolution of an old existing pattern, an aspect or attitude of the personality, or an old painful complex. Whatever sick entity exists must be destroyed in order to create something new, a secret attempt by the Self to destroy the dis-ease, making rebirth possible. Through these "little deaths" of fundamental life changes, a new identity is in the making. The dream often overdramatizes its content in order to shock our rather insensitive or ignorant consciousness, to incline us to at least wonder *why* we had this dream, rather than simply thinking our end is near. By considering dream series more than the single dream, its meaning will come to light (as the phoenix rising from the ashes); most often a "death" dream represents a transformation process in the dreamer, some future probability that is likely to signify a rebirth rather than a finality—a favorable prognosis, although no doubt such a dream will rattle most patients. Patience is required from the therapist and the analysand: further dreams in the patient's dream series will bring more clarification.

Another symbol of rebirth, resurrection, and self-renewal is "pulling off dead skin" (like a snake, which renews its skin every seven years).

Other examples of *life-threatening and life-changing motifs* are expressed by dream images depicting floods, storms, hurricanes, massive fires, tidal waves, typhoons, earthquakes, or other natural catastrophes, as well as outbursts of passion or panic. Is this a warning for the dreamer of impending death? Only when these events actually destroy the symbolic image of the dreamer's Self, or when animals get killed by these events (representing the dreamer's instinctive life), or when images appear depicting the destruction of one's house, bed, or a tree (representing the Vital Force) for example. But destruction in a dream may often be followed by rebirth as the dream has a happy ending by showing how the dreamer was able to escape the imminent danger. For instance, the dreamer finds a safe spot like the cellar of the house in case of hurricanes, or he manages to find an island in the middle of the ocean, or amazingly, he can now stay afloat even when he could not swim before. These dreams are warnings that the dreamer must examine the basic problem in his life, a life-threatening (to the body or psyche) motif, illustrated in an ominous dream in order to avoid a further spiraling down of his life circumstances ("burning the candle at both ends"). At the same time, the dreamer can receive a positive message of encouragement from the unconscious at a time when defeat seems near.

Here is such an example from a female patient. It is only part of her dream, and my assessment is without explanation of all the symbols, for I wish to show only the concept above.

Dream

Suddenly we (she and her young son) are in a huge river that runs in between two banks, the river is extremely wide, with lines of people walking on both sides. After talking to someone right next to us on the boat, my son is suddenly gone, and all of a sudden we are about one hour north of our starting point. How could I have lost him, I am filled with dread and think: if I had just held onto him tighter! I know he has never been taught how to swim and there is no way he could have made it to one side of the river or the other. My heart is broken. I fear the worst. Everyone on the boat tells me to keep going and I am stunned at this terrible advice, no one wants to stop and no one will help me, and they tell me that in my condition I cannot possibly make the swim to try to find him in the vast waters; he is un-locatable and I must save myself. At that, I am incredulous, and I just decide to jump off the platform/transport barge. I start swimming downstream, which is oddly the opposite direction the water is flowing, as the river flows upstream, so it requires a lot of effort and I am being powered by my thoughts and desire to find my son, whom I am wishing I had spent more time teaching to swim. I swim for an hour, the whole time thinking and panicking about my son. Suddenly I see a boy face-down, bobbing up and down in the river; it is in an unusual, fetal-like position, yet he is also treading water at same time. I cannot believe it. He is alive. He has taught himself to tread water, and he transmits to me the thought that he has been *holding on, treading water, which he taught himself to do.* (This is a conversation we have silently as I come closer to him.) It is a true miracle, and I have tears flooded with gratitude. He immediately throws his arms around me and hangs onto me with an embrace, and I have a surge of relief and energy, digging deep to get him to shore. I swim, and swim some more, and make it to shore with him.

Analysis

What is a possible explanation of this drama, and is it favorable? This dreamer was understandably taken by episodes of sadness and hopelessness. The favorable part of the dream is that the dreamer plays an active role and does not remain idle, as a mother in real life would never remain idle in a similar situation. The libido (which stands for psychic energy in general, not just sexual), withdrawn from the conscious, causes a "depression," or as Pierre Janet[1] called it, *un abaissement du niveau mental* ("a reduction of mental level"), and this withdrawal of energy is expected to accumulate in the unconscious, producing the dream material. But this patient can withdraw part of her unconscious creative energy and incorporate it into a conscious content, as seen in her active participation. Now in reality, this dreamer does have a child with developmental challenges who is her fragile and unique link with the outside world, as she is withdrawn from society (objective translation). But the boy in her dream is also the symbol for her newly developing animus (subjective translation), which is the relation to her unconscious. That she is active in the dream reveals a positive movement of her unconscious, a tendency to integrate the deposited libido from the unconscious, emptying the vast stores of unwanted material. Therefore, she is gaining more control in her conscious as the conscious horizon is now expanded, broadened, and extended by including the unconscious content (the activity of her animus). This promises a future change of personality, if the process evolves in the same favorable direction (from unconscious to conscious, rather than the opposite). Such a process of conquest stops the autonomy of the old animus, so rather than being possessed by the animus—where it can exert its independent and disturbing power—a beneficial relationship to her changing, developing animus is established. It is the first step to becoming "complex-free."

But what if serious pathology presents itself?

Warning Dreams in Serious Pathology

The following patient was a 45-year-old woman who had a long history of severe fatigue and concentration disturbances after head trauma, and many different psychological traumas such as recurrent grief. There was initially good improvement on *Carcinosin* and *Nat-s*, when she had a dream of retiring in what she called "a light cloister or monastery" (see drawing, p. 122).

In the drawing of this dream, we see lights all over, with bright colors and the cloister sitting on an island (=the conscious) in the middle of a stormy ocean—"ocean" being a multi-faceted symbol from time immemorial of the deep or collective unconscious, and of the unexplored depths within the Self. "Storm" stands as a symbol for the spirit, the force of life and Nature. The stormy waters represent also the "anger" and rebellion of the unconscious. In her dream, her body was an oil lamp which stood in a room with mirrors. The light of this lamp lit the room and was strengthened through the mirrors and transmitted to the outside (=connection with the conscious).

In her next dream the oil lamp is still in the cloister, but the oil is almost finished. The flame is just a red glow, and only dark smoke comes from the candle. The mirrors and lamp are now blackened. There is a draft in the room.

Her present conscious situation: An MRI showed a big white spot, diagnosed as a polyp by the neurologist; forgetfulness and total lack of concentration (syphilitic); mistakes in spelling (syph.); forgets appointments and what she planned, and time goes too fast (sycotic). She sleeps through three different alarm clocks, and forgets what day it is; gets lost in well-known streets, as she cannot find her way to her physician (syph.); always forgets what to do next, makes plans but then forgets them immediately (syph.); puts milk to warm up in a pan and puts the empty pan back on the fire. She can't find things where she put them, like her toothbrush, appointment book, etc. Her therapist tells her she is a malingerer, which brings her to the brink of despair (syph.). What does it make us think of when we hear this? An Alzheimer-like disease; disconnection. As seen here, most of the expressions are syphilitic in nature, no longer sycotic, so there is progression to her disease.

Here is the drawing of her first dream, and on the following pages, some symbolic explanations of the figures that appeared in the dream.

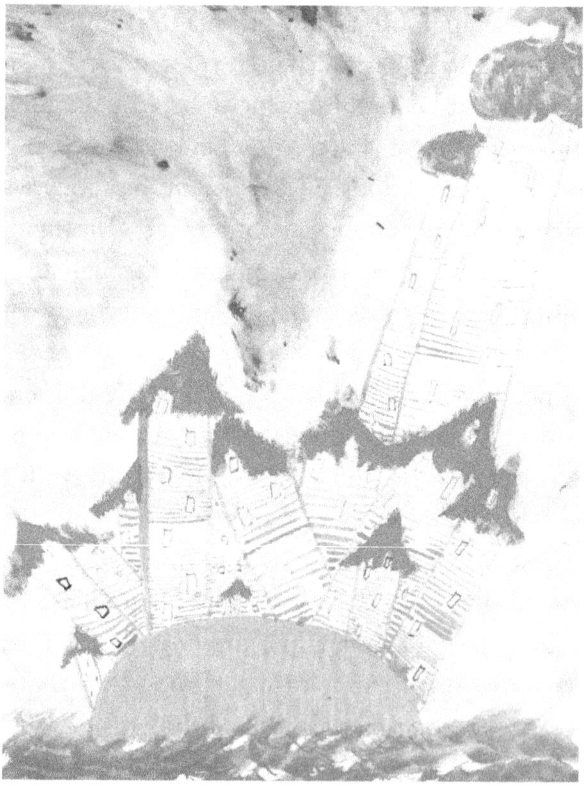

Cloister: A symbol of protection; isolation; silence to meditate; introversion; and examining the unconscious.
Light: The symbolic equivalent of consciousness, conscious direction, also the symbol of the male principle.
Fire: The basic symbol of life.
Storm: This symbolizes an unruly unconscious with **wind**. Wind stands for air, which is life, an archetype of the breath of the living spirit. Wind is also spiritual power, the spiritual quality of the conscious. It is the breath of a god-like force, used for good or bad. It also stands for the Greek word *pneuma* ("vital spirit, soul, or creative force of a person"). When we think about wind, or Fong in TCM, it is all those emotions belonging to the Liver element—anger, suppressed anger, and frustration—creating "internal wind" and upsetting emotions. Such wind (or emotions) makes the flame burn faster and consume the oil—contrasting to a calmly burning flame not excited by wind.

Accepting the fact that she could not wake up from three alarm clocks, she decided to sleep when she was tired without an alarm. Sometimes she slept three hours, sometimes one hour. Then she could do some spiritual exercises which she could not do before, and noticed she had more "air," more space and more acceptance for things as they are. In this way her despair disappeared, and she even repaired her bike where she had no energy before. She can now go for a walk, meet a perfect stranger with her dog, have a nice conversation, and enjoy life again.

As we can see, a certain acceptance, made clear by her dream to avoid "wind or storms" and go with thc flow as much as possible, gave her the impetus again to love life, even without a remedy for the moment. By accepting reality and not forcing the issue, she will react better to a remedy when she takes it. Accepting and doing what you *can* achieve (an adjustment to the present situation)—not feeling frustration with what you cannot do—is the key to healing. Again, the dream just told the patient where she was in life, what she was doing, it did not tell her *what* to do or offer any solutions. Her dreams brought more clarity to her situation, and it was up to the dreamer to find the "Aha" explanation to her dream—which she did, transforming her life.

To say one more word about the storm/wind/draft: creating "wind" or a "storm" within her being will use up the oil in the lamp much sooner, blacken the mirrors in the cloister, and block the radiation of her energy to the outside world, thus restricting joy and Nature from coming to her, keeping her holed up inside and surrounded by blackness, a prisoner of the unconscious. If not lifted, this will give way to utter despair and depression. I think, indeed, it is good to not "live by the clock" (which was frustrating for her), and better regarding her energy, as it is also better to avoid negative people.

Another example of a warning dream was seen in a 55-year-old woman who had a recurrence of left-sided breast cysts. This was each time followed by aspiration because of the size, but the cysts kept recurring. Then, one week before a new mammogram diagnosed a left-sided ductal carcinoma, she had the following dream.

Another warning dream

I am driving along a road quite quickly when the road falls away down, down, down, for a long way and I can see flashing red/blue lights at the bottom indicating danger. I realize the car is out of control, scream, and then wake up.

Analysis

The warning in this dream was evident. Because the situation was not corrected adequately before and the journey of her disease was not changed, and as the theme of her life was lack of nourishment and respect by her own family members, a last stand was taken by the unconscious to send her a message: to not let others invade her boundaries. Although she was at the wheel of her car (usually positive as it shows being in control of one's own destiny), she went too fast and all of a sudden the road fell down (slipping into the unconscious) with flashing red warning signals. The car (the symbol for her Self to go forward in life) was out of control. This is analogous to the cells of her body growing out of control, an accelerated mitosis (replication) of cells, the definition of cancer.

Dreams of Flying and Falling

Especially dreams of falling can sound alarm bells for the dreamer. Climbing a mountain is not necessarily an act that needs to be discouraged because there is too much danger involved. Its positive symbolism refers to the male aspect of animus—power, energy, and the higher Self—as we move towards light or consciousness (positive direction of cure) where we can reach a higher place to see what the problem is in the unconscious (far below), which is to achieve increasing ego-consciousness. It suggests also the determination that is needed to reach the summit (or set goal in conscious life, of which the summit is the self-realization), and to conquer the difficulties and obstacles encountered while climbing the mountain, reflecting the challenges the dreamer will meet in his daily life. Remember the idiom, "I have a mountain to climb." In other words, to get to the top (reflective of the ambition for business) by his own efforts, the road ahead will not be easy and the dreamer will have to muster much courage and effort to achieve what he wants, the ultimate triumph!

Often though, such a dream also contains plenty of warning, and can be dreamt by people in different conscious situations, pointing towards tendencies of which the dreamer is not aware of: metaphorically speaking, putting himself in situations where he will "fall off the mountain." One such situation is where the dreamer in his conscious life overexerts himself to reach a goal—most likely a materialistic goal, the obtaining of riches and becoming a slave to things which rule him, typical for a *Nux-v* personality. *Nux-v* is a money-maker who appoints no value to honor and engaging in truth, unless it has cash value. It reflects an unbalanced lifestyle, being at the mercy of uncontrolled passions and a reckless, controlling, power-hungry attitude of his unconscious, as seen in the rubric reflecting *Nux-vomica's* life: *businessman, worn out* (*Nux-v* 3).

Nux-v is a person who uses words to make the unreal appear as real when he says, "I am rich," when the word poor would be the correct designation of his situation, reflecting his inner poverty. He is reduced in spirit, and his only way to measure the value of life is by the single-minded accumulation of wealth. He is the fool who loses the *inner* man in order to gain the *outer*—splendor and goods—till he suffers early deterioration from illness he will not recover from, ultimately will die, and be remembered no more. He considers richness only in pomp, ostentation and show, and possesses greed incapable of moderation. Such a person does not understand that what a human really has is *within* him; what is outside of him is of no importance. His inward nature shows no sign of genuine happiness, only a thin veneer of it, glitter that conceals unhappiness with his lot. It is the mind's balance, not the financial one, that matters! However huge his mansion might be, he will still only have one puny body. Why so many bedrooms? He will only lie in one of them. His riches are stored in bank vaults, but it is his mind that needs to be filled. He never understood that without health one can do nothing, but with health there are few things one cannot do! As Diogenes proclaimed, "I don't possess in order not to be possessed. My days of moneymaking are over. Moreover, I do not need money" (Kaplan, 2011, p. 22). *Nux-v* would react incredulously to this with questions like, "But what do you gain by this? What is your richness?" Freedom is the answer!

There are two kinds of poverty. One walks the streets like the Greek philosopher Diogenes of Sinope, the cynic, living a very simple, careful life. The second type is lack of connectedness to other fellow human beings. Such an impoverished man walks on stilts, figuratively, fooling himself that he hovers above everyone else. But let him show himself in nothing but his shirt. How is his body? How is his mind? Although rich in goods and luxury, *Nux-v* loses sleep, stimulates himself with drugs, rich foods, and alcoholic drinks (*madness in drunkards; madness from mental labor; desire for coffee; desire for alcohol*), but at the end of the day finds that he is reduced, forced to socialize with a servant or his submissive wife, who are only staying with him to catch the little luxury he is willing to share with them. At night his poverty remains: he can't sleep like a happy man does, closing his eyes in satisfied peace, for thoughts about business torture his soul. He is never removed from care and fear, and has no true contentment (*Delusion, someone is in bed with him; someone has sold his bed*), making him captive to demonical forces. He seeks nothing but illusions and vain deceits. What he deprives himself most of are genuine friendships and joyous conversations, in which humans find the sweetest fruit of life.

In describing oligarchy, where wealth is the only thing that matters, Plato wrote:

> The further they go in the process of accumulating wealth, the more they value it and the less they value goodness. For

> aren't wealth and goodness related to two objects in a balance, so that when one rises the other must fall! (Plato, 1955)

Nux-vomica's cravings for power, fame, and possessions are damaging factors and such a person, suffering from an overly heightened level of confidence and even ego inflation, can dream that he is climbing higher and higher and then falls suddenly from a precipice to his death. Usually he will wake up in a cold sweat before he hits the ground, which is a kind of lysis of this anxiety dream. As he does not fall on the ground but plunges towards it and wakes up before it happens, it means the matter is not yet determined—there is still possibility of change, but it warns this person that an unchanged lifestyle could lead to cardiovascular disease with stroke and heart attack, along with a plenitude of ailments such as stomach ulcer, heartburn, obesity, diabetes, and a nervous breakdown.

A dream of falling not only reflects the busy materialist, but also the person Jung describes as one who "overestimates himself," or as we call it in homeopathy, *delusions of grandeur*, which a great proportion of the male population suffers from today. Hence, a dream of falling occurs more frequently in men. Delusions of grandeur refers to those who have unrealistic ideas or overly high opinions of themselves—out of proportion to their real capacities. Modesty—the ability to take correct measure of oneself—is not given to many.

The *I Ching* or *Book of Changes* in TCM defines it well in hexagram 15: "Modesty shows the handle of character, gives honor and creates success. Modesty that is honored spreads radiance. The superior man reduces that which is too much and augments that which is too little" (Wilhelm & Baynes, 1950, p. 64).

There is of course also the opposite of delusions of grandeur —feeling one's self to be a statistical cipher, one of the mass—

which could lead to a loss of meaning of life. Life is indeed a balancing act to not topple into one of these extremes. Elucidation, remaining faithful to the truth, and the desire to be more complete are the solutions.

We know the idiom, "falling from one's throne." That is the fate of those who plan grandiose ideas out of proportion to their real capacities, and as such lose touch with human reality (*psychic inflation*). It reflects the dark side of the Self, because the Self represents the greatest power in the psyche, even endangering the ego to the point of fracture, leading to dissociation where the conscious can no longer control the unconscious. This is obvious in people who always take themselves too seriously, who have lost a sense of humor and cannot laugh at themselves.

A third party subject to these falling dreams are those in danger of losing status, respect, honor, security, or emotional stability, reflected by the rubrics *Ailments from: wounded honor; pecuniary loss; business failure; egotism; embarrassment; indignation; mortification* and *loss of position.*

The most outspoken remedy in our Repertory that has *dreams of falling from a height* is *Thuja*, which represents yet another aspect of this dream theme. It reflects more the sensation of *vulnerability* as expressed by *Thuja's* cyber delusion *he is made of glass*, also expressed by delusions that the *body: is delicate; is brittle; is thin;* and *Delusion, of emaciation*. To compensate, such a person will create an excessive persona, a false power complex or Adlerian complex, a "pseudo ego" expressed by the delusion *appearance of building stones*. A very similar theme is seen in *Lycopodium*, a complementary remedy to *Thuja*.

Dreams of falling or riding a roller coaster can also happen to those caught in an unfortunate situation, or as TCM calls it, a "noble misfortune." The following dream of an adult woman reflects this situation.

Conscious situation: A 45-year-old female, a practicing

homeopath, received the news that the government decided that homeopathy could only be practiced by medical doctors and dentists, and even they could only use homeopathy after regular medical care was administered. In other words, even for licensed physicians, homeopathy was pushed to the background. This caused tremendous confusion in her and made her very unhappy as she wanted more time to study other medical branches such as psychology, dream work, and Traditional Chinese Medicine, useful for the homeopathic practice. It also created a lack of confidence in her to start this new journey. She wondered if her recurrent dreams had anything to do with this dilemma.

Dream

I dream that I have to go upstairs through a busy building with many rooms. In these different rooms, children are taken care of. Once I arrive upstairs, I have two choices of entering a door. I choose one door and arrive in a roller coaster that makes me descend with great speed against my will downward. I do not want to descend. I go upstairs again and arrive in the same door, again, on the same roller coaster. Then I wake up.

Analysis

Going upstairs is an attempt to get to a higher form of consciousness, gaining consciousness step by step. This dream brings her to consciousness to enlighten her (if the ladder or stairs would miss one step—a hole or open space—this would stand for a state of unconsciousness). The building represents the dreamer (Self), and there are many rooms (the different levels of her psyche/Self). In the rooms, children were treated: children in this case are potentialities or possibilities that have not matured yet, or maybe in her case cannot mature because they first need to be treated as they are not well enough to continue on their own. It reflects the choice between the potentialities (the different professions she needs to tackle to continue what she loves to do (homeopathy), becoming a nurse or something else), but obviously these children are not strong enough yet to go out in the world (in other words, her self-confidence needs to be bolstered) and once she reaches light (consciousness) she has a choice between two doors or ways. She chooses one door which leads downwards (=going towards the unconscious), telling her again to investigate her unconscious to find an answer. If she neglects to do so, this dream will recur.

The turmoil in her unfulfilled conscious naturally feels like a roller coaster. She really does not want to descend into the unconscious because it is too rough of a ride, so she goes back upstairs (refusing to be caught in this turbulent unconscious), to arrive again in the same situation. In other words, she cannot reach further enlightenment because she is becoming a prisoner of the conscious when she really needs to face the stormy, treacherous investigation of the unconscious. This additional *hearing bad news* about her profession caused her building (Self) to crumble, creating isolation and paralysis; she does not know what to do. Further guidance will come from the unconscious, helped by the simillimum.

Dreams of Failing Examinations

How can it be that dreams of failure in school examinations occur so frequently, even to those who have all their life passed every test from high school to university? Why does this theme show up with regularity and stubbornness in some people's lives (creating puzzling questions)? "But I am already a physician," some say. Their outer life might be successful, but their inner life can be in shambles. Is there a special message involved? Indeed!

Such dream communications are most likely disclosing how we pass the "exams of real life," not academic tests. The fickleness of life provides plenty of challenges, and dreams will tell us if we pass these exams with flying colors, or if they lead to an "F" grade with stagnation and regression on the individuation path, no matter how successful we might appear outwardly! The business of life is an entirely different enterprise, with unexpected problems showing up that require deliberation, good judgment, empathy, and love for mankind—in other words, a working union between animus and anima (see further chapters). Most often these dreams appear when either a big change in life occurs or when we are confronted with a looming ordeal of responsibility in the upcoming days, leading to butterflies in the stomach (who has not experienced those during real university examinations, even if well-prepared?). Here is such an example.

Dreams

An adult male (45 years old) dreamt on several occasions the same theme: he has to take an examination, and either arrives too late, has not enough paper to write on, has to borrow scraps of paper from other students around him, has studied the wrong things, feels he has to sit next to someone that he can ask to help him, or even must resort to cheating. In fact, at one point in the dream he had such a male "friend" who acted very intelligent but was so arrogant that the dreamer could not feel anything but aversion to him, so unsympathetic was that figure.

This same dreamer had another recurrent dream that somewhat reflects the same theme:

He goes to the airport to travel and is hurrying up to the gate. Once there, he is in vain looking for a boarding pass while strewing all his money on the floor. He knows he is going to miss his airplane, as the gate person does not allow him to board. He wakes up in a cold sweat.

His first reaction to these dreams was the usual one: "Thank God it was only a dream," not understanding that his dream was a sure indicator that a matter of great urgency was brought up. In this dream there is no lysis, therefore the dream will recur until a more favorable solution is found.

This theme was also seen in a following dream, where he had to join some friends for a long journey, and first had to take a bus to get to a train. "But when I tried to buy the bus ticket, I was too late, and I actually forgot the name of the city to which I needed to take the train. My reaction in the dream was, 'Then I am going home.'"

Analysis

Bus, train, airplane: These are vehicles of motion, and of power; symbols of libido, Vital Force, and/or progression on the path to individuation (see Chap. 3).

Journey: A voyage of discovery takes us to unknown territories; previously unvisited lands mean our unconscious is inviting us to make their acquaintance. The destination has not yet been reached in this dream. The dreamer tries to see glimpses of his true Self, but he has not let it become what it ought to be; something stops him from exploring further.

Home: This reflects the original home, the womb, which personifies also the unconsciousness. In other words, the dreamer was not yet able to make conscious the contents of his unconscious; something stops him, mainly himself. He is not ready yet to make the separation from his home, not ready yet to mature and become more independent. He is still attached to the Mother archetype and craves to be released from the risks of responsibility and freedom, of awareness, and of taking initiative. He wants to remain in an unconscious state without responsibility. It can also express a desire to lose his individuality, to become one again with Nature. Such a deep regressive desire and withdrawing in a cocoon conflicts with the wish to live. To be in the womb is to be removed from life and severed from the environment, which is an isolation from consciousness, a refusal to participate in life.

Male friend: In the first dream, this friend is the alter ego or shadow side of the dreamer, as it was represented by another man (see Chap. 10, "The Shadow Side"). It contained what he did not like about himself, hence the aversion to acknowledge him.

Examination dreams: The prototype of this kind of dream is exactly as it is in this case—taking an examination and finding that the questions are incomprehensible, or you've studied the wrong thing, cannot find a pen or it does not write, the allotted time is inadequate, and the examination becomes impossible to pass. Sometimes the dreamer arrives too late or is not able to find the place where the exam takes place. The *common denominator* is that the dreamer feels poorly prepared in knowledge or techniques to live life, and therefore fears the judgment of an authority figure or his peers when he fails. This shows that the dreamer is still ill-prepared to meet new challenges in life and prefers to avoid the responsibilities that come to people at his stage of life. It can be positive, as the dream sends a message to change direction in life rather than choose to live life directed by someone else.

Money: This is a symbol of psychic libido and psychic energy to move forward. When we put or have money in the bank, we have psychic energy or psychic capital in the storehouse of the Self, the unconscious. In this dream, the money is strewn over the floor, denoting a loss of psychic energy and lack of orientation to move forward. We need "money" to be able to become an adult. Money means power to change things, to do things.

For Schopenhauer,[2] who inherited much money from his family to the point that he never had to work for a living, money was considered a gift that protects one from all the nuisances of life. But he also considered it contemptable for a person born into riches to remain merely an idler and thief of time. He stated that inherited wealth reaches its greatest value when it falls to the individual endowed with mental powers of a high order who is resolved to pursue a life of genius by producing some work which contributes to the general good. He was of the same opinion as Socrates, who said upon seeing many luxury articles spread in front of him, "How much is there that I do not want!'

What is the common theme of all these dreams? The theme is reflected by our homeopathic rubrics: *fear of being unable to reach his destination; dream, his boat will founder; fear of appearing in public; fear of others approaching him; fear arousing from stomach;* and *anticipation about an upcoming event.*

These, just some of the expressions seen in his dreams, reflect the excessive persona of a *Lycopodium* person. There is recurrence of the dream because there is no lysis. Consequently, he will get the same message over, and over again, until he understands its meaning and makes changes when being confronted by this issue posed by the unconscious.

A similar dream of the same patient

We are waiting on one side of a canal to cross a bridge that is up to let many ships pass. We are waiting a long time and on the other side is a bus that will depart at a certain hour. Once the bridge was finally down it was too late, as the bus had already departed. We decided to go home.

Analysis

As we can see, the same theme is repeated with the accent on the archetypal dream aspect—that is, the theme of discontinuing on the individuation road, common to many races and people besides this dreamer (the dream starts with "We," not "I"). Again, a retreat to the unconscious is seen as the only solution, as the bridge (between conscious and unconscious) was drawn up, and as a result they quit the journey.

Embarrassing Dreams of Appearing Naked or Dressed Inappropriately

Clothes (of all kinds), or no clothes, or being inappropriately dressed in a dream, refer in general to the state of the persona (excessive, inadequate, or identification with the persona—see Chap. 7), the state of the dreamer as he appears at the present time. Being naked in dreams can refer to different situations. What is our specific reaction in the dream towards being naked? Are we ashamed and trying to hide, or is there instead a feeling of freedom and closeness to Nature, a state of bliss, a return to paradise where protection, love, and happiness rule? Most often, our embarrassment contrasts with the *indifference* of other people in the dream, as they don't appear to be surprised, astonished, or disturbed by our nakedness. In that case, it is an invitation from the unconscious to take a close look at our hidden feelings, stored tightly away in the shadow side. Appearing naked—"the Emperor without clothes"—is a quest to be more ourselves, without the usual hiding for appearance's sake behind a persona crafted to be what is expected from others, a far call from who and what we should be. Undressing is quite natural in children of a young age as it feels like freedom, bringing with it an intoxicating sense of happiness. (This frequent desire to "exhibit" can also be observed in many children suffering from autism, even at a later age.) Dreams offer us the same freedom, an opportunity to appear naked and regain that feeling of paradise, even if only in a dream.

Being naked in a dream also points possibly to the conscious state where we are dominated by others, leading to a state of vulnerability (naked!) and an inadequate persona in which everything pertaining to life is dictated to the victim. This is the negative side of being naked, as opposed to the positive expression (above) of lowering our guard and letting the world see who we are behind the mirror.

Being dressed inappropriately for an occasion shows the dreamer's approach and adaptation (or lack of) to the setting. One of my patients dreamed: "I am on the beach wearing a business suit."

No doubt, this clothing is inappropriate and unfitting for the situation. We would like to shout to that person, "You forgot to put on your out-of-office suit!" What it reflects is an implication that the dreamer seeks special attention and respect —he is not able to "let his hair down" so to speak. It reflects an excessive persona (see Chap. 7).

Theme of Being Chased or Chasing Someone

When we are unable to flee from a threatening figure despite great efforts—a theme occurring frequently in nightmares—it reflects a sense of helplessness and ineffectiveness. If we are being chased, it is probably that we run away from what we are afraid of, either in our conscious life but more commonly, in our inner Self (our unconscious), as our ego is not in control. We are, in a real sense, pursued by what we have created with our thoughts, emotions, actions, or inactions. What we are avoiding might be sexual feelings, responsibility, our true feelings in public, fear of death, guilt, emotional pain, or grief (considered "love with no place to go"). We can never escape from ourselves.

If we are chased by *animals*, like a raging bull or a lion, this expresses our passions and anger: either a wild rage we are not aware of, or natural instinctual feelings. It means that an instinct (by which we are made nearly powerless due to its fierce and autonomous character) must be readmitted or integrated in our life, otherwise it can become dangerous. The "animal" must become our friend, not a nightmare. Very often in such dreams there is a process that turns the terrible monster into a milder form, or suddenly a magical helper appears, or the dreamer is given some magic with which he can face the monster or animal. If that is not the case, the feeling of anxiety usually increases to a state of horror and we wake up from the excessive oppression (nightmare).

If we are the one *chasing something* it is probably our conscious ego chasing some part of ourselves that frightens us. Trying to chase it away means disowning it, although it might be better to try to integrate it into our conscious. It can also mean we are pursuing something in life or someone we want.

Toilet Dreams

Another rather bizarre dream theme—often recurring—is the need to go to a toilet. It depicts variations of trying to have a bowel movement and not being able to because the toilets (usually multiple) are blocked, overflowing, or utterly unappealing because they are unclean or open to view (no door, no cubicle, lined up holes in the ground, etc.). The dreamer always wakes up from these dreams feeling disturbed as well as frustrated because the meaning of the dream has eluded him. What is the symbolic meaning of such dreams?

Excretions and toilet dreams usually represent the dreamer's public anxiety or shame, or his urgent wish to unburden the

Self, whether for creative or cathartic reasons. Defecation refers to potentially transformative urges, assertive expressions that will have to find proper channels. To dream of unsuccessfully searching for a toilet may indicate a conflict between the need to express oneself in public (symbolizing the urge for self-expression) and a fear of doing so, almost like an *Arg-nit* expression, which is a well-known remedy for someone in this anxious state ("What if this (or that) happens?"), who suffers from urgent diarrhea and must know, for real, where the toilets are when he leaves home.

If someone avoids talking about something which he *should* talk about, he might have a dream in which he suddenly has to go to the toilet and can't find it. Causing a toilet to overflow or having diarrhea indicates fear about losing emotional control, or failure to discipline creative potential. Finding a stopped-up toilet refers to a situation where the appropriate disposal channels or self-expressive urges are impossible to access because of obsessions, neuroses, and/or ailments from domination where other people's expressions (feces) hinder self-expression (as in *Alumina*, known for its severe constipation). A plumber (therapist/remedy) is needed to unclog the toilet (integrating unconscious elements into consciousness). If in the dream we must clean up a room full of excrement (the Augeas stable), it indicates that we must become conscious of our shadow side, the "dirty and most repelling" part of ourselves (see Chap. 10).

As a relative fixed symbol, the toilet is a gloomy place, symbol of the collective unconscious, full of dangers and considered a haunted place. For that reason (besides hygiene) in the past a toilet was built away or separate from the main house. It is a place where the spirits of the dead appear. Even today this place is mysterious, taboo, private, and forbidden, expressed by the rubric, *aversion to company during stool*, strongly indicated in *Nat-m.* Erotic fantasies start there, which is quite normal since the beginnings of sexuality lie in the cloacal area where the natural functions are exercised.

This chapter has covered different themes in dreams. Although dreams are always the result of individual conscious situations, and any theme can be found to be an individual expression—reflecting a conscious situation—I have focused here on the most common recurring themes in dreams. Although already alluded to in these pages, I now proceed to discuss in detail the different important classes of dreams: recurrent dreams, series of dreams, and archetypal dreams.

5

DIFFERENT CLASSES OF DREAMS

Acknowledge your shadow, or your children will be compelled to live out your dark side!

Recurrent Dreams

It seems recurrent dreams are the only ones the homeopathic world has had any encounter with—albeit on a very superficial level and without much understanding. The homeopath might ask his patients about recurrent dreams, but consequently, more than not, to the patient's surprise he then passes over this important information without paying further attention to or commenting upon them. Other important dreams—series of dreams and archetypal dreams—have not yet reached the radar of the homeopathic world.

For many years now, dreams and their vivid imagery have accompanied us, gradually becoming a more integrated part of our daily life. It is imperative to take the first steps in trying to understand and follow the hints pointed out to us in dreams of all kinds, especially recurring ones. As when we get a postcard with an exotic stamp on it, addressed to us from a faraway country, we should likewise be as eager to listen to the latest news from the "land of unconscious!" This does not mean we always know how to interpret the varying forms and shapes therein—far from it—but kindly enough, "the sender" seems to react to our lack of insight and interest, and sends us a "new" message, maybe slightly modified or somewhat altered and amplified, so that we cannot shake it off before at least trying to make some sense of it. If we are on the right track, our dreams will usually let us know, or at least let us know otherwise. They are like a benevolent correspondence between two dear friends —with the unconscious being a friend that can always be trusted for genuineness, honesty, and acuteness. The endless creativity of dreams and their benevolence humble us in many ways, and we should be very careful not to overlook or reject any dream before giving it our full attention.

As much as we in conscious life run away from unpleasant relations and situations, more than likely because the root cause was never investigated, a repeat of the same escapism will continue to have the same disastrous results, such as quarrels, divorce, and neuroses. This is no different than with our dreams: no matter what the urgent message is, we usually refuse to listen and to ponder it over. Instead we take the easy solution, laughing at our dreams and proclaiming them "nonsense." Yet a recurrent dream is like a song, heard in fragments, that has been playing in our mind ever since. The unconscious seems to have not only enduring tenacity and patience, but also a psychic energy forceful enough to pierce the hardness of even the strongest conscious resistance. "Leave me alone," we say, but over and over the messenger of the unconscious proclaims, "I am here to stay till you hear my voice!" Indeed, why do certain dreams, for instance nightmares (in almost always the same form or with slightly changed features), recur at regular intervals, endlessly disturbing the dreamer's sleep?

Most of us have had encounters with dreams that recur from a young age on through adulthood with remarkable regularity, as if they insist on bringing a forceful and urgent message that needs to not only be heard but *acted* upon. These dreams point to a conscious and important defect in the personality of the dreamer, to a vital or basic life problem often introduced at a young age, sometimes triggered by ailments from domination, failures, rudeness, indignation, mortification, and countless other emotional traumas that have left an indelible stamp on the patient's psyche. The torture and tyranny of such dreams may seem inexplicable but look at them as a debt to be paid before they will cease! In these circumstances, an understanding of the recurrent dream, and adequately dealing with it—considering that it is an urgent message from the Guiding Self, or the Inner Healer—becomes desirable, for it is a present to move the patient forward in his individuation and life struggles. We need to ask, what was the psychological individual situation that created this inner constellation?

For sure, *Ailments from domination* since childhood (a *Carcinosin* situation) will create an inner configuration of self-doubt and low self-worth continuing in adult years. If consciousness fails to respond and assimilate the dream's message, or if the therapist's interpretation is unable to touch on the core of the dreamer's problem (and therefore is therapeutically ineffective), the dream contents resurface at regular intervals. They carry the same motif to emphasize a particular blind spot of the dreamer, until the problem posed by the dream is solved and outgrown as the content or pattern has slowly changed through the homeopathic simillimum, correct analysis, or acceptance and acknowledgment by the patient—which then leads to a *series of dreams*. As seen in some of the examples in this book, whenever the psychological situation seems to be deadlocked, a dream will appear showing possibilities of development, often with more information about the posed problem. We must follow the lead of the unconscious patiently. Although it is unpredictable, it must be met with great understanding. Refusal to do so leads to mental disharmony and, yes, physical disorders including cancer.

An example of a recurrent dream, pointing to a conscious situation, is seen in the recurrent dream of the late TV personality Anthony Bourdain, who traveled around the world visiting eateries with the most exotic and strange foods. A description of this recurrent dream (one he had for years) was published in an article, "The Journeyman," appearing in the magazine *The New Yorker* (Feb. 2017, 13-20, p. 64).

Dream

I find myself in a Victorian-era hotel, wandering through well-appointed hallways, unable to find the front desk.

Analysis

A hotel is a symbol for the Self, a symbol of transience, a place where we stay temporarily before moving on again. But he is wandering through this hotel, not able to find the front desk to check in. So, in his case he does not even find a temporary Self, far from a structured one like a house or apartment where one stays for a longer time and settles down. This of course was the message to him, as he still, at age 60, was running around the world putting himself in uncertain situations, with a restlessness that pointed to fear of being bored or being settled in one place. He was a jujitsu fanatic, visiting alien places and cultures and stating, "I am pretty sure I'm incapable of being a patriarch, always there, with grandkids running around." His dream told him, warned him, to slow down, to settle somewhere rather than roaming the world 200 days a year. Unfortunately, he committed suicide in a Paris apartment (not a permanent home), having not heeded the warning in his recurrent dream.

If there is no lysis (or solution) in the dream, there will be reason for perpetual recurrence. "Inadequate interpretation of the therapist or understanding by the dreamer is likely to call forth repetition of the same dream theme, often in a more numerous, more drastic or more dramatic form" (Whitmont & Perera, 1991, p. 14).

Not every dream without a lysis has an unfavorable prognosis, although naturally a dream without a lysis always leaves an unsatisfactory if not frightful impression on the dreamer, particularly if it is of catastrophic character. If the content of the dream is meager, it often has an unfavorable prognosis. As soon as a dream is no longer acute—that is, it is solved and outgrown—the dream vanishes from memory. If it persists in memory however, the problem has not been solved, or the dream touched on something that we perhaps have not understood yet or never will. Individuals who *resolved* recurrent dreams and the underlying issues that caused those dreams were able to achieve a higher level of well-being than those who never experienced a recurrent dream. So, a recurrent dream is like a *present* if we listen to it and try to resolve it for progress in our individuation. After all, *dreams come in service of health and wholeness!*

Here is another example of a recurrent warning dream. In her book, *Memoirs of Halide Edib*, the Turkish novelist and social activist (1882-1964) shared the following recurrent symbolic dream she had (Halide, 2005, p. 216).

Dream

In the large grounds of the Sultan there is a raised mound with thick clustering trees, looking over the sea. There among the trees a tall and half-naked woman in white drapery, her black hair streaming and a torch in hand, walked up and down. I woke up with a strange anguish and feeling that something happened to my young son.

Reality: When Halide came home, her 3-month-old son had suffered a severe attack of convulsions. These attacks recurred daily over the next month, and each time they were preceded by this lady appearing in the dream, "half-naked, usually appearing at the seashore and sometimes she would be swimming … her eyes black and she stared hard at me" (Ibid., p. 217). Then for ten years the dream stopped and so did the seizures. At that point her son had an attack of pleurisy but seemed out of danger, at which time she had her final dream. In it, the lady appeared and was dressed. But this time she sat there with a mocking smile. Three days later her son had a very severe attack of typhoid fever from which he escaped death by miracle.

Conscious situation: In order to understand these warning dreams, one must know her conscious situation at that time. Halide was born into a well-to-do family and at age 16, ahead of children her age, finished college. She was, as I can see from her story, a *Sulphur* girl, always eager to go to school and get into lively discussions with her teachers, offering her own critical opinions. Then, in the same year, she graduated and married a man nearly her father's age. Now she had to follow the old Turkish tradition, being a submissive wife with no other aspirations other than giving him a child and obeying his wishes. For an independent woman, this was too much to bear. She first suffered a nervous breakdown (a deep *Aurum* depression), at which time she was tormented with this recurrent dream, and her newborn baby started to suffer seizures.

Analysis

No doubt, this half-naked woman was the "lady of the night," her anima, appearing at the seashore and sometimes swimming (respectively at the border of the conscious/unconscious and sometimes immersed in the unconscious), trying to wake her up with hard stares: she needed to pay attention to her feeling function, not just the thinking function. In order to gain more insight to explore the unconscious, she needs to go with this lady in her dreams. As she was not in tune with her feeling function, the "punishment" was her son's seizure attacks, recurring for many days. After ten years of marriage, and at the time of the last seizure attack, her husband married and brought another wife home. She then made a conscious decision and finally divorced her husband. This was shortly after the last illness of her son and subsequent last warning dream. Apparently, that time she followed her feeling function and used her anima to explore her inner being (unconscious). Her "debt" was then paid, as she took care of herself, her own being or created Self, the one not imposed on her by her husband.

Another recurrent dream, that of a 45-year-old woman, also pointed to a vital problem and blind spot, warning her to pay attention. Her dream follows, with proving symptoms in bold/italic.

Conscious situation: She suffered from migraines for many years. Her recurrent dreams were different versions of a scenario of being "dissociated" from her luggage while away from home, due to an occurrence of some natural catastrophe. These dreams were always about trying to "reconnect" with her luggage, and the ensuing confusion and frustration in that failed endeavor. She was a practicing homeopath, a very feeling, intuitive person who was also hypersensitive to environmental factors. Her migraines had started when she found "a new technique" to investigate the unconscious, with the use of a pendulum, which made her very excited. She became obsessed on working on her Self, and was highly inspired with creativity (***Delusion, is under a powerful influence***), saying:

> "I could get enlightened; I knew I had the answer! I could set myself free from my demons. But at the same time I felt outsmarted (***Del, in the hands of a strong power; Del, is under superhuman control***); there was a sense of being sabotaged and toyed with (***Del, charmed and cannot break the spell***). I realized I had undermined my health (***Del, being injured by her surroundings***). I felt defenseless, had a nervous fragility, tremendous fatigue, and felt guilty and embarrassed."

She went through a deep depression and isolation, sleeping for three months as she felt very vulnerable. She was very eloquent, with sophisticated speech (***speaking in well selected phrases***):

> "I lost my creativity and lowered my performance standards. I felt sabotaged in my attempts at creativity (***Delusion, there are conspiracies against her***). I wanted to do something but could not achieve anything (looking for an outlet for her creativity and passion but not being able to find one). I felt ***despair about my religious salvation*** and got really paranoid about anything that was suggested as a remedy for fear it would harm me (***Del, remedy is poison; Del, she is about to be poisoned; refuses to take the medicine***). This thought was fixed in me since I am highly sensitive to the environment and medications."

During my conversation with her, she was loquacious, with a very refined vocabulary, using expressions such as "my imminent disintegration" (***loquacity, in selected expressions***), and showed great insight into her situation, saying, "I have been waiting to go there all my life," referring to a four-month depression. She had become very sensitive to situations in which people tried to dominate her, making her feel like exploding, leading to possible violence (***rage, fury; kill, desire to***). Her speech was full, and passionate (***loquacity, excited***). It is as though she had two worlds: she felt fulfilled in her work but suffered from the demons in her personal life (***wills, has two***). There was no doubt about the simillimum (*Lachesis*) and by taking into account her sensitivity, the 5th edition split-dose method was chosen (6c, in an 8 oz. bottle, 2 succussions, 1 tsp. from the second dilution cup). Her dream, after the first dose of *Lachesis*, was as follows.

Dream

I am at a human-potential type workshop that was being held in the basement of a hotel. The first evening of the workshop, for some reason I decide to move my luggage to a different location upstairs in the hotel. That night there is a huge flood, and in the morning the whole basement is under 15 feet of water. The workshop continues upstairs and, strangely, everybody seems oblivious of—or at least not bothered by—the fact that all their luggage and stuff is under water. But for once my luggage is secure. During the day I leave the class and go to check out the flooded basement. I am standing at the top of some steps looking down into the 15 feet of water that now looks like a huge swimming pool. As I am bending over, my brass pendulum falls out of my left pocket and onto the bottom of the pool. I want to retrieve it and I look around to be sure that I am alone, and I start to strip so I can dive down to the bottom of the pool and retrieve my pendulum. But as I am doing this, I notice that my brass pendulum is floating back up and is now sitting on the top step under a few inches of water where I can easily reach it and pick it up. At this point in the dream there is a feeling of great relief and celebration, as I knew that all this is an indication that things have finally turned around . . . knowing where my luggage is and it being secure and my pendulum coming to me in this auspicious and intentional way.

Her comment: "I have only a superficial knowledge of Jungian psychology, but from what I do know, this dream seems to be loaded with Jungian symbology. I thought the dream perhaps suggests the potential of the simillimum to reverse the trend of my life, to free myself from the bondage of delusion, and to reclaim my wholeness (luggage!!!). By the way, *Lachesis* is going very well—no more migraines!"

Analysis

There is a good lysis, as we can see, indicating that a step forward was made with the correct dose of the simillimum, finding the consent of the dreamer with an "Aha."

Let's look further, at the different important notions in this dream, and translate them into relative fixed symbols.

Workshop/seminar/lecture: This is a place where people go to look for solutions, to continue their way in the individuation process; for self-understanding or realization, more awareness. Ask: "What skills do you wish to develop to release yourself from the bondage of your suffering?"

Basement of the hotel: A building, house, or hotel are symbols of the dreamer herself, of her body or the various levels of the mind, the psychical space in which she resides, the psychological framework of which she is living. Basement stands for a deep level of the mind, if one has not explored the unconscious. It is the *first layer of the unconscious*, the underworld, which is also represented by the abdomen of the person, where the unconscious and the unconscious emotions reside. What is usually the last thing we visit when we buy a house, or live in a house, or stay overnight in a hotel? (Has anyone visited the basement lately?) The cellar represents the dark abyss, the place of dark powers, the yin in Chinese medicine. Beginning to explore the cellar will be to begin to explore the parts of our unconscious that we have not yet inspected. What part of her unconscious is ready to be seen? Cellars are dark places, and so are the unemployed layers of the unconscious, since they have not been illuminated by the light of consciousness. Because cellars are dark and because they may harbor spiders and other creepy-crawly things, cellars may be frightening places.

As I remember my old family house, it had steep steps going down into the basement. It was strictly forbidden to go there; my father told me there were ghosts and spooks in there. Of course, the only thing that it contained were his precious bottles of wine. One day he forgot this message about the forbidden part of the abode, as I had done something "bad." He locked me up in the cellar and forgot all about me. Lo and behold, I found heaven! I discovered wine bottles half-opened and drank from all of them. I was 5 years old and it was the only time in my life I became drunk, having been invited by Bacchus (the Roman god of wine). This aberrant discovery shocked my father so much that for once he lacked the vocabulary and moral category to apply to the situation.

It was from a dream of his parental house that Jung formulated his theory of the collective unconscious, with the revelation that the house represented himself, his life and world. He used the different structures and levels of the house to convey his concepts, calling the cellar the "world of the primitive man," which he termed "the collective unconscious." The cellar (also named "cave" as a relative fixed symbol) is the place of birth and rebirth and change, and when we remain in the cave, afraid to venture out, it means we remain in the maternal womb, looking for security, anchored in that vast, underground world. The main floor, he believed, stood for the personal level of his unconscious, the upper floor for his current state of consciousness, and other parts of the house, attic included, represented consciousness.

It is also important to ask about the state in which a house appears in a dream: is the house in disarray (the Self)? Does the house resemble a shack (the Self is in shambles, ready to fall to pieces)? A **hotel** might also represent a *transitional* aspect of identity. What part of the dreamer is in transit?

House/city: These depict the Self, or the body.

Luggage: 1. This stands for what you need to get rid of: old habits, opinions and attitudes, and old conditioning. It represents the habits of attitude, or the emotional environment we have created in life; also, the past we still carry with us, what we can't let go of in life. Unfortunately, we bring this luggage ("baggage") into future relationships. **2.** Sometimes luggage expresses a need to get out of some present situation: "It is time to pack your bags! What am I ready to leave behind, and what do I really need to pack to move on?" Going on a trip, the journey of individuation, we need to take luggage or tools along. Such was the case of the dreamer in this dream.

Moving luggage upstairs: To do so is to make old habits conscious, being aware of them and trying to get rid of them; it stands for the integration of unconscious contents into consciousness. In this case, the dreamer is the only one who is in the process of becoming conscious, the rest of the people in the dream are unaware and oblivious, reflecting what is really going on in the world: most people are oblivious of their shadow, a collective trait. But for her, "connecting with her luggage" was a positive step, having integrated dark forces from her shadow into consciousness!

Flooded basement: Water is the unconscious, and the cellar is the first layer of the unconscious. Hers became flooded with 15 feet of water in this dream, larger than any human, meaning that the unconscious had become larger at that point. Her long-time suffering and suppression led to an ever-increasing unconsciousness with receding consciousness, until the homeopathic simillimum reversed the process.

Top of stairs: The top of the stairs signifies entrance to the unconscious where conscious meets unconscious! This can also be represented by a pier at the ocean or lake, or by an entrance to a tunnel or metro.

Swimming pool: A pool stands for personal unconscious (the sea=collective unconscious).

Pendulum (brass): This dreamer divulges that she uses a heavy pendulum in her practice, and for her it is access to the unconscious, and at the same time, the main instrument of her feeling function. Indeed, it falls out of her left pocket (left=feeling—the feminine, yin, protective, and unconscious side).

Being naked; stripping: (See Chap. 4, "Common Themes in Dreams.") This denotes going beyond outward appearances, "the Emperor without clothes." In her case, it stood for her desire or readiness to explore the dirt in her unconscious. It may therefore be accompanied by an anxious, vulnerable feeling; making sure one is alone (private), as in this dream, before exploring the unconscious.

A happy ending (lysis) occurs in this dream, as the pendulum comes back up, floating. It did its work and she is relieved things have turned around. The remedy has made the first step towards homeostasis in her life. She eventually got rid of her migraines with *Lachesis.*

Recurrent dreams alone do not give us the solution to find the simillimum, but understanding the message brought forth in them, coupled with the conscious situation, can shed new light on the nucleus of the patient's suffering, even when the simillimum has not yet been found.

Have you ever encountered a patient who, despite well-chosen remedies, and after resolving the miasmatic overload and using remedies of the rubric *"lack of reaction,"* still does not respond in the direction of cure? What to do? It is here that dream analysis can give you a glimpse behind the curtain without having to consult the Oracle of Delphi. Following is an example of such a perplexing situation made clear through dreams.

In this difficult case, not only one but four recurrent dreams plagued the patient for years, pointing to unresolved issues and the cause of his unhappiness. He never responded to any remedy, not even in the subtlest way, despite going up in potency (up to 10M of any remedy tried). Over a period of several years, he received a total of 26 remedies from different homeopaths. Unless he had no pulse or VF, he should have reacted to some of these remedies, even with new symptoms (when the remedy was wrong), or with accessory symptoms (if the potency was too high)—but none of that happened! What could this mysterious X factor be, that interfered with the patient's Vital Force, keeping him imprisoned in a tight harness? Were suppressed emotions somehow being maintained, and if so, how does that happen? Was there difficulty in achieving insight, for whatever reason, including into his constitutional and temperamental make up? Let's see if dreams will give us a clue and possible direction! According to the compensation law of dreams, we must first examine his conscious life. Here, the patient is speaking (rubrics in bold and italic):

Conscious Life of the Patient

> "As a child I was rather a happy, free spirit with natural free-flowing energy. I felt good, enjoyed games and sports with friends, sometimes was mischievous in an innocent, playful sort of way. When natural instincts were thwarted at school or by parents, I used to get angry, irritated, short-tempered, but not so often as a child. I had found changes unsettling, and I did not enjoy the change from primary school to high school. After puberty, going to an all-boys private high school

> with lots of rules and regulations, along with pressure from parents (particularly father) to study and do well, I felt less free flow, more restriction, limited, pressured, boxed in, thwarted, frustrated, and gradually unhappier. It affected my confidence and I became more indrawn.
>
> "So again, it was like there was more thwarting of natural energy/instincts, along with caution and control of my behavior (rather than free flow), fear of rejection, underlying anxiety, confidence decreased, energy indrawn, head pressure, and low-grade depression all the time. I really didn't want to go to law school; however, I didn't know what I wanted to do at that age, felt confused, and no one seemed to be able to understand and guide me. I really wanted time off, a break from the pressure, maybe travel overseas and just enjoy (probably seeking to recapture that free flow I felt as a boy)."

At age 17, he felt like a worn-out businessman. He needed, as he states, "a repose which I did not get." This brought him off track, unstable, syphilitic: OCD, chaotic life, not focused, loss of control.

> "However, in the end I chose law school (even though I felt I wouldn't enjoy it, which was in fact the case), thinking I could always do something else later. Relationships have always been an issue and difficult, and not having been married, I have felt a lack of free flow and relaxation, tense, inhibited, awkward, with fear of rejection, especially around attractive women. I guess it's been like a push-pull. One part of me wants to connect with others in general, and particularly with a woman, to create an enjoyable relationship. Another part, maybe it is younger, is in conflict, feeling distressed and overwhelmed by that thought. There is a strong seeking to resolve the unhappiness and inner conflict and distress."

Family life can be metaphysically, incomprehensibly intense —an inherently conservative unit bristling with the potentiality of being the most widely imaginable conduit for the transfer of misery, and at the same time, the source of all joy. It stuns, it stimulates, it overwhelms, or paralyzes. Often it resembles a battle between David and Goliath, as the social genetics of family inheritance keep bequeathing unhappiness, indifference, expectations, hatred, or pleasure upon its members, or the family follows a path of tyrannical, socially imposed contingency. This is such a story, as we let the patient (a 40-year-old man) continue to do the talking.

> "I have a sister and mother who surely have had influence in my life, but not in a way that I could say they were real role models or great positive influences from the point of view of encouraging natural abilities. My mother (and father) looked after all my physical/financial needs; however, it was not natural for them (and me) to express feelings, emotional support and love. I could feel that my mother loved us underneath, however due to her own personality restrictions she could not express it, she could not properly nurture us, and didn't protect us from father's criticism and harshness. So, it was hard to feel secure, encouraged, and to grow in that environment. Rather it built just the opposite—anxiety, lack of confidence, having to protect myself and change natural inclinations just to avoid disapproval and punishment. With the state I'm in, there is tremendous constant anxiety, and physically I feel a very strong inner tension in the body, especially in the head. It's like a protection, fear and vigilance have taken over (***fear of the fright remains***). I can't relax and my system is on high alert, and I do not feel (connected to) my body (***Del, body separated from mind; Del, floating in the air***). My mother was rather unassertive, and even though she didn't like the

harsh way my father acted towards us, she would seldom stand up to him, allowing him to be a patriarchal figure of absolute authority whose judgments were not challenged. At age 17, a girl who I was interested in laughed at me and told me my nose was too big: this was devastating to my self-esteem (***Del, some part of the body is deformed; Del, being laughed at, being mocked; Del, people looking at him; Del, he is being watched; A/F vexation, from mortification, from mental shock and emotional excitement; Del, being observed; fear, people will observe his confusion***). Becoming a lawyer was not something I really wanted to do; it was more encouraged by my parents. I was more a free, boisterous spirit when younger, mischievous, enjoying adventure, and I did like art and sports when younger, but was pushed more into the mind/intellect by my parents to achieve success academically—especially by my father who was a scientist and wrote/published many textbooks. I also found out a few years ago that he always wanted to become a lawyer, so I seemed to live out his desire. I wasn't that interested in academic or artistic pursuits, more physical energetic activities. However, when I did go to a painting class as a young boy, I really enjoyed it. I didn't come from an artistic family and it was never really encouraged or pursued much further. Academic activities became more important to those around me, and the increasing family pressure to fit into their model of who I should be—to do well academically—caused a lack of balance with other pursuits, which created stress and inner conflict. I did not suffer from physical ailments when young. Gastrointestinal symptoms are the more prevalent now, especially to emotional stress (author's comment: in TCM, this represents suppressed anger and frustration).

"Presently, the OCD type symptoms are the same since I was 17 years old: obsessive feeling and thoughts that my nose is too big and chin too small and especially a dislike for my profile (***Del, some part of the body is deformed; Del, parts of the body seem too large***). I have constant underlying anxiety/fear (since it is constant it borders on ***Del, anxious***) and don't like looking in mirrors or photos being taken, especially in profile, and try to look straight on when I am photographed (***Del, being laughed at, being mocked; Del, he is being watched; Del, he is criticized; A/F rudeness of others; A/F mortification***). Linked to this is the constant fear of being emotionally hurt, humiliated, and being rejected (***self-depreciation***). I always feel very tense, scared, on guard, and unsafe; the world is dangerous, and I have to be vigilant for the unexpected attack (***Del, he is about to die; fear of the fright remains***). I am wary of people in general, and have fear of public speaking and relationships (***anxiety when in company***). I feel stuck and trapped in this state of anxiety/fear and feel desperate to get out of it (***despair of recovery; Self, at odds with***). It feels like I'm in an intense life and death struggle (***fear of the fright remains; Del, is about to die; despair of recovery; terror; unbearable pains***).

"My (psoric) need: I think (I'm suffering from) lack of encouragement / appreciation / emotional warmth and nurturing / not being understood and heard or listened to, how my natural inclination was growing up. Many of my ways of being did not fit into my parents' expectations—especially my father's model of how I should be. So, I was disapproved, criticized, or punished, sometimes with public humiliation (**A/F mortification**). It felt like I was forced against the grain to change myself to fit their image, to gain approval, for them to be proud of me (as it felt they weren't), or at least to not be punished. I felt I could not be myself, nor relax for fear of parents' reactions. However, it never felt good to change from my natural inclinations. It

> created inner conflict, resistance, anger, and emotional suppression. Associated with this, I felt a lack of guidance, especially around my teenage years—that is, a parent or role model who understood/listened to me, to what I wanted to do and how to help me grow, develop, and be strong (emotionally) naturally. Not speaking up, fearful, and not as strong underneath as I present on the surface, I do not do well with domineering, critical, judgmental people. I react with anger, irritability, and impatience, especially with trifles."

As we can see, everything that reminds him of his father, real or imagined—discipline, forcefulness, and attitudes—repels him with an intense affect response.

In order to treat the "man and not the disease," a further intake analysis is conducted.

So far, we know we need a remedy for a person with the following characteristics:

- Introverted and reserved at this point in his life, suppressing his emotions (anger especially)
- Genetic nature: not so timid, as he reacted violently to hurt as a youngster and still now, gets irritable and angry about trifles
- Lacks confidence and has a feeling of deprecation
- Reproached and not truly loved by parents and female figures in the family: he wants an emotional bond with family. Not nurtured by his mother/father, only nourishment. A/F disharmony in the family
- An equal relationship and to feel accepted is very important
- Creativity/art: more of a free spirit, more interested in the "new and mysterious," like holistic healing

methods, rather than strict "scientific" ones; in other words, he is right brain dominant (vs. left brain)
- Responsible, dutiful, conscientious, and diligent
- Rapid thoughts, hurried (*thoughts, rush, flow of; intrude and crowd around each other*)
- Chilly and moderately thirsty
- Affected tissue: skin (lipomas, blepharitis, dry skin: P and S); stomach (gastritis) from stress; nerves: Level 1 and 2 diseases,[1] sycotic physical diseases. Mind: predominantly psoric-syphilitic reactions
- Very sensitive to rudeness

Psoric need: only his basic physiological needs (food, liquid, shelter, and sleep) were fulfilled in childhood. His *safety* needs are already in question, as he did not live in a predictable world: he always had to live according to family standards, which led to anxiety and insecurity, especially in relationships—still present today. His tensions and apprehensiveness are indeed the result of "safety-need frustration." What he did not receive from his family was true *love* and a sense of *belongingness*, and *self-worth* or *esteem*. Above all, a child has two basic needs (besides physiological needs): the need for love, and the need for self-worth. This is where his festering life problem started. He was not accepted, loved, respected, and encouraged as he was, according to his innate temperament, something psychologically desired by any child. He lived under the shadow of an imposing but distant father whose approval he longed for but never quite won. His father was ambitious for him but showed little affection. He was only his father's pet and project. Such a relationship often leads to veiled resentment of the domineering father. Needs for love, approval, reward, and respect can only then be satisfied by other people, creating dependency on one's close environment. It is interesting that his physical complaints are limited to stomach pains (gastritis). It is well-known to psychologists and TCM practitioners that those cases in which symptoms are primarily gastric are in nearly every instance found in persons who seemed to have an inordinate desire to be loved—a craving to be taken care of, loved, and protected (Earth element in TCM). Keeping feelings locked up and concealed is like a suicide wish, often starting with an upset stomach or continuous constipation. Such a small illness, according to the Ko or controlling cycle in TCM, also points to how he is overwhelmed by suppressed or half-expressed anger—oftentimes masked as a low form of depression (*sadness, dejection, anxious*) and continuous anxiety.

In the name of convention and birthright, the family mask of repression has been forced upon him, making him a well-adjusted slave, while his psychological bones were crushed, and his own true inner nature violated. The father's love for a son is unique, different than the unconditional love of the mother for all her children. This father "loves" his son only in that he wants him to live up to his expectations and become the real heir to the father's worldly position—to *be like him*. It is sad to see that his father's authority relied more on force than on being associated with true love. Unfortunately, his father wanted submission to his wishes, making the patient function in his non-dominant conscious function—thinking (see Chap. 8, "The Four Conscious Functions"). It was a command to his son, "This you ought to be and do." His father only showed a frowning face full of scorn, so his son believed that he was unable to be loved—something that has become the legacy of his life. His father chose everything for him, and experienced everything, so his son (the patient) can find nothing for himself. This is called the negative aspect of the patriarchal complex. What is *healthy* in such circumstances *is to react* and protest while this crime is being committed, but can we expect such a courageous stand from a young person? How did he react? "When younger I used to feel and express more frustration and anger, like have temper tantrums, kicked and broke a glass door, even picked on my younger brother and sister (***anger, violent***). This stopped a lot/was suppressed as I got older and when I went to high school."

So initially when his psora was injured/not nourished as a child he did not accept this but reacted violently. He went from psora to syphilis. He was also naturally very active, energetic as a child, and that energy had to be used. He couldn't just sit quietly at home as he would get bored and into mischief, so he had to get outside to use up the energy—walk, play outside in the mud, play on swings and slides in playgrounds, etc. What he lacked, above all, was familial love, which would have drawn him into the realm of being a full human. He became confused about his own Self, as it was overstepped by others. He felt neglected and became a slave who does not know what his role in the world is supposed to be (***contradiction of will; Del, is about to die***—figuratively speaking). He became trapped in a world of fancies for the rest of his life, unable to overcome the power of his unconscious, wandering on the border of dreams (***Del, of fancy illusions***). When he was 17, he had to submit to discipline as cold as that of a monastic rule. The dreariness of his life was created by his father, who brooded over his son's mischievous and joyous fancies, clamping them down. Displaying any affection towards him was deemed inappropriate, as his need for affection was looked upon as that of a silly child who had to be put in the paternal frame of mind. To his father, this man always remained 10 years old, a youngster that needed to be reminded what his future should be: a duplicate of the feared and "successful" father. The son consequently has a feeling of powerlessness which pervades his whole life. We also must consider if hate for his father—always stronger than love—is blinding and paralyzing him, overshadowing his love for other beings. Love and hate cannot live in the same abode, in the same soul.

Why does he accept the atrophy of his heart and mind that his father imposed on him? As we see, years later he pays for it with neurotic and psychosomatic symptoms, when he realizes that he missed the true fulfillment of promise and failed to discover a life that can be thrilling. Although on the surface he thought he had arranged his life according to his own plans and will—really, deep down, he is filled with resignation. He is convinced that he could not do what he wanted and had to conform to what was expected of him.

This is reflected in his dreams with failure in exams, as well as his lack of desire to function as a lawyer (due to the repression of his real wishes and adoption of expectations of others). His original wish to follow his natural instincts was replaced with a pseudo wish (lawyer). What we might look for in his dreams are feelings that he has not experienced all these years: feelings of hatred towards the father, feelings of being liberated, or messages where he feels stuck in his situation, unable to go forward.

To throw the yoke off his neck, and to try to experience the delight of being himself, he started to travel later in life as a compensation, to exotic, third world, unconventional countries (***travel, desire to***), which became more of a *wandering* (***runs about; desire for light***—symbolic), looking for a solution to the increased anxiety that took control over his being, and to still the ever-present torturing thoughts in his mind.

Lack of self-knowledge can only lead to lack of self-understanding, a curse for most of this man's life. He is flooded with memories of feeling that his father runs through him like water. The damaging effects of such a dictatorial, authoritarian father —controlling, squelching, and overprotecting him—are still part of his present life: deficient of some of the basic emotional needs, he has become afraid of his environment since there is always a possibility it will disappoint him. This hinders his autonomy and self-direction to take any risk in relationships, and worse, makes him unsure of what he really wants or what his true vocation should be. Non-love and non-acceptance led to anxiety, self-doubt, feelings of worthlessness, and a catastrophic need for safety, certainty, and perfection (OCD). His existence was and is as unstable as a stream, changing in every way. He developed contempt and resentment for his parents, especially for his father who frustrated his need for esteem and self-respect.

The insult at age 17 by a girl about his appearance (his nose), a most important and vexing event (***A/F mental shock***), caused him to remain shy and unskilled in the jargon of relatedness towards women (lack of Eros). This insult was received like a branding-iron seared onto a convict's shoulder, leaving a mark which he has never been able to erase, leading to fear to have his picture taken in profile (***fear of the fright remains***). In spite of the totalitarian upbringing by his father—or rather because of it —he was incapable to react rationally to this insult, as his Eros, or art of relationship, was crushed resulting in the syphilitic symptoms of OCD, a loss of control of his will and emotions. There were no guard rails left to protect him from the force of fixed syphilitic ideas: ***Del, parts of the body seem larger; Del, some part of the body seems deformed***. He was dissatisfied with himself, thought himself ugly, and was ashamed of his looks. Only in his 20s did he stand up to his father, but outside of the family he cannot retaliate. The lack of love, approval, and fairness has stifled his growth and development of potentials. He wades in quicksand (he calls it obsessive-compulsive), stuck in how he looks and where he fits in (an unsatisfied psoric need of belonging), asking himself if he ever can find someone who will love him unconditionally (psoric need for love) and understand him, without introducing strict, rigid, domineering rules. As a child he felt (and still feels) as if lost on a lake in the fog. Days spill over one after another in a muddle. He remembers only snippets of things, aside from a constant feeling of misery,

irresolution in acts and projects, and insecurity. At the same time, the world is seen as a dangerous, threatening, humiliating and unpredictable place (***fear of the fright remains***).

The danger exists because of his insecurity and helplessness, causing him to submit to another authority figure as he is still looking for security and relief from doubt about his capacities and appearance (***magnetized, desire to be***). Being insecure, he shuns intimacy (***misanthropy; social meeting aggravates***), withdraws, and is shy. His shyness, an expression of his insecurity (***timidity after fright***), makes people dislike and reject him —making him even more insecure, leading to a vicious cycle, as he wonders if this world will ever be a place where he can find happiness and acceptance (***despair of recovery; Del, has an incurable disease***). Despair is indeed the denial of hope. No wonder he has not been able to climb up the ladder towards self-actualization and esteem needs, causing him to withdraw (***absorbed, buried in thoughts; misanthropy***), always on high alert as if a great catastrophe is about to happen, a PTSD situation (***fear of the fright remains***). This is a warning to many, that a secret psychic death in childhood can become such an obstacle and hard to "outgrow," an impediment he is dangerously close to. If he is possessed by a complex—a father-authority complex in this case—it is exceedingly difficult to know how this feels in him. What does reason demand of him? That he lives according to his nature, his dominant conscious function. But even now in his adult life, his dead father pushes him forward on a path least desired.

So far, besides *Carcinosin*, *Bar-c* and *Aconite* are indicated, *Aconite* the most indicated. Remember, *Aconite* is the acute of *Sulphur*, which can complete a cure begun by the former.

Let's see if his dreams give us any more information, especially about what his unconscious is trying to tell him through its messenger (dreams). Is this idea of being stuck, not being able to move, of being threatened and feeling lost in a forest (collective unconscious), seen in his recurrent dreams? He has had at least four different themes of recurrent dreams.

1. Recurrent dream of being stuck in a ditch, filled with mud. "I am making enormous efforts to lift my legs out of the sticky mud so I can climb up the bank out of the ditch. It is so difficult to lift my legs out of the mud. I feel really exhausted and stuck from the effort."
2. Recurrent dream of being chased by dark mafia type figures who want to kill him. "I feel like I have done something wrong and they are after me because of this. I feel a lot of anxiety, terror as I am trying to escape from them. Sometimes I manage to get away, sometimes they shoot me."
3. Recurrent dream of sitting for exams in high school or college. "I feel a lot of anxiety because I haven't studied enough for the exams and feel a lot of anxiety/fear at being unprepared."
4. "Sometimes I dream of jumping and flying from a high place, like a mountain or high lookout or ledge. I'm fearful as I am not sure if I can fly or not, however usually it is OK, and I can fly or glide with my wings. Contrary to the three previous recurrent dreams, I have not had this dream in the last three years."

Analysis

First, without amplification of the real-life situation, we analyze these dreams just through relative fixed symbols. Second, through **amplification**, we will find out if our interpretation is correct.

Analysis of each element
First recurring theme: stuck in the mud

- **Mud:** At the bottom of the unconscious. He is stuck in the mud to his knees, and despite enormous efforts is not able to get loose. He can't lift his legs (***Del, he walks on his knees; Del, his legs are cut off***). He is not even "swimming," which would be at least "exploring" the unconscious. Instead, he is stuck in the deepest part of the unconscious, close to the collective unconscious, reflecting the search for the eternal Divine Mother and indicating that in real life he is stuck in a regressive infantile state. He is so unconscious that the dream tells him he cannot make psychological progress unless he frees himself of his complexes (father-authority complex especially). All his efforts lead to exhaustion. The directive posed by the unconscious is therefore: identify the factor that bogs you down, that makes you stuck in the mud! This can be emotions that cause one to feel bogged down, or past experiences, or a complex holding him back. Looking at his past, this theme is self-explanatory.
- **Bank of the ditch or river: 1.** A border between unconscious and conscious. **2.** A barrier or safety measure to stop the river from flooding. **3.** A difficulty to overcome, not being able to integrate unconscious elements into consciousness.
- **Legs:** Support; motivation; the emotional and physical strength we use to go forward in life, to evolve. Expressions: "I don't have a leg to stand on"; "I can't stand up for myself." To have "one's legs knocked out from under him" means loss of

confidence (think about *Bar–c, Del, he walks on his knees*).

Second theme: chased by mafia

- **Mafia:** Stands for a tight-knit secret community ("omerta!"—extreme loyalty) that conducts criminal activity hiding behind a bona fide business, and in fact often gives the appearance of doing good in their neighborhood like buying gifts for the poor, for weddings, paying for college, or providing food. In other words, they have an excessive persona: they appear friendly and generous, charming, and look like they have only good intentions, appearing to look out for others, take care of and protect others, etc. But of course, this is just appearance. Really, they are ruthless, demand complete obedience, and anyone violating the omerta is on the dead list. They have professional killers to do their dirty work and kill all those with a dissenting voice and those they consider a threat. These mafia figures are chasing him. Sometimes he escapes, sometimes he gets killed. Mafia figures also stand for maleness, or animus. Who are these mafia people for this dreamer is the question!
- **Being chased:** When we are not able to flee from a threatening figure despite great efforts—which occurs frequently in nightmares—the cries of the mind leap out of its lodgings. As such, this reflects a sense of frightening helplessness and ineffectiveness. Sometimes this dreamer escapes, sometimes he is killed. What is "killed" is his individuality, his Self, by a sinister identity, dressed as the mafia. Often, we must turn around and face the one chasing us, and

demand what that being wants from us. This way we have a chance to incorporate what we need to, if we are to escape the clutches of the unconscious (see Chap. 4, "Common Themes in Dreams").

Third theme: failure in exams, the *earliest* of his dream recurrence

- **Failure in exams:** Not prepared enough, no confidence (very common dreams). His dream tells him constantly that he is unprepared to take on the challenges (exams) in life. He fails and keeps on failing. This theme fits in with the first two, and indeed these three themes alternated frequently, in no special order, throughout his life and even now.

Fourth theme: flying

- **Flying from a high place: 1.** Dreams of flying represent a longing for freedom and joy. It might feel like a liberation, getting rid of shackles and traditional taboos stemming from childhood experiences such as *A/F domination.* "The Sky is the limit!" **2.** Flying from the Earth, or body, can also be overreaching in your goals. Your dream will *warn* you against projects that are too grandiose or not in accord with your fundamental constitution. This may mean that in entertaining wild fantasies you have overlooked your real capacities and gifts (like Icarus, who overreached and fell to his death when the wax on his wings melted when he flew too close to the sun!), representing a person who is not "grounded" but inflated. It is like building a house on the wings of a big bird that never settles. The

Greeks called this situation *hubris*, which is an ego inflation, an arrogance always punished by the gods or by a compensatory reaction of the unconscious. "Looking down" could also refer to "looking down" on people, being in a position above the regular crowd and ordinary relationships (delusions of grandeur) **3.** Bright sky symbolizes consciousness or pure reason, spirituality, and represents a male symbol versus the "Mother Earth" female symbol of feeling/intuition. The dream proposes that he needs to extend the range of his consciousness by bringing unconscious contents into his conscious mind, or that his previously neglected feeling and intuition-feeling function need a fuller role in his conscious life. By creating a higher standpoint, we obtain a higher point of view. **4.** Sky is an age-old symbol for God or transcendence, so flying might be a symbol of coming closer to your authentic Self or true Self or to the meaning of your life. We will have to decide what it stands for in this patient once we amplify it with his conscious life!

- **Wings:** A symbol of transcendence. A winged creature or person may represent a part of the dreamer's psyche beckoning him to a higher perspective—more spiritual or more detached, a higher level of consciousness or liberation from an oppressive situation.

Before we even look at the amplification, we can already conclude that the message of all these dreams is to create more awareness in this patient (and also the treating homeopath), to illuminate what makes him stuck at this point in life, by investigating his unconscious.

Further interpretation through AMPLIFICATION with his conscious situation

Theme 1. Stuck in the mud, close to collective unconscious: This was a 40-year-old man, very sensitive, who early in his adolescence was laughed at by a girl for his nose being "too big." He always longed for a relationship, to be married, but never did. So, he could never connect to the Divine Mother, she was elusive since adolescence as his mother was not an encouraging person when it came to the formation and support of his anima, his feminine side, that was thus relegated to his shadow! And subsequent feminine figures were not positive in forming his anima, including his sister, and a girl who refused to go with him to the prom, and later, a female who laughed at him.

Theme 2. The mafia: The father archetype can appear negatively in dreams as a dictator or a mafia boss. The first example of animus for a male is always the father (see Chap. 12). His father was a scientist, very Logos oriented, and he wanted his son, whose dominant conscious function was feeling, to become a "successful" person according to his plans and opinion, to mold his son in his own image, violating his son's dominant function. He had impressed upon his son that it was through rational scientific thought alone that a real man in society should function, and it was not difficult for the son to take on his father's idea about the value of professional life and of a college training as part of the equipment of a successful person. He lived in a patriarchal family where the son is subject to the father's will, and being the only son, he was destined to become the heir and successor to his father's worldly position. In order to please him, he had to submit to him, obey him, and replace his own will with his father's. Even later as an adult he did not have the power to rebel against his domineering and authoritarian father, never to secure his independence and unfold his own capacities. His father loved him on the condition that he fulfilled his expectations. Alas! Fulfillment of duty and financial success are poor substitutes for the capacity to enjoy life with one's natural strengths and the inner security of being loved unconditionally. As it was the only path to have contact with his father, he followed his father's pattern faithfully, trying to become like his father but unconsciously rebelling. Oppression usually leads to hate, to a wish to liberate oneself from the oppressor and to eliminate or kill him. Such an oppressive demand for obedience is nothing but an undermining form of "benign" *Ailments from domination.* The patient came to see life through his father's eyes, and to think with his thoughts—a form of father identification and father-complex—an archetypal image of masculine authority, demanding masculine success in life. His father's wish to control and to pronounce "what is best for him" was destructive love, a kiss of death to the son's true personality. There is no protection of the law against paternal force delivered from self-interest and misplaced love. When the patient suffered an indignation situation at age 17, his repressed undeveloped childish emotional side took control and never left (*childish behavior in old age, Bar-c*). It interfered with the trust he had put in Logos, taught by his father, setting into motion a strong neurosis still present at this time. The tool he used so far (thinking) was directed by his father's traits, which he was unconscious of, and by reducing himself to the status of the tool, this unnatural superior function has become itself his master. A renewal of his life will have to come from the apparently dead and untrained inferior feeling function.

So, the mafia person in the dreamer's life was his father, a threatening figure from which he could not escape or find peace, undermining his confidence by forcing his son to operate in his non-dominant function. His father died when the son was 36 years old. At that point he threw off the yoke (a classic symbol of submission) and went on a different path from the prescribed paternal one. He went to the Amazon looking to discover his real Self, the symbol of totality (*self-realization*), and took some drugs from a Shaman, an invitation to dive into the unconscious and seek answers. This was the only time he felt liberated! During that time only! But he cannot just stay in the unconscious, he must come up again, hopefully with some discovered gems in order to conduct a real life. In his dreams, sometimes he is killed. What is killed of course is his own projected life, the life unlived! He is not at the wheel of his car; someone else is driving his car, before and now! This forced, over-rationalized masculinity has killed his anima, his sensitive side, while forming a pseudo animus. Even as an adult he never found his own car to drive, neither did he find a spiral staircase to liberate himself from the shackles of the father-complex.

Theme 3. Examination failures: Why these dreams? Of course, he fails in any situation as he was forced to operate from a young age on in his non-dominant and even archaic conscious thinking function because of his father's demands! The part of him that wants to live (his natural dominant feeling function) is killed by the other side of him (thinking). There was *no lysis* in these dreams, just like in the other dreams, so this theme will resurface in further dreams. Indeed, "rebirth" can only come through the release of the neglected function, his feeling (as we will see further in Chap. 8). It is apparent that this man operated with an underdeveloped thinking function and is going through life with a crippled animus and a weak, non-exercised anima.

Theme 4. Flight to liberty: Which one of the possible translations of the symbol "flying" will create an "Aha"? Getting rid of shackles and traditional taboos stemming from childhood experiences! It is the equivalent of a "magical" flight, resulting from exceptional psychic powers. This was certainly the case in this patient when for the first time, after the death of his father, he went to the Amazon for spiritual experiences (something his father surely would have disapproved of). He threw off the yoke and followed the road less traveled, towards the Self! Flying as a free bird is related in his case to the feeling realm of spiritual uplift. This dream started only since his trip to the Amazon and stopped about three years later. Obviously going to the Amazon, cutting his legal career and then stepping into the spiritual world, was in tune with his feeling function. It felt like liberation to him: finally, free as a bird! Unfortunately, this dream ended when the father-complex took hold of him again —he was now a soldier in the mafia again, his wings had been cut. Freedom lost once more!

Another possible explanation of the **4th dream theme:** In his case, it meant also that he needed to extend the range of his consciousness by bringing up unconscious contents into his conscious mind, or *that his previously neglected feeling and intuitional feeling functions need a fuller role in his conscious life!* As well, it can have yet another meaning for him. Sky is an age-old symbol for God or transcendence, so flying might be a symbol of coming closer to his authentic Self or true Self, to God in him, or to the meaning of his life.

Looking at the message of these recurrent dreams, with the exception of the relatively brief recurrence of dream theme #4, there is a general feeling of being stuck in life, not prepared to grow or be self-assured enough to climb the ladder to self-realization, as basic needs of love and self-esteem are still unrealized for this patient. The theme of the mafia, sadly, repeated itself, crippling him now with a neurosis late in life where everyone (especially people trying to impose themselves because of their own shortcomings) can become a threat, an enemy. So, the fear of the fright and the danger of a spiritual death remain, halting his progress. He feels danger everywhere, so insecurity and danger at home, or within the Self, is always lurking, creating continuous, strong anticipation anxiety, which does not attract females like moths to a flame.

After the analysis, I asked questions regarding the meaning of the elements in his dreams, and he answered accurately. His only question was, "Can you give me a remedy?" The real answer: "Not until you get rid of any relationship that imposes its rules on you, purposely keeping you in an infantile state to be controlled and be held as a slave." (*Tolle causa*, "remove the cause," first!) He has not realized he "needs to grow up," to follow his true dominant conscious function, and to try to fulfill his basic needs first, as mentioned before, as a free individual. But even if he understands the NWS, the causality of this complex operating in him, it does not automatically stop the complex from operating. It is here that psychoanalysis, and even more the homeopathic simillimum, can bring relief and dissolve the ever-growing power of the CD, so that his energy can be focused on constructive goals, rather than the CD continuing to rule his conscious. A homeopathic remedy will be important, as it works also on the unconscious energy field through the process of integration. This translates into the slaying of the old reigning king and the son's accession to his throne—into building up his desired Self, not a pseudo one! In order to not be possessed by the complex, he needs to confront it, not run away from it, based on the homeopathic law of similarity.

Conclusion: From what has been discussed, *Aconite* seems to be the indicated remedy, as the fear of the fright remains, a PTSD situation, still roaming in his unconscious, and further dreams always point to an emergency with fear of death. Also, *Sulphur* (*A/F embarrassment*) is the chronic of *Aconite* and might be needed at a later point, more than *Bar-c* or *Carcinosin* for now. Positive dreams for this patient would be the appearance of a female person, pointing to a psychic need to include a feminine principle, complementing his forced-upon excessive masculinity.

Addendum: After taking *Aconite*, there was no positive

response. Why a deadlock? Why a logjam? I re-examine the case, as follows.

His dreams are animal-like and compulsive, destructive to his Self. He needs awareness that could dull the sting of this destructive drive. But understanding and good will are not enough, as awareness can increase his compulsion. And certainly, repression is not to be done. He needs to have a dream in which he can crush the conscious reasonableness (Logos) and imposed ambitions, meeting a female, meaning getting in touch with his own feelings, so his anima can now become an ally. The father-complex got ahold of him, and this is not under control of the will as it has a psychic autonomy. He unconsciously created a state of identity with it, a primitive destructive drive. He now projects his drive on anyone who he feels tries to control him on any level, mentally and emotionally especially. An intense affect reaction is inevitable, and he reacts with anger and resentment. Is this how he reacts to any relationship, female or male? Running away from discipline, authority, and responsibility? This will be to no avail! He needs to find a source of renewal. If he can draw water from a tap in his room, it is a waste of time to look for a well somewhere else: he has to come to his senses by applying his sense, to achieve genuine contact with the other sex in lieu of pseudo contact with his projections, to stop his rumination (OCD). Is he still incapable of finding the key to the door, understanding and integrating this father-authority and inferiority complex? Is there a constant brooding on the past, of looking at things that cannot be changed now, a faulty adaptation of moral, intellectual, and aesthetic values?

He suffers from stomach pains: *what* can he not stomach? Will he finally confront his pain in the present moment, rather than dwelling and obsessing about the past or future time? He needs to realize the importance of the moment, focus on externalizing his inner conflict. He has a crippled animus and a weak anima, a sick hero and a hurt child. He needs appreciation by feeling so he can distance himself from the dominance of his dead father. Does he need to pick up painting again, go to art exhibits, stop sacrificing his creative desires? When branded like a convict at age 17 by a female, unable to withstand this assault because of his archaic anima, he is now hypervigilant towards any female he meets. Fritz Perls, father of the Gestalt therapy (the German word implying "wholeness"), would have astute advice for him to deal with actuality and not fantasy, and would have said, "Well, let's have a look at your nose," and then would most likely say, "It is an ordinary nose, so let's move on and embrace the here and now."

This patient needs to elevate his feeling function from the unconscious, in any form, the positive and negative aspects alike. His early humiliation has become a barrier between himself and all other women, causing him to feel that he might again be rejected. His loneliness might draw him to others, but his paranoia—his fear of getting hurt should he love too dearly and then be betrayed—made him keep all others at a safe distance. Therefore, a sense of disconnectedness—looking for and fear of connection—keeps him in a private limbo, unable to bridge the gap with others. The more he tries to find a solution, the more he creates an obstacle. He must rediscover the perpetually flowing present, a feeling he had known before only under the influence of psychedelic drugs in South America. It also would be rational to transfer his disposable libido to new interests or a useful activity, not transfer it to a physician, a guru, or another controlling male. Only then will he be able to truly continue living, rather than mournfully living in the past. Is he doomed like Cain to wander homeless upon the face of the earth, unable to enjoy the warmth and intimacy of a relationship he so desires? Unexpressed (suppressed) feeling—his natural dominant function—is trapped in his body, creating chronic tension. The future is unknown: we can only see what we have left behind. Blockage also starts in the chakras (centers of consciousness, where there is flow of energy in the body). Is there a damming up of libido?

In his case I think it is a blockage of the 4th chakra, *the anahata,* or heart, and the fourth element in TCM, air, represented by the lungs, which take in and expel energy, relating the inner and outer worlds. The Self is found in this chakra, as it is in the heart that thought and feeling are joined. Obviously ascending through the next chakras is not possible when there is a blockage—so the 5th chakra, or throat, where we learn to own the projections that we place out on the world, and the 6th chakra, or third eye, where the psyche is able to fly, as well the 7th chakra, or crown, self-actualization, are never achieved by him. Childhood and adolescent injuries have created an armored character of the body, a false Self, besides his unexpressed or undifferentiated part or shadow that must be integrated. He is caught between his shadow image—hating his nose—and his ideal body image, and such a swing creates in him despair and disgust. What he must correct are his internal images, his anima and animus, his female and male nature, so he can leave the past behind. He must perceive himself in the here and now, be liberated from and accept his shadow elements. If we do not see our shadow, we drown in it just like Narcissus did!

The rubric *impulse, to run* can be used for him. He is "running away" literally with frequent travels to visit meditation and yoga centers, but even more, figuratively, running away instead of confronting the father and inferiority complexes. His previous analytical therapy sessions have not brought contentment and solutions, not worked enough to alleviate him from his hatred towards his father and his injuries caused by the cruel insult by a young female. Even now when his father has been deceased for several years, salvation can only come from meeting this dis-ease in him upfront—this father and inferiority complex. Rather than doing acts of escapism, he needs to find the courage to wipe clean the slate on which his father and the girl wrote his life story.

When he was younger, before entering university, he *desired repose and tranquility* (*Nux-v*, *Sulph*). Why is there a logjam? In legal trials, when there is such a standstill, the prosecutor asks the advice/guidance of the Grand Jury, to have a second look at the problem. This corresponds to a wise counsel, representing the animus voice. Looking at his history, he indeed needs to listen to a renewed animus voice in order to free himself and decide what direction this process must go. Why remain in the never-ending struggle to be perfect?

As I get older, I sometimes ask myself questions about things that happened in the past, and rather than dwell over them, I only ask myself, "What would I have preferred to happen, and above all, can I still change this now in my life, at this old age (74), and can I transfer my energy to things which are still possible?"

I posed the following questions to this man, and I think his answers are very insightful, as it seems that the incident with the girl at age 17 has created this standstill.

Q1. When you think about the past and now, what emotions have *permanently* stayed with you?

A. The feelings from the incident at 17 years of age when people laughed when the girl made a comment about my nose —when I was taken off guard/surprised/shocked, shamed, rejected, embarrassed; feeling that something is wrong with me that needs fixing. Anxiety, wary/vigilant of criticism.

Q2. What is it that you think keeps you from going forward? What is the string that holds you to the past, as right now, apparently nothing is rationally holding you in a stagnant place, like your father or old business partner?

A. It seems to me like this is the central thing holding me back (answer before).

Q3. What in life do you still want to accomplish, career wise *and* relationship wise?

A. I don't have any grand outer career ambitions, more like inner ambitions. I've become more interested in creative interests, like Indian music, learning Indian tabla and pakhawaj drumming, holistic health, chanting, the mind/consciousness. (*Author's comment: I really hope he will follow these interests, as they all belong to the mystical, the female and feeling side.*)

Q4. What especially stops you from having a relationship with a woman? What handicaps you in your Eros capacity (art of relationship)? Usually when you meet a woman, what goes wrong in you or her?

A. I would like to experience a long-term warm connection/relationship with a loving woman. This inner feeling since age 17 seems to hold me back—as described above. I can't seem to relax and open up; fear/anxiety are triggered, so the relationship does not progress.

Q5. What is your dominant conscious function: feeling, thinking, sensation, or intuition? Meaning, which one gets the upper hand in any situation you encounter in life? And which one is "the hair in the soup," your Achilles tendon, bringing out uncontrolled emotions, evoking unexpected reactions?

A. I'm not that familiar with Jung's dominant conscious functions. Even though I was raised in a rational family and education, I seem to be most controlled by feelings, which are just under the surface and easily triggered as mentioned above. I also feel the intuitive function a fair bit. (*Author's comment: indeed, his natural conscious functions are feeling-intuitive, although not allowed to blossom early on.*)

Additional comments from this patient:

> "I did try Frits Perls Gestalt therapy and also a Gestalt offshoot called Voice Dialogue (with PhD Jungian

psychologists). They still didn't seem to address/resolve the issue for me.

"I read your summary. The Jungian interpretations and conclusions resonate to some extent, however I'm not sure they address the full spectrum of my experience. For example, what became obvious to me (esp. when taking psychedelic plants) is how much tension is held in my body. In fact, the first thing that happened when taking the plants is relaxing of this strong tension in the body, especially breathing. I could actually take a full relaxed breath, feel a release and flow of energy through my body, good feeling and relief of this inner state! I experienced the energy system in the body, which, once freed and flowing, seemed to be the key or doorway to freedom. This is all recognized by TCM and other Eastern yogic traditions, which may be why I'm so drawn to them."

Instead of pursuing many avenues, rescue could come from telling him to look at the complex that holds him prisoner, the father figure, to observe it, to get rid of this evil spirit that he carries on his back. Or does he remain a child, not able to look in a mirror or in the camera lens, as it reflects imperfection? But who is perfect? Of course, most of us are more imperfect on the emotional level than the physical one.

There is another remedy to be considered, depending on the answers I get from him upon further questioning, and that is *Hyoscyamus.* It has the *Delusion, parts of body are enlarged; he is injured by his surroundings; he is about to receive an injury* (when meeting women); *he has suffered wrong* (by father and girl at age 17); *childish behavior; A/F disappointed love; foolish behavior; jealousy* (stalking a previous girlfriend on the phone), and *despair from disappointed love.*

Series of Dreams

As much as homeopaths have vaguely heard about recurrent dreams as important to take into consideration for the "total" patient's investigation, Carl Jung paid even more attention to series of dreams, as they provide interpretations more accurately. Series of dreams point to different aspects of one and the same situation in such a way that one dream gives one aspect and another dream another, so that through the series the situation becomes clearer and more revealing through continuing translation of the relative fixed symbols. In this way, series of dreams can find confirmation or corrections of our original analysis through the dreams that follow.

In series of dreams there is usually a lysis, although most often an incomplete one. If by any chance we would have dream series without a lysis, it would of course signify that the dreamer's personal conflict persists. In this case we might instead call it "a recurrent dream that tries to bring more clarification and elaboration" so that the dreamer finally understands the message and the problem is solved (lysis). Only then will this recurrent dream finally disappear. At that point, the next dream surfaces as part of a series of dreams, usually presenting a new problem. Something has happened—maybe someone is dead or is dying or sick—and then we have to ask ourselves, "What will happen next? What can be done?" It is like we have finished reading chapter one of a book, but the story is not complete. We don't know the outcome yet! The second dream takes the problem up again in a different form, attempting to give the dreamer more insight or considerations, so we can go on to the next chapter in the book of life. So, dream series are a sequence of interrelated events, like the chapters of a novel or long text, and can reveal the continuity of the unconscious with surprising clarity as the motif is repeated. Interpretations of dream series provide a check on one another, so that we are less likely to get a one-sided view of the dreamer, as when we only have one dream to work with. The content of a neurosis becomes more apparent through analysis of several dreams, versus interpretation of just a single dream where assumptions are made about its psychological content, constituting the blunder of pure conjecture. It is not surprising that Jung had a famous patient who he analyzed for years (from November 1928 to June 1930) with a multitude of dreams, repeating the same motif in continuity (Jung, 1984).

We can also recognize in series of dreams the basic theme and problem posed by the unconscious. And dream series can be useful to assess progress with our therapy and simillimum, providing another measure of the direction of cure according to Hering's Rules (rules in homeopathy determining that true healing happens from within-out, from more important symptoms to lesser ones). Can we be certain if an interpretation of a dream is correct? We can answer this in the affirmative, for if we have missed the meaning or found it only incompletely, this will become evident in the very next dream. If the interpretation was wrong, the earlier motif, theme, or message may be repeated in still more definite extended form. And if the second interpretation also misses the mark, both the homeopath and the patient will be stymied by doubt. A right interpretation is rewarded by its animated effect—the "Aha" we look for in the patient—which is the final court of appeal. We see in the evolution of these dreams the fragmented parts of the original dream mirror, worked on and repaired, leading to a restoration of psychological balance.

We can conclude that the interpretation of dreams can become relatively certain *only* in series of dreams, making them even more important than the recurrent dream. Each successive dream corrects the mistakes made in interpreting its predecessors. The unconscious does not care about time: series of dreams do not form a book with *consecutive* chapters, a chronological linear progression, so it might be difficult to tell what chapter comes first and which one comes later. It can happen that the true order of series of dreams only becomes clear much later. The situation of a previous dream can be taken up again after some other dreams, amplifying the message of the dream again. The various single dreams of a series deal with one and the same problem and thus group themselves around this problem, shedding light upon the central theme. Interesting too is that the final thought in a long series of dream images, after going through the ever-renewed symbolic disguises, contains precisely what the first image in the series was trying to represent. If the dreamer in the initial dream wanted for instance a close relationship to someone, in the last dream she might be pregnant with the child of that person in her dream, so that this string of dreams is not senselessly disorganized, but rather is an orderly process. Sometimes, to our surprise, we remember two dreams the same night. In that case both dreams should be looked at as a single whole, as they often complement each other, trying to put more light on the obscure points of our ego awareness and enhance the totality of the unconscious message.

Examples of series of dreams come later, after discussing elements of the conscious and unconscious. Let's proceed to discuss the third class of dreams, the archetypal dreams, full of mystery and symbols!

Archetypal Dreams

Although Freud talked about "archaic vestiges or remnants of old experiences," a term he used for thought forms the dreamer could not explain as they were not at all related to anything in his present conscious life, it was Jung who introduced the terms *archetypes* and *the collective unconscious* in a psychological sense —dream images and living symbols, not of an individual but of a collective nature. In other words, these are symbols not only traceable to experiences in the patient's individual life, bringing a certain message to the dreamer, but also to the rest of mankind, regardless of race, gender, and color. Personal dreams arise from the superficial layers of the unconscious, while archetypal dreams originate from the deeper collective layers, the collective unconscious. For Jung, all humans have common, inherited patterns of emotional and mental behavior which he called *archetypes*. Contrary to what the average person thinks when a child is born, it is shallow and naïve to think that a child starts on a *tabula rasa* or "clean slate." St. Augustine claimed rightfully that we are all marked in our very origin with evil. Indeed, we are not a blank sheet on which life writes its text. Augustine called it a *massa pecati*—a "mass of sin." Besides collective basic needs such as those for love, harmony, and freedom, the genetic or miasmatic predominant family traits already have filled several chapters in the book of any and all humans at birth.

Jung, practicing unconsciously as a homeopath, was aware of a newborn having *a priori* existence, born with marks of the collective unconscious. But according to Hahnemann, newborns are also settled with parental miasmatic heritage. The homeopath knows that the child will already be additionally "infected" by transgenerational traits or miasms (which are *not* the same as archetypal inheritance), and aside from this heavy *individual* familial inheritance, every newborn inherits a tendency to form *universal* archetypes or mythological motifs. Therefore, from the moment he is born, a child is already an individual with instincts to react as a human being without being taught by the parents to behave in that way. The ancestors are not "dead" and gone forever from the earth, but still exist in the form of these archetypes and miasmatic traits. A logical, exact definition of archetypes surpasses our rational mind, but it is clear and visible to all that human behavior and experiences and reactions to typical occurrences—since the very beginning of humanity—are somehow deposited in all subsequent generations (collective traits).

Just as human physiology shows *common* anatomy and functionality, transcending differences of all human races, when it comes to physiological and psychological needs and basic desires (psoric needs), life as we know it now is the same as it has been for the past hundreds of thousands of years. The collective unconscious is made up of archetypes, which are collective traits and patterns, a combination of the most beautiful and despicable of the many psychic experiences of humanity—the good, the bad, and the ugly—and are as old as human life. They vary from the desire for love, for close relationships and friendships, for shelter and protection, but also include our insecurities, acts of revenge and hatred, greed and materialism, incest, and desire for power and domination followed by unspeakable acts. These are all archetypes forming the collective unconscious, or in other words, the true human foundation of every individual psyche. As Jung said, everyone carries in him a murderer and a saint—an *Anacardium* figure with the devil on one shoulder and an angel on the other, both whispering in man's ear, and it's never known who will get the upper hand. Which one will surface depends not only on circumstances like a war or natural catastrophe, but more often depends on the dominant family hereditary miasmatic background, constitution, temperament, and the degree of spirituality—a word misused in homeopathic practices, as spirituality is nothing but having the courage, sincerity, and willingness to visit our unconscious (especially the garbage can), and to not identify with the shadow side. This should be our moral guide in life.

That these archetypes extend to all kind of patterns, happenings, characteristics, etc., is easily observed in animals too. The building of a bird's nest, the unfolding of the peacock's tail, the migration of the caribou herds, the migration of the grey whales from Mexico to Alaska along the California coast, the migration of the birds southwards, salmon swimming upstream, and the urge of the beaver to build a dam from the instinctual reaction to the sound of water, are just some examples. We can call these patterns of behavior ritualistic behaviors, serving the purpose of preservation of the species.

Another aspect of archetypes is their dual nature, just like there is no yang without yin, or no darkness without light. Likewise, any archetype (discussed later in detail), be it the anima, animus, shadow side, the Self, the Hero, the Divine Child, etc., can exhibit either, or even both sides, in the same dream. It is important for the dreamer to assess what role and effect (positive or negative) this archetype plays in the dream, in order to get further guidance for his life. Other interesting archetypes are the *trickster* and *the child.*

The *trickster archetype* is hard to define because he is always one step ahead of us. As mentioned further (see Chap. 10), with some effort and courage as well as education, the shadow, closest to the conscious, is the archetype that is the most easily accessible to the personal conscious, much more than the anima and animus. Who is that devilish trickster? Most humans are prone to pursuing goals that find no correlation to their physical or mental capacity. The trickster in their unconscious leads them in a merry dance and they are all too happy to follow pipe dreams, not steered by common critique or a rational mind, as at night any inhibitory mechanism is silenced, allowing their unconscious the most incredulous desires while playing sly jokes and malicious pranks on them. The trickster is the Pied Piper, the Lord of the Dance, the jester at the king's court, a monkey who offers us delight and pleasure, but if we follow his call, we might end up a laughingstock. Although blessed with cunning and great mischievous power, and full of malicious pranks and playfulness (he is the mischievous *Tarentula* of homeopathy!), his antics can be corrective (if we escape from our unawareness) as he can prick the balloon of our inflated sense of Self, mocking our vanities, lofty ambitions, and desires which are often the subject of delusions of grandeur, not based in reality. As any archetypal figure, this figure is powerful when on our side, and baffling and disturbing when not. We must not forget that the trickster gives us the opportunity to transform and change our journey, from a side road to the main avenue to the Self. In emergent situations in dreams—showing the positive side of this archetype, because of his semi-magical powers—he will lead the dreamer to safety.

The *child archetype* equally shows the duality of the opposites, the yin and yang side. On one hand it is a symbol of innocence and purity, the Divine Child or *puer aeternus*—embodying the birth and growth—a figure that possesses enormous transformative, creative powers and potentialities of life. The growing of such a child in further dreams is a very positive step in our individuation, as the old attitude "dies" and there comes the "birth" and growth of the new one. The Divine Child is the return to innocence, a readiness to be reborn without the mask, to appear naked—an important step on man's individuation path. The negative side is when the dreamer is stuck in his childish fantasies, in a life full of frivolities and play, a person who never will grow up, an immature child-man, the typical Peter Pan (*Calc-c* comes to mind). He is a happy-go-lucky guy who knows all the answers to life and can afford to play forever. Such an adult refuses to work hard, lacks maturity, commitment, and responsibility (*aversion to and inability to take responsibility*), often a reflection of a mother-complex, making people remark, "When is he going to grow up?" He needs an intervention through the lightning bolt of Zeus, a sudden onset of depression (to which the *Calc-c* person is very much prone) or a sudden debilitating physical disease. Always relying on God (*religious affections, wants to read the Bible all day long* and *metaphysical concerns*), he should be reminded that God helps those who help themselves, for doing so stimulates self-growth. The appearance of a child in his dreams confronts him with his existential situation which he fails to understand. Refusing to listen to such a dream will keep him stagnant and withdrawn in childish fantasies and inappropriate dreams. The opposite archetype, *senex*, meaning "old man," has the positive characteristics of working hard and responsibility, but if we are totally shaped by the senex, we become rigid, inflexible, stiff, and far removed from our feminine side, losing heart and our youthful, playful spirit.

Archetypal dreams are rare and of great power, shocking the dreamer, and were called "big dreams" among the primitives and tribes (*arche* means "principle or beginning"). Among the Native American Indians, dreams of the chief, medicine man, and shaman were guiding principles for the tribe as they had an important message for the whole tribe, not just the dreamer. Big dreams have a powerful influence and baffle their possessor, who feels compelled to share them as they are mysterious and feel important. They are also called "numinous" dreams, from the Latin noun *numen*, meaning a presiding deity or divine majesty, carrying words with the power of the gods (because they carry so much psychic energy). When a dream is numinous it means that it must be respected and listened to, treated in a special way, its urgent message acted upon. The problems or challenges posed in these dreams are not unique experiences but have been faced by many people, of all races and countries throughout time, transcending all personal life experiences. As mentioned before, in archetypal dreams, persons unknown to the dreamer appear, and little appears in the dream about aspects of his everyday life, which indicates that these dreams stem from the deep layers of the collective unconscious.

When do archetypal dreams occur? They often occur when important changes happen in our life, when we are undergoing major life events or crises—what Jung called "periods of turmoil"—when a major new personality development must be attained. Typical instances include the terrible twos and puberty, menopause, marriage, midlife crisis, pregnancy, divorce, children leaving home, taking up a new job or moving away, when dying, when looking for the meaning of life in the second part of life, leaving home for the first time at age 18, and at age 5 when going to school for the first time. Unfortunately, they occur also in instances of rape, incest, or near-death experiences in murder attempts. Other instances they occur in include times of great social, political, and religious upheaval—like the outbreak of war, or a religious scandal as with the Catholic Church pedophilia crisis—often leading to disorientation and confusion but not pathology. "Another situation in which the collective unconscious becomes active is through a crisis in an individual's life and the collapse of hope and expectations" (Jung, 2009, p. 210).

For the child under 5 years old, being close to the collective unconscious, we should not be surprised to see such strikingly mythological dreams, which provide us great material and insight for their investigation. When the collective unconscious replaces reality and forcefully tries to assert itself, the danger for dissociation (infantile schizophrenia) is always present. This splitting off of the unconscious can have different triggers: when there is a conflict between the parents of the child (*Ailments from discords between chief and subordinates; quarreling*); when there is a psychic trauma like sexual abuse or incest, and when there is a dominant syphilitic miasmatic predisposition in the family and in the child. Many sources of an archetypal nature are to be found in dreams of early childhood, from the third to the fifth year, as the normal development of the libido can be arrested or distorted by the impact of environmental influences. An example is seen in the following archetypal dream of a 5-year-old girl.

This case was presented by an excellent pediatrician/homeopath to a congress as an example of a "*Sulphur*" type girl, treated "successfully" with *Sulphur* for her chief complaint—allergies—but did not include the sudden onset of incomprehensible change in her temperament, going from outgoing and joyful to a choleric state, in which she exhibited mood changes and temper tantrums. She had the following dream before consult, a dream which during the lecture was casually mentioned by the homeopath as if it was a sign of a *Sulphur* personality. To my surprise (or not), none of the attendants asked what this dream really meant. The treating homeopath should have been alert to the fact that the initial complaint, allergies, was of psoric origin, while clearly the change in behavior, and especially the theme of her dream, reflected the destructive character of the syphilitic miasm. The entry point of her case to find the simillimum should have been a syphilitic expression, discovered with the help of the meaning of her dream. Here was her archetypal dream.

Dream

Once upon a time I touched something inside a castle, and I was transformed into a snake with two heads as I was catcn and killed.

Analysis of this dream is presented later, on page 196. Before getting to that, I wish to share more about the significance of the girl's age, and archetypal dreams.

Firstly, think about the horror if *you* would be faced with such a dream! And what would it make you think, if your child pronounces this nightmare to you? Are you going to say, "Listen dear child, it is just a dream, forget about it"? Looking at this dream, it has no lysis but ends in catastrophe, being eaten by a snake. Additionally, the dream content is meager, often a sign of an unfavorable prognosis. This dream is an impressive example of inner psychical activity, archetypal in nature. Many of the symbols in children's dreams are direct expressions of material from the collective unconscious. The images in this one particularly must come from the collective unconscious, as we are sure that parents or fairytale books would not present material of this kind. Certainly, its contents have nothing to do with aspects of the child's daily life, or do they? Children's anxieties and fears during the day, caused by emotional or traumatic events, often find an outlet in dreams, and we must remember that we discover in children fear of life and death equally, represented in dreams, also symbolized here by the duality of the snake.

Interpretation of such a dream is always difficult, but it is the task of the conscious mind of the therapist to understand the hint of the dream, otherwise the child's developmental process could be halted, or she might become the victim of a thwarted individuation process and dragged along to an ominous fate. First, archetypal dreams with their amazing image-making faculty shock the unprepared conscious of the dreamer, creating confusion, horror, astonishment, and disorientation as well as incomprehension. Additionally, this is a child; we cannot expect personal associations or amplifications, which creates considerable difficulties in the dream interpretation. We depend on others in the family to know about her conscious situation, and sometimes, if that family member wants to keep secrets, such important information is not forthcoming. And what if the situation of the child—the crime committed—is perpetrated by one of the parents? It can also be unknown to parents when, where, and by whom the crime has been committed (coach, teacher, priest, physician, scout master, etc.). It is left to the analyst to exercise his *own amplification* as nothing can be deduced from the relatively meager visual language of the dream.

Furthermore, as seen before, a single dream expresses only a partial aspect of the dreamer's psyche. But here, further dreams were not available, as it never went to a series of dreams, but only a *recurrence* of this single dream with different aspects. The dream did become a recurrent dream in the following years, indicating that a vital problem was not addressed or corrected, as the treating homeopath was not able to understand this dream and use it as a tool to confirm the needed simillimum. We also cannot call on the ultimate judgment of our interpretation, which is the agreement of the dreamer with the "Aha" moment, impossible to obtain from such a young person. An interpretation on the object level also seems impossible, as this dream contains no figures that are in vital and immediate relationship to this child, such as her mother or father. But the first step for the homeopath is to question family and friends to see if this dream deals with a *personal problem* (objective analysis) before delving into subjective interpretation. After that, the best way for the homeopath to understand such an archetypal dream, because the child cannot, or fears to give associations (repression), is to go to the bizarre world of the collective images as found in fairy tales, myths, poetry, and religion (among others).

Also note the sparse and symbolic content of this dream, which is not uncommon in such a young child, as her ego is still close to the collective unconscious. However, such a cosmic dream reflects a deeply disturbing actual conflict, which her conscious mind cannot understand or resolve. Because of the great susceptibility of children, there is a threat to her inmost Self of disintegration and splitting, pointing to the danger of the burgeoning consciousness being swallowed up again by the instinctive psyche, the unconsciousness. A meeting of the child's archaic consciousness with the expanded collective unconscious always causes the risk of disintegration of this developing consciousness—a possible destruction of the unity of her personality. Although the language of fairy tales, as expressed in this dream, is a language in which children are used to as they are close to the collective unconscious at this age, if there already is a predisposition to psychosis (because of a familial hereditary syphilitic predisposition), it can happen that the archetypal image represented by the snake in this dream will escape from conscious control of the archaic ego, producing a state of possession, leading to dissociation—as can be seen in infantile schizophrenia—a danger present in this case, as the archetypal situation could become overwhelming. In such a young child, where consciousness is rather weak and still growing, unconscious contents can fall below the threshold, overwhelming the ego. Let's try therefore to first analyze the dream without any additional information regarding her conscious situation. Being an archetypal dream, having a personal and collective significance, we need to ask ourselves what it means for the dreamer, this young girl, and what it means, or says, regarding the whole human race.

In order to help you, the reader, understand this dream, let me first give you a rough scheme of important archetypal dreams during the lifetime of a human being. The primary important fact to note is the age of this girl: 5 years old! Before age 5 we have the *participation mystique* with the parents, or mystical participation, where children even dream about the stresses and discords of the parents. It is important to say a word about mystical participation. It is present strongly from the intrauterine stage (day one of pregnancy!) until age 5. So when conducting inquiry of a case of disturbed development of a child, as often seen in cases of autism, not only the intrauterine state of the mother needs to be investigated, but also the time between age 0 (birth) and age 5, to see if the mother was under any emotional stress. The following example points this out.

A child of 18 months had seizures and twitching that were unresponsive to any allopathic medication (a combination of at least three medications was given) and the case was called "resistant convulsions," cause unknown. An operation on the brain was considered a potential solution to these convulsions, which often result in status epilepticus. On my careful inquiry, not one factor of distress in the mother's pregnancy could be found. The onset of these seizures was at 11 months. Upon questioning what happened just before that, the mother told how she had traveled to India to visit her mother and was only told then that her own mother needed an operation for cancer. This shocked her greatly and she wept for one week, looking for emotional support everywhere. The child started the convulsions within three weeks of this news. Although parents think that their own emotional state would not affect their children (especially if they try to hide their grief or discord), this child *knew* and reacted to her grief with seizures. The homeopathic remedy had to be found in *hearing bad news* and *Ailments from grief* and *cares*, besides the following other syphilitic rubrics: *anguish after hearing horrible things; despair with fear of death; horrible things and stories affect her greatly; desire to be magnetized* (looking for support)*; taciturn* and *despondency.*

Calc-c was chosen successfully as the remedy (dd. with *Nat-m/Ign.* was necessary), based on the previous rubrics ("the person with the disease"). Reading about *Calc-c* in Hering's Materia Medica revealed many proving symptoms with seizures under the heading "nerves": *chorea, involuntary motions; convulsions in a little boy; tonic spasms; epilepsy before the attack of something running in arms, or from pit of stomach down through abdomen into feet, worse at night and at full moon; epileptic attack without consciousness* and *epilepsy of three years standing, eight or ten daily.*

The other archetypal kind of dreams are the ones due to the proximity of the child to the collective unconsciousness. From age 5 on is when psychological separation from the parents starts, where the child has to perform a heroic effort to liberate himself from the father or mother complex; it is a change from the prenatal psyche to the process of ego consciousness, an age to differentiate him/herself and move out into the world. It is a very important developmental stage, well known in allopathic science, when the child evolves from a primitive ego to a more developed one.

Let's return to the archetypal dream presented in the seminar.

Analysis

Looking at this 5-year-old child's dream and its catastrophic ending with being eaten, as well as her change in behavior, we can deduce that the child's development did not proceed undisturbed. Considering her age, this is the time that she starts becoming female, so to speak, the *beginning of the female instinctual world*, when often animals such as snakes appear in dreams. The two-headed snake, two signifying a duality, as we have seen, points to an unconscious process trying to become conscious and fused—in her case, her female instinctual world, leading normally to an expansion of consciousness. This dream is also like a fairy tale ("once" as in "once upon a time") as her subconscious is still close to the collective unconscious. It is her language, the language of fairy tales she is comfortable with, despite the horrific ending. After all, there are many fairy tales which show the struggle of the biblical hero of Jonah's story: Jonah was swallowed by a "big fish," likely a whale (the monster or animal from the unconscious), and was overcome by the sea monster—a kind of death—but after he prayed (struggled from the dark towards the light) and gained new awareness, God commanded the fish to spit the hero out, and we have the hero reborn. Yet for this girl, the integration of unconscious content (the instinctual female process) into consciousness was obstructed—and at a precious moment of evolution in this child, a period of important transformation—as she was eaten alive. This is as if she was swallowed by the unconscious content, harming her—evident in her change in violent conscious behavior, following the rule of opposites and compensation and the recurrence of this dream, pointing to an unresolved important aspect in her life. Why did she change into a snake? What was the obstruction in her developmental process? And why was she killed and eaten? What stopped the process of psychological separation and growing up, the formation of her femininity?

Looking at the symbol of the snake (see Chap. 2), the image of the snake, appearing in many myths and dreams throughout centuries, can be a collective symbol for sexuality (its common interpretation in a dream is a sexual one) and therefore can be a sexual dream, and in fact "being killed and eaten" shows the dangerous aspect in this dream that this young girl will be overtaken by a sinister entity/person destroying her life or the Self. The unconscious has an ambivalent nature and is often symbolized in dreams by a snake. To be bitten by a snake—an archetypal image signifying the awakening of sexuality—is becoming vulnerable to the collective unconscious, to the natural instincts (i.e., sexual ones). This girl is not just bitten, but devoured, implying a greater danger, a threat of being engulfed by the collective unconscious! This could lead to infantile schizophrenia, often starting at age 3 and often confused with ASD. The release of these unconscious contents, possibly fracturing the fragile archaic ego of this 5-year-old girl, can lead to a dissociation that is a real and great danger for her. Now we see clearly the need for understanding this dream in order to protect her and as an important tool in remedy selection and management, as it carries an important message.

We must therefore look at the conscious life of this girl and hopefully receive the help of close relatives if available (she came on consult with her grandmother, with whom she lived). Then there is the *castle*. As a symbol it stands for different things: it can be a safe place or home (certainly for a *Calc-c* person whose home is his castle); it is a medieval place with little roads and a labyrinth of rooms; it is a fortress difficult to get in and out of; and it also stands for a male symbol. A black castle is a place of darkness, representing the powers of the unconscious, and it is in the unconscious that people need to find "the answer to all questions," by integrating the unconscious elements. But any dwelling—house, hotel, castle, city (is the city in ruins, in construction, or new?), barn, houseboat, etc.—refers to the Self, the total psychology of the individual, the sum of the conscious and unconscious.

As mentioned before, since personal association and amplification in this young girl is not possible, we need to get more information from the grandmother. Jung stated: "If there is a neurosis in the child (as we saw in her change of behavior), first examine the parents' relationship!" The girl's mother was schizophrenic and hospitalized. The father sexually abused this girl, and thanks to the pediatrician was put in prison. This situation fractured the growth of her archaic anima/femininity and it was killed before it could be fused to grow further. The child was treated with *Sulphur* for allergies until age 8, and this dream kept coming back on a regular basis till that age. Besides *Sulphur*, the homeopath administered a dose of *Staphysagria* each time she had this dream. In my opinion, *Staphysagria* was the remedy she needed initially, not *Sulphur*. By age 8, this recurrent dream stopped. But much time was lost, years in which she continuously suffered anxiety and disturbed emotional behavior, with the danger of a psychotic break or schizophrenia always lurking.

We must also remember that if incest occurs, it will remain a family secret and the person, often a child as in this case, will be plagued by nightmarish dreams for the rest of her life, not understood by most physicians and homeopaths, and therefore *Staphysagria* might not have been given, only *Sulphur*. And most incest and rape victims would try to put the memory in the garbage can, plagued by recurrent nightmares forevermore. Incest victims have *an ill-equipped feeling conscious function* (see Chap. 8), as they are overwhelmed by *guilt* and *self-reproach* often for a long time. And imaginary pain no doubt is more painful than a so-called real one, as it is accompanied by moral suffering caused by the secret self-accusation, "It must have been my fault." Luckily this girl's grandmother could provide protection and feed her anima since the real mother is schizophrenic. By age 8, this recurrent dream stopped. Why? She most likely had received enough *Staphysagria* (after three years) to deal with this incest trauma, plus the father's imprisonment, and the grandmother's protection and love, helped of course. At this time the homeopath deemed her treatment was finished. Or, was it?

Now she is 10 years old and still lives with her grandmother. Is there still danger, or are we done with treatment? The good thing now is that her grandmother has taken over the role of the mother to cultivate the formation of her femininity or anima. What is the next dangerous period in her life? Puberty! Because of the strong syphilitic background in *both* parents, this girl might exhibit character disturbances in the future around puberty, when the dominant family miasm might flare up from its dormant state—puberty always being a period of turmoil with sexual awakening. And her miasmatic syphilitic character already became apparent before, not only in her recurrent dream but also in her aggressive behavior and withdrawal, going inwards. She should be monitored closely by her homeopath as she approaches menarche. If not, if the roots of the syphilitic miasm are not sufficiently eradicated, besides being overcome with all the negative characteristics of the syphilitic miasm, she will grow up to be a woman that hates men, as her anima remains injured, giving birth to menstrual disturbances, vaginismus, yeast infections, and honeymoon cystitis, representing hate for men as sexual intercourse is perceived as a violation.

This case teaches us how understanding dreams warns us about the actual situation, and although it was recognized by the grandmother and intervened upon by the homeopath, treatment of the patient was not correct, and the future of this child was still in danger. The syphilitic miasm could still explode in her any time, leading to different forms of psychosis like schizophrenia and hallucinations.

Another archetypal dream occurred in an older male (68 years old) during an episode of a severe acute flu, in the following case.

Conscious attitude: This was an intelligent man, with good psychological insight and great interest in the unconscious messages of his dreams. He was driven and ambitious, very psoric in character, a worrier more for others than himself, who always "found an excuse" not to take a rest period in his hectic life, to stop for a moment and smell the roses. Something or somebody always intervened, so that he "had" to perform first this or that before he could even think of taking a rest. The "excuse" seemed to always win the battle. When this flu hit him, the discomfort started with a light impression of fatigue, but nothing was going to stop him. He just felt he was slowing down a little during his tennis match. Regardless, the next day, as "he could not refuse his good friend to play," he played again, not listening to any warning signs like some dry cough and increasing fatigue. The third day he *had* to pay attention. Suddenly he could not muster the strength to move at all, as if the wind was taken out of his sails, not wanting to move as he lay listless in bed, too tired to lift a hand. It was the most severe weariness and general dopey feeling he ever felt in his life, pinning him in bed for the next five days. Other symptoms were complete lack of thirst, aching on moving the eyes, shivers going up and down the spine, and a dull, disoriented, and dizzy feeling. With the slow onset of this illness, any homeopath should recognize the feared *Gelsemium* flu. If anything will flatten you, a *Gelsemium* pathology will! During his disease (the third day) he had the following dream.

Dream

I have to return from a foreign country (where I have worked) to my home country and have to take a bus, which would take me to the train station. I am accompanied by an old looking man I do not know but who seems to tell me where to go for the bus. In fact, I ask him if I need to change trains before reaching my destination and he confirmed this. Upon seeing concern in my face, he promised to accompany me on this trip home, which relieved a lot of my anxiety as I had a hard time figuring out the directions. We are waiting for this bus with many other people, but as the bus does not arrive on the scheduled time, everyone starts walking in the direction of the station and no one seems very concerned or surprised. Coming close to the station, there are food stands and a lady seems to put paper bags (3) on the side to be picked up and payment should be done in the station. Only 3 people (my older companion is one of them) do so, and each bag seems to contain 3 sandwiches. Before reaching the rail station, several different roads all come together, with many people on them, making the entrance to the station somewhat of a struggle to overcome. I, together with my companion, squeeze through and push forward. Then I wake up, relaxed and thinking, "What does this all mean?"

Analysis

The first thing to notice in this dream is that *many* people seem to be going on this journey with him, always pointing to a problem or goal posed by the dream that is not just a personal problem but one that belongs collectively to mankind—hence a representation of an archetypal dream. What was this message?

The other outstanding person in this dream is the old man, who seems to be the one he turns to for advice; in fact, the elderly man will accompany him on this great journey homewards. We recognize one of the more common archetypes, the wise old man, ready to be a spiritual guide and one of the representations of the four animus images (see Chap. 12, "Animus"). The dreamer is at once put at ease for what seems to be otherwise a very difficult trip, as he has a hard time figuring out the directions. No doubt this journey, this trip—not only undertaken by him, but also by the masses in his dream—refers to the path to *individuation*, a path to become a more complete person. That this is not a straight road is seen from the different stages in this dream, where he must take a bus, walk, and then change trains while traveling. It refers to the many obstructions and challenges we will encounter during our life journey. But the dreamer has come this far in his life and in his connections to the unconscious, and he is now accompanied by the wise and powerful old man, which is a reassurance to him for the rest of his life journey. Why did he have to walk when the bus did not show up? Buses, trains, and airplanes are all transport, taken by a lot of people, and it is someone else, pilot, driver, who is bringing him to a certain destination determined in advance and impossible to change once set in motion. This is opposite of driving our own car, where it is important if we are at the wheel of the car. This dream indeed tells not only the dreamer but many people (humanity) that on the individuation path, we need to walk on our *own power*, not always depending on others, and that it will take personal effort. Also, that we are to make the unconscious our friend, where we will meet other helpful images and characters (people, friends, and animals represented by archetypes) to guide us on the way, the journey *home*, which can stand for security, compassion, finding peace to relax, and comfort. The message, in view of his conscious situation, seems to be very wise advice: "Slow down, reap the fruits of your labor without feeling guilty, you deserve it."

There is only one thing left. The number **three** shows up in this dream, and I refer the reader to "Numbers Appearing in Dreams," found in Chapter 2. There is lysis and certainly a step forward, as he will be ready to board the train, ready for further destinations in his life, but certainly this "acute disease" was a good imposed "stop" in his lifestyle, where the wise man tells him where to go (home) and what to do. No wonder he woke up relaxed, a good sign!

We have brought our discussion up to the important different aspects of dream examination, and will now proceed to discuss examination of the elements of the conscious world: the ego and its production, the persona figure, and the four conscious functions, all playing an important role in many dreams.

SECTION TWO

Elements of the Conscious

6

THE EGO FORMATION

The move away from the dominance of the ego to the acceptance of a larger context of the Self, enriching the consciousness, is the road to self-actualization.

Stages of the Development of the Ego

Jung states, "The ego is a complex of representations which constitutes the center of my field of consciousness and appears to possess a very high degree of continuity and identity" (Jung, 1990, CW Vol. 6, para. 706).

How does such an entity come to be, and what role does it play in a human's life? Is the course of life only and mainly governed by the ego, are there no other forces at work to guide humans in their life journey? Is the ego responsible for *all* human actions and decisions, or is this just wishful thinking? To what extent is it responsible? If it forms just *part* of the psyche—does it form the most or least important part? These are all questions coming to mind that need to be answered.

Let's talk about the normal child first and investigate what normal childhood development is—including the function of the ego and the four conscious functions—so I can contrast it with the child with autism (ASD). By seeing how the application of Jung's principles are prescient to a child with ASD, we can identify the stage of development that needs to be addressed and treated, to appropriately recognize what part is stuck. Jung extensively studied philosophy, Greek mythology, religion, folklore, language, alchemy, and oriental medicine in order to explain the individual. This should not come as a surprise to the reader as all those modalities were and still are necessary to examine the psyche, dreams, and the unconscious of man—the often neglected but influential other half of one's life.

By first examining ideal and healthy development, Jung then examined where things went wrong and where assaults took place. According to Jung, size and growth of the shadow run parallel to the growth and size of the ego. The child gradually develops out of the infinitesimal unconscious state into a conscious one, and usually the first impressions of life are the strongest ones. From the time of conception, the child is moving towards individuality and is prepared for an independent existence. Progressive mental development means extension of consciousness. In the case of a normal child, such consciousness is shaped initially like separate islands, which gradually and slowly integrate to form a continent gaining on the vast sea of the unconscious. The primitive ego-consciousness is like a flickering light that comes and goes. Much depends on the predominant miasmatic family hereditary state—not understood by allopathy—which often shows its influence early on by flooding the growing consciousness with sudden and strange contents, such as jealousy (sycosis) or self-destructiveness (syphilis), which hints already at the abnormal future development of the adult he will become. As usual, allopathy is totally ignorant of this powerful development and consequently is baffled by the unexpected abnormal behavior of young children we often witness in present society. Whenever a horrible crime is committed by such a youngster, everyone seems to grasp at straws for a possible trigger, but these psychological mishaps are never sudden. They find their impetus and nucleus in the ever-growing, abnormal miasmatic influence, reaching a strong acceleration at puberty.

A child's life begins with the goal of striving for growth and authority as he absorbs his environment like a sponge. He lives solely in the pleasure or pain of the moment—a capacity to exist in the moment—something an adult like *Calc-c* is quite able to retain. While he retains childlike immediacy (an immediate response to simple objects), he can also be thrown into despair if the object of delight fades, just as the ancient Epicureans exhibited in their lives. What the child and the *puer aeternus* ("eternal boy") do not understand is that life not only yields many flowers but also weeds, so the search for the pleasurable moments can be short-lived. Ego growth depends on the way communication between a child and his environment is possible. The first opportunity for communication between a child and his environment takes place in the womb.

During these first stages of development of a fetus, the ear is the first organ to develop in the embryo and becomes functional after only 16 weeks. Active listening starts at 24 weeks. The mother's womb is the perfect resonant sound chamber to receive messages from the outside world—mom's soothing voice, her excitement, stories, rhymes, the music of Mozart and Vivaldi (but alas, also disarray and family conflict is received with great clarity). As to the benefit of music, it can be considered a pre-linguistic language which is stimulating and nourishing, affecting the whole human being, as soothing sounds calm the child. After all, while swimming in the amniotic fluid, the relative peace of the womb is ideally only disturbed by mom's heartbeat, respiration, and intestinal gurgling, as well as a few songs delivered with love. The fetus already has a memory from early on. Some investigators even think that consciousness exists from the very moment of conception. Most scientists (neurologists, biologists) agree that from the sixth month on, the unborn child can remember, hear, learn and even act on his mother's feelings. The brain is in a critical stage of development from the ninth to the eighteenth week.[1]

This is all the more reason to pay attention to any physical and emotional trauma happening during that period. Until birth, the child's body and mind are part of the mother's body and mind. And even though the child becomes a separate physical entity when the umbilical cord is cut, the important psychic cord remains. Not that the child is an exact psychological duplicate of the parent, as the child has his own constitution and personality, but each child remains affected in his development by the attitude of the parent and those in the close vicinity of the home.

In normal children, language develops slowly in the first year of life. A child gradually becomes competent in the use of language and other communication skills through observation of, and interacting with, other people. Over the first year of life the normally developing child uses vocalization expressively and communicatively, to indicate needs as a means of expressing feelings, and even to socialize before developing verbal communication. Turn-taking in vocalization interaction occurs at an extremely early age (approximately 1 to 2 months old). An infant is sensitive to acoustic features, which for a typically developing infant act as the mechanism to identify the speaker. The normally developing child is also sensitive to visual features (recognizing and interpreting facial expressions of mom), which communicate direction of movement and helps to identify objects by the end of the first five months of life. Further, and crucially, the very young normally developing child perceives and uses those linguistic and situational features that communicate intent: gestures, actions, and objects in their immediate environment. These features Jung would consider being part of the typically developing primitive persona.

The condition during the first two years of the child's life is more like a primitive animal state from which a child will grow slowly into a more civilized conscious state. By age 5 the ego has steadily grown, and verbal humor and make believe already have surfaced. Till this age the psyche is still close to the collective unconsciousness or psyche. As personal attributions with the appearance of inner contradiction arise when the child's world expands after this age, now being in school, this child must make a differentiation between good and bad—the question of responsibility and morality. The *process of becoming psychologically an individual* (the individuation process) is now in full force and encouraged by caring parents. It is evident, and generally accepted by scientists, that one of the most important tenets of early normal development is the creation of a world for the child where there is a sense of security created by parental love, which includes courage and honesty in facing the problems of daily life. In such an environment the child can grow normally with his psyche firmly rooted in a spirit of love. We must think of life as developing from within as well as from without, a notion confirmed by epigenetics.

In the child, *projection* is one of the earliest forms of thought. He projects his own attitude into things animate and inanimate. When he bumps against the wall, it is "a bad wall." When he is angry, "Mommy is bad." Another infantile adaptation for Jung is identification in an unconscious manner with those around him. The child takes over the manner of another (sibling, parent) as if it was his own. As the conscious mind comes into existence, he uses "I" instead of "he" or "you," and although this growth is throughout life, from puberty on it becomes slower as the growth of ego is also connected to the plasticity and hardware of the brain. This makes recovering the autistic child before puberty (rather than age 5) very important, although the plasticity of the brain remains intact under *individual* adequate treatment—an investigation that has a quantum (vitalistic/energetic) approach, rather than a rigid and linear Newtonian (mechanistic) approach. So even after puberty, recovery and cure are possible, as everything depends on the continuing growth of the ego and increased size of the conscious world of the individual. Between the first and fourth year, consciousness is nothing but a conglomeration of small islands, as a child still lives in a state that is a combination of factual observation and fantasies.

The building up of the ego starts when the child reaches school age, when he comes in contact with his environment and is confronted with situations unknown till then. Depending on his constitution and miasmatic hereditary prevalence, he will blossom or withdraw. For example, being away from the protection of the home, encounters with others will present painful shocks and feelings of sadness for the introverted *Nat-m*, or a chance to be taken with open arms to augment one's circle of friends for the *Phosphorus* person. Others retire into a fortress from a sense of vulnerability, like *Thuja* (*Del, appearance of building stones; Del, he is too thin,* and *diminished*). The results are predictable. *Nat-m* feels very different from others and her development of consciousness will be disturbed, as she escapes in a fantasy world (*Delusions of fancy illusions*) and dreams of retiring in a cocoon or castle or the womb, or of finding herself in the middle of the magic protective circle, to avoid facing the stern reality of life. *Nat-m* thinks back too much, creating appalling gaps of unimproved feelings, which is like swimming against the tide, making life for herself and anyone else in her environment difficult and stressful (*dwells over past disagreeable events*). Contrary to the contractive world of *Nat-m, Phosphorus* shows expansion and opens her ego filter to all stimuli from the outside, vastly expanding her ever-growing ego conscious. A *Calc-c* child already seeks earnestly for higher protection and the meaning of life as he is invaded by *religious affections* and *metaphysical concerns*: "Who is God? What happens when I go to heaven? Will it hurt? Are you always going to be there for me?" For *Calc-c*, God will always be the permanent protector, and at the same time he does not accuse God of being responsible for any mishap in his life. He is an escape artist to avoid unpleasant duties, and if his infantile mentality is nurtured and tolerated, wishful fantasies and a paradise-like existence can begin to grow luxuriantly with all the dangers of making him stuck on the future individuation road, rather than strengthening his ego. How can we help to strengthen the ego of our children when they are somewhat apprehensive in new situations (like going to school, or a medical consult)?

Strengthening of the Ego

I remember a mother dressing her child in a fire chief costume or a cowboy uniform, guns included. If needed, she could say to him, "Well, you are the fire chief and fire chiefs don't cry when they are faced with a new situation!" Such projection amounts to hero or model figures for a young child—someone he wants to become growing up. The need for a hero figure arises when the ego needs strengthening; when such a child makes this momentary transference it reinforces his ego, drawing on the inner strength that such a hero archetype presents. This is especially the case in children who are afraid of life (the carbon personalities like *Pulsatilla* and *Calc-c*) and might keep dwelling on childish fantasies even in adulthood.

For adults, another function of the unconscious and its messenger dreams is to strengthen the ego by bringing the unconscious contents into the conscious, more easily achieved by an introverted person. This can provide the psychic energy and libido needed to become more mature, transforming one into a responsible yet individual person who has no fear to commit to the challenges of life. Quite different from a young female I knew, who even when married preferred to take vacations with her mother, and after the inevitable divorce, went to live in the same house as her mother. This strong mother-tie reflected a fear of commitment to life, its responsibilities and difficulties, keeping her a lonely unrealistic youth with a desire to remain in the cocoon of the well-protected security of the mother presence, held in a strangle-hold of the mother-complex, more of a prison than any incarceration. In order to respond to the inner urge to grow up she will have to detach herself from her mother, an event that seemed more and more unlikely as time went by. Such a person is attracted to the world yet fears it. Her inner maturity does not at all match her years of age, and by the time I met her she had regressed to a *Bar-c* state, with immense fear for reality and outer life. It is here too that a careful, steady dream analysis will give her valuable insights into her vacillation and ambivalence towards life as well as her stubborn attitude to remain passive under the protection of the mother-bond. Because of the compensatory nature of dreams, she often had dreams of her mother appearing as a witch and sucking the blood out of her, which was simply the compensatory reaction exercised by her unconscious.

I remember a classmate from my youth who was always driven to extreme cleanliness, isolating himself so as not to get dirty during the little games in the school yard. Such strange content of his unconscious hinted already at his abnormal future development. His compulsive behavior, this pedantic sense of order, became so ingrained in his personality that it was like a character trait. In both big and small things, he lived his life according to a preconceived irrevocable pattern. When he was married with two small children, the obsessive-compulsive demon hit with a vengeance. He subjected his family to lunatic commands and scrupulous cleansing ceremonies; it took him three hours just to hang up the coats of his little girls, a result of the ever-present penchant for circumstantial ruminative thinking. He would put every object in the same place exactly and cleaned the interior of his car for hours, until deep into the night, as he could not disregard the superficial aspects of his actions—unable to focus on what was rationally important. Obviously, he created a hellish existence for the entire family, driven by his syphilitic miasm (*washing the hands, always; Del, he contaminates everything he touches; Del, he is engaged in some occupations*)—his search for total control being nothing but fear of losing control, coupled with *irresolution*, *suspicion*, and *doubt*. This "perfect" father was in fact a demon for the poor underlings, and only the simillimum (*Arsenicum*, and *Syphilinum* come to mind) could erase the evil that dominated in the background. Not surprisingly, dreams in which he killed his children (which upset him greatly) were the reason he sought help, as he considered his cleanliness a virtue to be taught to his children. What about the ego growth in children with autism, each of them presenting so differently in the practice?

Lack of Ego Growth in the Autistic Child

For the autistic child, saddled with a lack of communication which makes true conversation impossible, along with inconstant perceptual input (either too much or too little), the quantity of stimuli coming to the ego is decreased, resulting in frustration, misunderstandings, and anger as the ego is banished to the background. The special limited world of a child with autism, linked to a restricted ego, does not tolerate elements once experienced (words, places, etc.) in a certain sequence or setting in any other way, hence the obsessive repetitiousness and the phenomenal rote memory in which even nonsense can be recalled.

When life comes up against an obstacle—and obstacles are numerous for the autistic child from young age on, and no adaptation of the primitive ego can take place because of lack of exposure to exterior stimuli—then the only recourse for an overwrought nervous system is introversion and escape in the unconscious (*exaltation of fancies; abstraction of mind*). There is no surge towards the new, only a pull back towards the safety of the old—the safety of the womb—a paradise of intimate contact with the nourishing source of love. Instead of a growing of the conscious under the ego in a teaching and learning position, the unconscious of such a child is growing increasingly parallel to the increased desire to escape the adult's world. So instead of working towards reality—to connect to the human world—there is an increased fantasy activity in the unconscious, which aims at removing the obstacle or at least removing it in fantasy (*Delusions of fancy illusions; absorbed in fancies*). There is no collapse of the conscious attitude as its formation never got off the ground! The original inborn psychic layers remain an autonomous functional system, as these layers remain close to the collective unconsciousness, universal to mankind while less individualized.

When the child is overwhelmed with what is presented in school, because of an immature ego and non-understanding, one possibility available is to escape to the dream world that was created in his mind through games, TV, films, and books. This action provides temporary safety, free from any intrusion as he reigns over his desired world. The child checks out or blurts sentences out that have nothing to do with the real situation at hand, startling the teacher and peers alike. Because his conscious world is minimal, this is a normal flight reaction to keep his fragile and undeveloped ego intact. Yet the outer world remains a place where danger and unhappiness lurk.

I want to paint a picture of what happens to the child in the ASD world according to Jung's teachings if the situation is not successfully addressed as time goes on. When the unconscious forces remain the ruling ones, there is a danger that the growing contents of the unconscious will burst like a tsunami into the conscious and overpower that primitive weak ego, leading to a psychosis or infantile schizophrenia. Such a transition depends strongly on the hereditary soil and the kind of trigger present in the individual child. Another possibility is that the child with autism accepts this world of vast unconsciousness as the real and safe thing, which a child with ASD might outwardly demonstrate through display of obsession with strange, stereotyped behaviors: lining up cars, flapping, and even verbalizing eccentric ideas, all which seem real to him, despite that these displays—examples of what Jung called fixed ideas—gradually cut him off from contact with others. This is often seen in the social isolation of many children with autism, including the high-functioning ones.

Much misunderstanding of the autistic child arises from people's expectations that a person with autism looks at things the same way we do. When the child throws an object at someone, it might not be reflecting misbehavior but an attempt at communicating, as throwing this object is the only way to draw attention to himself. He wants to be "involved" in a strange world where everyone seems to speak a foreign language. If such behavior is punished or ignored, it will only lead to further withdrawal from the adult world. Physical restraints are, sadly, used more on these children than we might realize. When the child with autism interrupts his mother on the phone by hitting her, it might reflect his intense neediness for attention and deep sense of insecurity and inferiority complex. Even when the child pushes another child and takes his toys, it can very well be to get a reaction from the other child, so they can "play" together. For the autistic child, any connection is better than no connection at all. It is a tough world for the autistic child when he cannot read social cues. He can interrupt you when you are busy doing something as he does not recognize a natural pause where he can ask for your attention. This leads to a series of rejections, painfully felt by the child, an enormous hurdle that even for the strongest normal individual would be hard to bear! Besides the homeopathic simillimum, extra patience and love is needed for these children. If your child is 8 years old but has the mental age of a 2-year-old, don't expect him or her to function as an 8-year-old and punish or isolate him with silence when he can't perform what you ask from him, which will no doubt reinforce the sense of rejection and isolation in this child.

Initially, even the child with non-conversational language tries to connect to others, but constant rejection by other children and non-understanding by adults pushes the child away from consciousness, at first to float in a position between conscious and unconscious, a dark borderland, and then with full force into the unconscious to "fix the obstacle." But pushing the content of an undesirable situation to the unconscious is not equal to disappearance of the painful or suffocating event. It will remain in the shadow side, in its primitive state, unchanged and always ready to overwhelm the ego. The habit of failure (in contact to others, in speaking, in being understood) starts with the autistic child in early failures which were beyond his control, bringing nothing but discouragement and lack of self-confidence and utter isolation. Disbelief and embitterment can follow, as the child sees himself as a victim of circumstance. Failure after failure leads to nervous tension and anticipation anxiety, and this in turn leads to more failure. After all, the human psyche is not a rigid and fixed system but a fluid stream of events which change kaleidoscopically, influencing the psyche at every turn. It is the unconscious of such a child that spins the fancy illusions his dream world produces, eventually imprisoning him in a cocoon from which escape can become impossible. What is unconscious remains unchanged, and a child with autism has increased difficulty in raising these unconscious contents to consciousness. Nothing is more obstructive to normal development than persistence and being frozen in a psychologically embryonic state.

The child with autism, in contrast to the developmental state of a normal child, is at this point unable—trapped and prevented by the state he is in—to exercise the extension of his consciousness or awareness, an exercise important to grow his ego, the root of consciousness. He is captured, arrested in a state of a dream world, continuously in search of Self. The autistic child has consciously or unconsciously put all his qualities in the unconscious which is like the vault of a great bank. The trouble is, he cannot withdraw the contents on demand, as he must wait until a guard appears at the door to open it (only the right therapeutic intervention has the key). And it is the guard who decides how much can be withdrawn. Consciousness and unconsciousness are a pair of opposites that need to be in balance and operate in a compensatory fashion for normal functioning of the individual. A child needs a continuous consciousness to learn how to interact with the outside world, hence for an autistic child any psychological relationship to others becomes hard if not impossible. This child cannot distinguish himself from others and has an incomplete understanding of himself and others. As he becomes isolated from his weak primitive ego he feels, and acts, disconnected from anything which might possibly have meaning and importance. I want to bring to the attention of the reader that I believe that the ASD child *has* capacity for emotions and that his actions and reactions are often created by how he feels—frustrated, forsaken, misunderstood, or rejected, whether real or perceived.

In fact, it is the subconscious that dominates our world, and only by understanding the unconscious—impossible for such a child—can we free ourselves from the conscious. Freeing ourselves from preoccupation with things in consciousness (stagnated on thoughts or actions) is a desirable goal for any adult, but not for a child with autism who has been detached from consciousness of the world, often from the beginning of his life. As a result, the child with autism, until he is freed from this state by a therapeutic approach that embodies mind and body, does not grasp the feelings of others, and even if he can speak, blurts things out that are offensive to his closest family members, sometimes without apparent remorse. Yet such a child yearns to relate to others with warmth and pleasure and communicate purposely and meaningfully.

This expansion of unconsciousness and stagnation of consciousness are not normal in children, who usually have an ever growing and continuous build-up of the ego, master of the conscious world. Normal children have few delusions, used as compensations and defense mechanisms, as the birth of these fixed ideas runs parallel with the size of the unconscious, but the autistic child is forced to live in a world of *delusions of fancy illusions* as a result of lack of communication and understanding. The consciousness cannot be recognized as a co-determining factor along with the vastly created unconscious of such a child in his growing process or individuation. For the ASD child, conscious and unconscious have become a pair of conflicting opposites! A dream example expressing the isolation of a 12-year-old child with autism is as follows.

Dream

I see my friends through a mirror, but they cannot see me. Afterwards I want to join them in a swimming pool, but they reject me.

Analysis

The dream is self-explanatory, as he looks through the mirror but his friends (alter ego) on the other side (the unconscious) cannot see him. And when he wanted to join them in the swimming pool (the personal unconscious) he was rejected. The two worlds, conscious and unconscious—which should already have come together—are still completely separated in his life.

Imprisoned in the Unconscious

The autistic child in this solitary world often struggles with becoming conscious, not recognizing someone (like family members) or something. He might just walk by his brother without acknowledging him, as if his sibling is just another shadowy figure of that other world. He seems to have no interest to invest in the world outside himself. He seems so withdrawn that sometimes even his parents think he is mentally challenged or at least deaf or hard of hearing, which is almost never the case. When parents call his name, he continues on as if he has earphones on to block out all communication. You wave at him, you hold him, you tell him to look in your eyes, and you are lucky to get a fleeting moment of focus or recognition. It is the *absence of presence.* There is no boundary between fantasy and reality. It can all become one, indistinguishable to his mind. A normal child knows the difference between the real world and dream world. Such a child easily says, "I had a bad dream," and knows that it is part of a different world—a dream theme most likely created by an event in his life (parallel dream) and more rarely by compensation towards a one-sided strong conscious state such as fear or a feeling of abandonment. This is different from the creation of a dream world for the child with autism: the creation of a fantasy world is almost imposed on this child if he wants to find some peace and connection to imaginary friends, things that are often sorely lacking in his conscious world.

However, once effective treatment has broken the chains in which the child is imprisoned, we often find that he understands our world to a much higher degree than we initially realized. Reading the cases in the book, *Autism and the Myth of the Person Alone* (Biklen et al., 2005), it is striking to discover how, when these children became adults and could finally communicate, often through computer and after working with devoted parents and therapists, they recalled the anger they had at being forced to do simple things which they had mastered years before. They were treated as an infantile idiot and had to repeat tasks which were infuriating and insulting to them, while no one could see the bars of their prison or hand them the key to open the door. Mind you, these cases were described as success stories, but I do not consider them cured in the real sense of the word. Gaps in socializing remained, but there was enough functioning to relate their levels of understanding and frustration.

The autistic child cannot pick up cues of expressed emotions, usually a function of the right brain hemisphere, cutting him off from social life. This is a lonely child in a cold and unfriendly world. Because it is a struggle for both parents and medical practitioners to understand what it takes to develop consciousness and the role consciousness has in the present ASD disorder, a clear diagnosis becomes rather vague because of crossover observable phenomena among disease names. I have seen many parents struggle with the diagnosis, raising to me on countless occasions the possibility of the child being wrongly diagnosed; could their child have brain damage, mental retardation, and or even be psychotic. My answer was always: you have a child with a special need, a need unique to your child, and once we understand through thorough investigation, taking in account the peculiar mental, emotional, and physical make up of your child, as well as the hereditary background and the pregnancy story, I will be able not only to understand what your child is thinking but supply him with the right tools (foremost the homeopathic remedy, the individualized diet, and guidelines for parents) to start the journey towards cure. Only in this way can we build up the child's ego and with that, the different personas man needs to move adequately through life.

What is this persona needed for humans to sail smoothly through life? And why is a specific persona formed, and what determines this, when so many people have either an inflated or an intimidated ego?

7

PERSONA: THE MASKED INDIVIDUAL

"Living unconsciously, you remain forever the same."
—Jung

Deceit and Value of Persona: A Dual Role

It is a fact that our face conveys "who" we are by telegraphing a kaleidoscope of emotions. The face is also a doorway to the sensory world, allowing us to see, smell, taste, hear, and feel the breeze. And are our eyes not the portal to our soul? But are we really our faces? Does a persona flaunt the way it "falsifies" life? Can the surface of anyone ever harmonize with what's inside his mind? Or are we always somewhat strapped in the life of a stranger? As if we were not complicated enough, we feel the need to create a vast world of Shakespearean drama to navigate through life's challenges: a persona, which can create a person who has erected a make-believe reality, one in which his significance is undisputed. The most we can hope for, it seems, is that both sides, the surface and inner Self, approximate somewhat a healthy (albeit a frail) equilibrium, while often struggling with high expectations for social conformity and molding ourselves to be the ideal person for our surroundings. Persona is a commanding collective trait that out of necessity creates masks, as we are by our very nature social actors—resembling what actors wear in Chinese opera. These masks express different emotions, and the role within the play, casting a cloak between our ego and the outside world. The persona represents armor against the stimuli and situations of the outer world and our repressed inner drives hidden in the shadow (see Chap. 10).

We introduce in our life masks and dances, purely for the pleasure we give to the eye of the beholder. Persona is an urge to self-display—mostly as we *want* to be perceived. It indicates a deformed Self, unseen by others and us; it does not bend back to the true Self (introspection.) Nevertheless, it is acknowledged and seen by others, as actors are in a Greek drama, integrating with others to mingle in the finite play of life. The creation of this persona is an attempt to fit in, in whatever profession and activity we choose, to find an adequate place and home in this world. Usually what appears turns out to be a mere semblance of our true Self, an error of perception of ourselves, mostly deliberate, and for some a Fata Morgana[1] that unfortunately does not resolve of its own accord but can only be resolved through courageous introspection. A correct estimate of our Self should be a prerequisite to guide our life, but typically we are glued to a desired persona, and thus are inclined to overrate our capacities and expectations.

We portray a predominance of outward appearances, not the "inner Self," forgetting that our inner life is more relevant to who we are than what appears on the outside in an illusion fabricated by the ego, master of consciousness. Except, we cannot avoid the expressions of our inner life due to its numinous strength. Emotions such as anger, joy, envy, disappointment, and hatred all manifest themselves unadulterated on the persona—by facial expressions, gestures of body parts, by the fire in our eyes, by "being besides ourselves"—so that thought and speech anticipate each other. This persona seems to be at the complete mercy of our inner life process in the most inopportune and surprising ways. Our emotions and feelings are even linked to physical expressions (*anxiety felt in the abdomen, anxiety in the stomach*), and our heart aches when struck by grief, all expressions of individual psychology. Maybe we should adhere to the TCM principle of Tao—not to get overexcited or too sad—so our emotions remain glorious, inside, and do not come forth.

Initially, this persona creation seems for most to be so accurate that no one can have any doubt about its realistic character and design. We know how important it is to present such a persona to produce certain dramatic, convincing, and useful effects. A persona can hide torments as well as joys from our face (as in the proverbial "poker face"). The picture projected is an *assumed* pose, not innate. The mask and appearance do not reflect our real essence. Persona can look like a new skin, belonging to the surface, but like every skin, it betrays something but *conceals* more, reflecting the saying, "skin-deep." But no one can hide for long behind a mask, as the pretense soon lapses into true character. Only when one's basis is truth, where the roots are solidly planted, will time foster real growth in size and quality of its owner, rather than following the tailor's philosophy that the clothes make the man.

As for the uses of personas, makers of disguise, instances are almost numberless. We enter the world prepared to perform roles and manage the impression of others, with the ultimate evolutionary aim of getting along, fitting in, and getting ahead in the social groups that define who we are. The persona can also serve as a mask for the pseudo character of our feelings and despair; putting our mask on, we can look like a buoyant, joyful person, but the moment we find ourselves alone, sadness and desperation may appear on our face, as we cannot further conceal our true inner state. We can heap layers of earth upon our heart, carefully hiding it from public view, protected by a mask of mirth brandished with the deflected wit of a mourning clown. And yet, the paradox of pain and creativity permeate our life and purpose, our inner dejection deeply in variance with the "joie de vivre" of the public mask. We cannot forget that when we deny the existence of sorrow and remorse, at some point in our life we will be forced to taste each of them in return. This will happen until we are no longer afraid to possess them, to confess that we are, to quote Nietzsche, "human, all too human." May we find a point of connection in citing collective vices and virtues, as a reminder that none of us is alone in this business of being human. Alas! For any human, how hard is it to forsake all masks and reveal the naked truth of one's soul?

The persona is the appropriate and convenient face shown to others, rather than the true face man meets in the mirror. Persona is mostly a relation—demanding, often absurd and extensive—but not the true relation with ourselves. The true relation with ourselves is with that which we really are, and not with the pseudo Self we have roughly created in our own shape and desire. All masks involve inauthenticity. But often, identification with the persona becomes familiar for all to see, white and polished like a dog's bone, a "perfect" mask. "Yes," others acclaim, "that is exactly who he is!" If only humans could cast aside the multicolored veils of the shadow side with which they cover themselves. It is precisely this mask, mainly of benefit for the carrier because it allows him to go unseen, that is often not only devastating for his psyche, but results in being an obstruction for the person's environment, friends, acquaintances, strangers, and physicians to "get to know" that person, and depending on the use of this mask, moreover becomes a hindrance to becoming the individual he should become.

We guard our persona very carefully, on the look-out for a thief at our safe, while knowing very well—if we care—that it contains little of importance, as our real treasure lies elsewhere, in our unconscious, our inner life. We are afraid of knowing ourselves fully, not being optimally aware of the processes inside and outside ourselves. On the other hand, these masks are useful to hide our inner states to cope with life and people, so that labile emotional states do not hinder us from fulfilling certain necessary daily tasks. Yes, we might feel in a rotten mood one day, but that does not mean we can bring this foul mood to work where our boss expects us to perform our task.

These striking masks we wear when going out to confront the world were named *personas*, a term used by Schopenhauer[2] (known for his cynical and rather pessimistic, or realistic, view of mankind), and further elaborated on by Jung. In Schopenhauer's *Essays and Aphorisms*, he mentions the notion of persona: "Persona really means an actor's mask, and it is true that no one reveals himself as he is; we all wear a mask and play a role" (Schopenhauer, 1970). What is the use of persona and how is it formed?

It will come as a shock to most parents that they teach their children from a young age on—around 2 years of age or somewhat later—not to express themselves as freely as they would like to. When parents start suppressing the child's spontaneity and increasing search for independence, the growing child feels more and more unable to stand on his own feet. Worse, parents conceal from him and lie about conflicts going on between themselves, and yet expect these same children always to tell the truth. Maybe in a court of law we have to make an oath on the Bible, "I swear to tell the truth, the whole truth, and nothing but the truth," but this seems not to be a universal oath when it comes to conducting our life or teaching our children how to conduct theirs. A child is taught to suppress the awareness of his rebellion and to lie to others, although children (especially the intuitive *Lachesis* child) have an innate capacity for noticing concealments. Of course, the parent says, "I want to encourage my child to become a good adult," or should we say, "to reach the 'maturity' of the average adult."

I have often witnessed this in my office. "I hate you Dr. Luc," some of the children would say, when I asked them to take their clothes off for the physical exam. The mother always retorted immediately with horror to apologize for the behavior of her innocent, honest child: "Don't say such a thing! You are not being a good boy (or girl)!" I am sure the child heard such reprimands many times in his/her early life, learning from a young age that there are certain rules to be followed to conform to society, or rather, that there is reward for being "good," not necessarily *honest*. But the child still had the ability to feel or think for themselves, and it was keenly expressed in the face. Parents do not always appreciate their child's honest and direct expressions, free from concealment, and prefer that they express the opposite feeling. The child, being close to the collective unconscious, is used to viewing everything as bad or good, black or white—never grey—just as any archetype has a dual nature, a dark and a light side.

At first, left undisturbed (a rarity) such a young heart opens to life like the petals of a flower unfolding in the sunlight. The immature intellect looks incessantly for nourishment in a world supplied with the appeal of novelty. But soon under parental guidance, the garden of Eden with plenty of beautiful images to behold—the initial world of illusions—gradually fades to real life, when his will is now shaped according to the environment (and miasms!), by readjusting his expectations. Soon the child learns that by following the desired rules, such a persona built by the ego has its special purpose: by putting a mask on he can hide his true feelings and somewhat distort the true nature of his ego, so that a reward instead of punishment is expected and obtained. During each such incident, the child's persona as well as the increasing size of his shadow starts taking form, finely chiseled and sculpted step-by-step. The specific conscious persona is formed by adaptations to what is expected and, of course, to what is beneficial for the individual, although such persona formation is built up by desired characteristics of the close family, first, and then by the conformity of the masses, rather than *who the individual* really wishes to be. Parents have expectations of their children and a child learns quickly what is required, approved, and rewarded.

The recipe is often simple. The child borrows sentences from grown-ups to make fake grown-up remarks, which are always received with high praise and thus illuminate expectations. But the child is stringing these words together without understanding them. The only goal is to obtain the desired: gifts, instant admiration, delicate praises, and to be the master of any situation. The child stores the praises away in his memory, thus developing a taste for unstinted praise, always ready to show off, and at the same time developing an increased need for approbation. "He is beyond his years, he is an old soul," the excited parents claim, not knowing that they only increase the burgeoning shadow of the innocent child, changing him into a fake, a liar and pretender. Parents are so happy to claim that such a young child is gifted—a present from Providence—and there is no hesitation to pay vast sums of money to have him tested by the "experts," believing that this young person should be treated differently than the "non-gifted" collective mass (which usually possess more honesty and virtue than their child.) Rather than focusing only on their child's achievements, parents would do well to nurture kindness, empathy, and generosity in their offspring, as these will nourish supportive relationships and carry over to adulthood. But often for parents, their child's accolades are considered a personal badge of honor, and teaching kindness is the first casualty in this increasingly fierce, competitive world. All too many foster the illusion of having a child that will make a mark in this world. And as that child grows, he adjusts to the expectations—

to be the next genius—and keeps recreating himself, with a shadow that overcomes the real Self.

What is so inhumane and terrifying is that all the "goodness," the make-believe, can turn into the darkness of hell later in life, when the young shadow side needs to find an outlet because it's become too strong to remain caged. Such sudden change of behavior elicits the cry, "What happened to my child? He (or she) is not the person I knew!" Of course, no one knew him really. When younger, he was the cornucopia of generosity and virtue in his family. However, few such children can resist revolting against the settler of their soul when grown up, against the succession of childhood ceremonies. It is inevitable. All those pious lies to make the parents happy! Of course, most would call the child loved, and lucky, but really, he is bored like a dog that does not get his daily walk. He is expected to be the subject of the family play-acting, making a false entrance in life. Growing up in such a sham paradise, the child is unable to use his real voice, waking up every day in a daze and realizing that such forced behavior—at least for the time—must be the path to eternal joy and fulfilling quests. But after he is grown, others don't seem to be so admiring and accepting as his doting parents. What a shock! How unexpected!

The child's natural inclinations were thwarted to immediately acquire, or at least as soon as society expects it, habits and opinions that fully obscured signs of his natural inclinations. That child became a disguised person in the name of conformity. I wonder how many children are deviated this way from their real purpose in life. As a consequence, the imposition put on children to function in a non-dominant conscious function (see Chap. 8), abdicating their birthright, has wasted many lives, when as adults they question whether their chosen path was actually one that followed reason rather than the heart. To their chagrin they find out that book-learning about a subject they do not really care about, but only supported the goal to make money and obtain external advantages, did not enrich them inwardly as a person. Their path to adulthood was paved with the stones of a *well-filled* brain, not a *well-formed* brain with a sense of worldly responsibility, critical thinking, and human character. Modern teaching often produces people resembling donkeys laden with books. Alternative schools like Waldorf do not make the child's mind work like a porter, slaving over long hours of homework, with topics he can and should forget the next day—topics which do not teach how to live life but waste brain energy—like continually eating indigestible foods, bringing not only discomfort but bloating. Standard education obscures the mind with frivolous and forgettable topics.

Ideally in schools there should be more conversation taking place, following the definition of education, where not just the teacher does all the talking, expecting to be repeated like a parrot, but the student should be encouraged to speak also, and should be listened to. He should be invited to give his opinion about a selected topic, as this will stimulate self-confidence and provide the armor and weaponry to go through the ups and downs in life. As Socrates said, "For those who want to learn, the obstacle can often be the authority of those who teach." Often when I lectured, during a "question and answer" interval, I answered a student's question with another question: "Does anyone know the answer to this question?" This was not done to expose the student's lack of insight—although some took it wrongly that way—but to stimulate other students' thought processes, as the answer will be better remembered than if I immediately gave the right answer. This course of action also guided me as a teacher to what I needed to explain more and what path needed to be followed to adapt myself to the ability of my audience. As a side note, speech therapy as it is done in the unfortunate ASD epidemic mainly consists in "repeating words," without finding out if the child has really grasped the meaning of them and made them part of himself. Book-learning is only an ornament, while forming an opinion about the subject is the foundation for further steps in life, an exercise in thinking, judging, and speaking in one's own voice.[3]

For any child, the mask identified with the ego ideal and its opposite, the accompanying shadow, the secondary personality, is built up as life goes on. Some can cultivate a careful persona from youth on, creating masks who amuse and delight their friends and infuriate their enemies and those less gifted. The question remains: Does such a carefully crafted mask reveal the truth about that person more than conceal it, or vice versa? All depends on how well we can see through the masquerade and how much we like it. Many people cannot see the truth beyond the facts; this is especially so if the mask has replaced the person and he is no longer in control.

The fight between the mask and the shadow can lead to painful situations in a young child. In my practice, I treated a 6-year-old child whose father was an abusing alcoholic who punished her cruelly for even quite innocent behavior. A natural reaction would be justified rage against this cruelty, but of course she was afraid to show rage towards her father. Crying too was forbidden, as "big girls don't cry." As a result, the child developed an *Anacardium* state, a split into two diametrically opposite character structures, with *Anacardium's* typical delusions: *Delusion, strange figures accompany him, one on his right the other on his left; Del, devil speaks in one ear, an angel in the other, prompting murder or acts of benevolence.* This continuous back and forth between devil and angel can become the end of the story when the person dissociates. Such character traits are mutually exclusive and incompatible, and the result is that this young patient kept one or the other of the contradictory structures continually in a state of repression while the other one ruled. Consequently, she feared the father while thinking of killing her mother, the good person in the family. Privately, when I asked this young person why she behaved this way, she answered, "*Someone* makes me do it," which represented the delusions of *Anacardium*, the remedy that saved this sweet girl.

The carbon family is the easiest in following these rules of conformity and morality, while types like *Sulphur* and *Phosphorus*, with their early streak of independence, show more resistance to molding expected social masks and are often called rebels, eccentrics, and dreamers. Especially *Sulphur's* motive to be unique trumps his motive to belong. While most people are groomed from early childhood on to conform to social norms, *Sulphur* belongs to a select few that seem uniquely resistant. The norm and wisdom of the crowd repels him like a charged magnet. Obviously the more extensively the mask is formed—whatever does not fit in that persona, whatever the child *really thinks but is not socially acceptable*—has to be put somewhere else, locked up and hopefully not released unless by accident or when caught off-guard. That place is found in the other world, the unconscious, where the child learns by force, or to please others, to put everything that is "not so nice," even if it is the truth or meant at that moment, in that hidden and secret vessel, the shadow side. From then on, there is no end to the extent of the formation of an ever-increasing shadow, the dumping ground of the human world.

In the course of our individuation—of psychologically becoming an individual—the content of the ego is not just the persona, which is only part of the ego. While growing up, a differentiation must take place between the ego and persona. The ego and especially its dominant conscious function (see Chap. 8) fabricate the persona, but the latter *is not identical to the ego*. As the ego hopefully outgrows its infancy, man must acquire a sense of morality, judgment, and responsibility, which makes for the difference between remaining a child or becoming a well-functioning adult. Why and how does man use different personas?

The Need for Different Personas, Archetypes of the Psyche

As mentioned before, a persona is created to facilitate negotiation between our ego and society, with the special accent on its formation by the ego as it is molded towards the expectation of society that an individual may have. It is also the part used by man to achieve goals, expectations, wishes, and ambitions. It is the part of ourselves that is shown towards others, just like the "clothes (that) make the man" and hide what is underneath—hide the naked body that must remain private, visible at best only to those closest to us. Just as everyone has a skin, everyone has a persona, which has a dual purpose: "How do I impress people to my advantage?" and secondly, "How do I hide who I really am?" What goes on behind the mask is then called, according to Carl Jung, "life behind closed doors" (Jung, 1966, para. 305). Indeed, man needs to be able to turn the mirror inward, to look past his persona, to perceive its dark twin, his shadow.

Just as man has more than one set of clothes, so he needs different sets of personas to play his varying roles on the world stage. A well-balanced person can change clothes to be professional, social, private, or among loved ones. In the latter circumstance he must try to wear a minimum of clothes—even be naked—as hopefully he can be closest to the true nature of himself then. Professionally, persona facilitates social interactions that require people to relate only through their roles, without personal feelings involved, as such a persona is a collective way (an archetypal pattern) of playing a role in the world by acting and behaving in the style belonging to this persona. For instance, the persona of the physician facilitates the examination of the body of the patient and the asking of private questions, while the patient contributes to the examination by adopting the persona of the patient. Socially, we must expect that we can change clothes appropriately to fit the situation. We may be a physician, but that does not mean to show up at a party in a white coat, stethoscope dangling around our neck, playing the role of a physician flawlessly in any and all circumstances.

Another example can be found in primitive cultures where the persona created by the chief (wearing the head ornament) serves to accentuate his role of leadership. The rest of the clan wants to confer this mask on the chief, as they play the role of looking up to the chief for guidance and advice. In Native American Indian culture, the chief and the medicine man stood out through their ornaments, expressive of their social role. These outward tokens differentiate the individual from other people, like a shell around him, which is another form of persona or how one must be perceived by others.

Northwest Coast Indians used animals as symbols of archetypal power and created totem poles, a sacred act that brought wholeness and balance to the tribe. The totem pole would portray animal images representing the spiritual forces that would protect the house and its inhabitants.

Even modern times have examples of leadership like those of primitive cultures. Ataturk, called the father of Turkey, and the Shah of Iran, King of Kings, for example. As we can see, such personas are built mainly by the ego, and therefore contain elements of the collective psyche. Thus, it cannot be said that persona is totally individual—as seen before in the example of the physician and the chief—as persona represents a role in society which refers also to the collective psyche. From human existence on, there was always a need for leaders and followers, each playing their role. We receive a title and exercise the function attributed to that title, something that can go back centuries. So, this persona is not as purely individual as it looks.

What makes the persona "individual" is the way one's dominant conscious function is determined or formed. It is here that the dominant hereditary family and personal state—the *predom-*

inate miasm, *constitution*, and *temperament*—will play an important role. A *Phosphorus* with her carefree attitude, her penchant for colorful designer clothes, hats and outrageous hairstyles, plus blessed with an animated and friendly loquacity, stands out from a *Pulsatilla* person, who is childish, eternally demanding attention, dressed instead with clothes decorated with childish motifs like angels and butterflies. Every homeopath knows *Lycopodium*, and *Silicea*, as "the angel at school and devil at home." *Platina* stands out with a huge and haughty persona. She feels it pointless to try to make others understand her motivations. *Platina* does what she thinks is best, without bothering to explain and see if others follow or agree. Hers is an imperious approach that belies the value of different opinions and the importance of forming connections with people. Her body is cold as ice and her heart has "ceased to beat" although there are no other signs of death. Proud of her beauty, and perhaps of her vices, *Platina* reigns, the queen of haughtiness, a mixture of sexuality and spirituality, two strange bedfellows. But then again, *Platina* has the *Delusion, she does not belong to this world. Platina's* inflation is nothing but an escape mechanism for the feeling of insignificance, so the world outside becomes small in comparison (*Delusion, things appear smaller; she is very tall; everything in the room is diminished, while she is tall and elevated; Delusion, inferior, people seem mentally and physically, on entering the house after a walk*). In other words, she is an atheist in the temple of true love, and it is very hard for anyone's heart to beat in unison with such a creature.

I will refer to two more characters, but the homeopath can see that each personality or portrait of a remedy (as described in my book *Discovering Life: Homeopathic Portraits*) can present its own persona as part of its dress in life. Look again at the *Pulsatilla* person. One of her characteristics is eagerness, waking up every morning with a commanding willingness to please and be loved, consuming her all day long (*fear of being neglected;*

craving for affection; submissive and yielding disposition; wants to kiss everybody). Even when this perishes at night, she is on fire the next day with renewed interest in finding the object and subject of her desire, even before she gets her clothes on. This goes on for 365 days a year, creating a life full of tears and joy, mottled from sunrise to midnight with alternating brilliant sunshine and black clouds (*mood changeable*).

Palladium on the other hand is a person whose existence depends upon intense lust for approval (*longing for approval*). This person is so eager to be approved by anybody and everybody, without discrimination, that she is commonly ready to forsake her opinions and convictions at a moment's notice in order to get the approval of any person who did not pay attention to her. Having too much deference for the opinion of others, *Palladium* gives up her own better judgment, establishing a weak ego. You can break her heart and spirit with a single word, but you can raise them up again to the sky with another one. Even a disapproving look from a dog would crush her heart. Just like *Lycopodium* who *desires to be flattered, Palladium* should understand that what one is in the opinion of others is generally much overrated, either from lack of insight or their interest in obtaining favors. But just as a cat purrs when it is stroked, few can avoid showing delight in their face when praised with sweet, palpable lies.

The predominant miasmatic state is of course also part of the persona, as mentioned. The syphilitic person will use persona to hide his real motives from people, which are always selfish and destructive. The sycotic person—who has the carpe diem attitude—will have offensive (at least to mainstream people) clothes, rings through the navel, lips and tongue, as his sole goal is to surprise and shock others at first impression. The psoric person is the follower, he who wants to belong, who follows the dress code in vogue, not standing out in a crowd—not through his clothes, vivacity, or nimbleness of his feet, as he is the rock planted on earth with an aversion to move. But he is always ready to be part of a joyous feast or banquet!

Every person also has a penchant to be one of the four Hippocratic temperaments. These temperaments are sanguine (enthusiastic and social—*Phosphorus*); melancholic (introverted, moody, quiet—*Nat-m*); phlegmatic (relaxed, peaceful, childish —*Calc-c, Puls*); or choleric (short-fused, fast, irritable —*Sulphur*), although most have shades of several temperaments. All this will color man's persona and often give a definite form to it, which can also hinder his maneuvering through society.

Persona does not only refer to the clothes literally but also to the *demeanor* and *speech* of a person. Many people, out of lack of self-confidence and self-worth, feel they must dominate the conversation by talking about their profession, constantly boring people around them. I have witnessed a physician who would show up at social tennis matches with his beeper stuck on his tennis shorts, to show how important he was. But I knew him personally, and he was not the kind of physician that ever had any emergency calls, so it was only for show and to boost his inadequate ego. He had to drag his privy position into every situation, his soul and speech inflated to the height of his "royal" seat.

Some personas are obsessively cultivated and finely tuned to a T. I had a patient who, although coming from an ordinary middle-class family, thought Providence had failed to bequeath to him the role of aristocrat. Adopting a fitting, exterior manner of living, he appreciated elegant gestures, social graces, frivolities, parties, and living like a dandy, being able to charm the pants off anyone with his refined talk. Upon second sight, he lacked the more serious virtues of the bourgeoisie (virtues he never even considered). Life to him was a theater, a play-acting ground, in which he always had the lead role, convinced that he was born to be an outstanding person, which comes automatically with all the virtues belonging to it: intelligence, wit, eloquence, and a hefty dose of self-confidence and ambition. Of course, this was only real in the life of fancies he inhabited, and he was often disappointed when no one recognized his obvious virtuosity. It did not help that he had a common name, nothing preceded with Sir, Baron, Duc, Compte, or at least a "de" preceding his family name. Indeed, he was no descendant of Michel de Montaigne (1533-1592) or Duc de La Rochefoucauld (1613-1680), two great philosophers. He should have recognized that ambition is very common and genius rare!

Since he did not have the means to live like an aristocrat and spent most of his money keeping up his excessive persona, his family lived in need of the most essential things. That did not deter him, as he clearly thought he was special, always scheming to obtain the pot of gold that seemed near. To tell you the truth, he should have become and remained a starving actor, without a dependent family. That way he could have ceased to be himself and transformed to any kind of impersonation offered him on a platter by the stage director.

Persona is sometimes a collective image. I think about Italian men in general. They are the most foppish representatives of their sex on the planet. They smear on substantial quantities of hair products and expend considerable mental energies on color-coordinated socks and belts, while zooming around the city on their Vespa or in their Fiat, with eyes wide open and passionate cries for any beauty that crosses their path. On the other side, a perceived and real collective image of women are Parisian women. Everything about them—their poise, their refinement, their cool dispatch, looking almost untouchable, their trim, tidy figures, their chic appearance, their purposeful glances, their hair, their scent—exemplify an ethos of personal expression, as they are the caretakers of a sensuous intelligence. And on the other hand, in forming the persona of the Arab desert tribes, they (the Bedouins) pride themselves on four things: their poetry, their eloquence, their horsemanship and finally, their hospitality!

The persona is easily recognized in the way we dress or use hair styles to show that we belong to a certain group of people, or sometimes just the opposite, that we want to remain an individual. An example is the contrary dresser *Sulphur*, who does anything but follow the latest mode. He often looks like a relic of the feudal age. Someone who stands out, he dresses with whatever he gathered at will at the neighborhood thrift store, and to his amazement, that piece of clothing can sometimes become the "in fashion" for everyone else! Of course, since a woman is able to change her desirable appearance easier than men, the persona for her can be a change in hair, or wearing an outrageous hat, or painting the entire surface of her lips—her mouth ending up like two big slices of tuna—expressing her passion and beauty. Men match their persona more often with their profession: he is the Judge, the Pilot, the General, the Physician, and so on.

Should we always look at how people present themselves as their true personification?

Never Judge a Book by Its Cover

As much as personas are used to guide us through life, they are also unfortunately used to deceive other people. After all, persona is only the outer layer of the personality, what is clearly visible and desired to be apparent, as it will and can be used for misrepresentations, lies, and as a disguise to fool people and take advantage of them, or worse, represent something they are not at all professionally. The many Reality TV programs like *Who the (Bleep) Did I Marry?*, *Women with Knives*, *Dates from Hell*, and *The Neighbors Next Door*, attest to the great extent to which humans have become experts at putting on misleading clothes, contrasting a dazzling seductive persona with a dark private life. A perfect example was the mass murderer Ted Bundy who had a persona of being intelligent, self-assured, cocky, and witty, but he murdered 35 women! He looked like a normal human being, the kind you meet everywhere who defends his point of view, and thanks to a dominant thinking conscious function, subsumed the incomprehensible so that every crime he committed became normalized. Sometimes, it seems as if the two entities, the unimaginable crimes and the man who committed them, were irreconcilable. He was ten percent cloak, and ninety percent dagger! Psychiatry would possibly say he was suffering from a "dissociative personality disorder" and a "narcissistic trait," a person filled to the brim with himself. How to recognize such a person?

Unfortunately, people bearing the stigma of the syphilitic miasm are prone to using deceptive personas to maximum benefit. Alas, the miasmatic theory is not taught in medical school, and therefore such a person is rarely shielded early in life from such a destructive path. The syphilitic miasm was clearly visible in Ted Bundy. As is often the case, his life was "a coincidence of unfortunate circumstances," and what he did was such an anomaly that it makes little sense to guard ourselves against it. He never knew his father (he was an illegitimate child), members on his mother's side were depressed and had violent characters, and his own mother told him she was his older sister and his grandparents were his parents. Later, upon finding the truth, he was very angry and reacted according to the syphilitic dominant miasm from his mother's side: he even had sex with dead people (necrophilia) and always murdered girls that resembled his first girlfriend who rejected him. Enough predisposition towards and triggers on the dangerous syphilitic terrain created that monster!

Another common example of persona deception are the preachers of God who are wolves in sheep's clothing, preaching by day and visiting prostitutes by night. *Lachesis* people with their *loquacity, intellect,* and *religious fanaticism* come to mind. It is a strain for them to hold their tongue, when they are full of desire to talk. Their pious attitude is nothing but a compensation for their hidden moral inferiority, as their animal instincts subject them to the worst temptations. These deep dark instincts are like wild storms of madness, desire, and passion, which erupt in them despite themselves.

How can dreams tell us something about the state of a human's persona?

Persona Representation in Dreams

The symbols of persona in dreams can take on many different forms: images of clothes, hats, dresses, uniforms, veils, armor, shields, and masks. An individual's choice of attire is an effective way to show rejection of society as a group, and clothing is often an incredibly accurate indicator of what a person thinks of himself and his life. It is a way of making a statement. The persona can also be expressed in awards, diplomas, or the characteristics of a profession or trade as well as a variety of status symbols (stethoscope, wig, etc.) or specific tools, equipment of various sorts and specific books, while other signs of recognition of the persona are in reference to performances on the stage or manners with which people behave (like the stiff upper class Britons). A common way of presenting our persona in life is identifying with our profession, titles, and business. This will also be reflected in our dreams in which we keep a commanding role, meet famous people, or appear as the wise old man. For Schopenhauer, persona is "that which somebody represents in contradiction to what he actually is."

The *state of the skin* is also a form of persona that will appear in dreams (healthy skin vs. unhealthy). For instance, when the skin in dreams shows spots, blemishes, pockmarks, bruises, moles, or looks unhealthy, this reflects a sense of not being as good, acceptable, and attractive as other people; a feeling that other people see us as unattractive or see defects in us. Another symbolic explanation for such defective skin is shyness or difficulties about being in the company of others. If we are shedding our skin in dreams, then we are in the process of changing old ways or attitudes. When we appear in our pajamas, it means we have *no persona* since we are in the garment suited to the unconscious!

To be naked in a public gathering or inadequately or inappropriately dressed (like wearing a suit on the beach) is a commonplace motif in dreams, and it shows the state of the persona or the desired projection of the dreamer. Sometimes a dream will reveal the real nature of the persona—through an actual image which may caricature it—as the world sees it, as in the next dream. We do not have to analyze every element to catch the meaning of this dream.

Dream from a man

I am naked from the navel down, but the upper part of my body is dressed in wonderful, colorful clothes.

Analysis

What does this dream tell us, and what is exposed here? It reflects his excessive persona: his upper part, wonderfully dressed, getting the attention. This is how he wants to appear in public—important and pompous, drawing praise from everyone. This overelaboration of clothes means pretension, or a weakness for worldly display. Flashy clothes may represent the knowledge of the dreamer that he is deceiving others in some way, establishing a persona at odds with reality. The lower part of the body however is naked. It is unmasked, exposing him as he is, "the Emperor without clothes," the naked truth. The lower part of the body stands for the sexual, instinctive, and primitive part of the dreamer, the unconscious. He can't hide his hyper-sexuality and hidden desires. Who are some of these types? *Fluoric-ac*, *Medorrhinum*, and *Lyc.*

Sometimes being nude in a dream reflects a state of being at ease with yourself and not feeling a need to apologize for being the person you are (this often relates to a person *completely* nude). The common dream of being naked or improperly dressed at a public occasion, as happens in this case, is often related to the fear of "exposure"—the fear of self-revelation as the mask of the persona is lifted. It is the fear of other people seeing us as we really are. It may therefore be accompanied by an anxious feeling of being exposed or vulnerability.

Although we should be urged to look beyond appearances, so as not to become prisoners of our unconscious, is there a need to adapt in life to different personas?

Switching to Different Personas

We always have to put a mask (clothes) on to meet the outer demand of the world we live in—to establish our identity at that moment, as this persona is the mediator between the ego and the outer world where anima/animus will serve as the liaison between our ego and our inner world (see Chap. 11-12). Depending on the roles that we must call upon, appropriate garments are necessary to suit different occasions. "How do I look? Do I look OK for this occasion?" We should wear an adequate mask or clothing to fit the role we are playing, pending we do not believe the mask needs to stay on for the rest of our life. For instance, when I play tennis, I put tennis clothes on, but I do not think I am a world-famous tennis player, and I take these clothes off when the match is over. Different constitutions, temperaments, and attitude types will have different adaptations to a persona. A *Sulphur* type has no need for more than a couple of clothes, as what he has to say is more important than impressing others with fancy clothes. Of course, his witty and commanding speech is part of his persona. A *Phosphorus* person selects and packs carefully different styles of clothes that she thinks she needs for every possible occasion: traveling in a jeep through the desert, the welcoming dinner at the beginning of the trip, the stroll through the souk to have tea with merchants, one dress for the farewell dinner, and then another set of clothes for "unexpected" moments. This is a natural gesture, belonging to her constitution. She is the traveler arriving with two big suitcases for a five-day trip! She is also the extrovert type, for whom it becomes natural to "put other clothes on" when the occasion demands it. It is just genuine for her and a formidable tool to attract the attention of all the possible friends she will make. "Stylish" is the name of the game. Under her gentle enthusiastic exterior burn inextinguishable fires of sympathy, energy, devotion, and limitless affection. Contrary to any extrovert who on the spur of the moment dives into some other garment, the introvert (*Nat-m* for instance) is very limited in choice of clothes and feels ill at ease in meetings unless the situation corresponds to her inner feeling. As the introvert is attracted to investigating the unconscious, she will feel at ease in the Friday night group discussing "Jungian interpretation of dreams." But if she gets caught at a festive party, where the topic is sports and travel, she feels like she borrowed oversized clothes and her unease is noticed by everyone.

The bottom line: when it is appropriate at times, we should change our representational clothes into something more comfortable and should be naked at other times (letting our guard down). We must use our social and professional masks in the right circumstances, and unwrap ourselves from an inappropriate persona when necessary so as to form an adequate ego and an adequate mask, rather than going through life as so many do, "putting on airs" to hide inadequacies well-entombed in their shadow! Many fail to form an adequate persona in their life—a convenient mask, used but also discarded of appropriately—and will therefore form a pseudo ego. What different persona malformations are possible?

Malformation of the Persona and Formation of a Pseudo Ego

A. Identification with the Persona (*Ars*, *Nux-v*, *Lycopodium*, *Lachesis*, and *Mercury*)

It is appalling to see how little these personalities are alive to reality, as delusions of grandeur are common to them. These delusions dull their sense of reality, reducing their capacity for self-criticism. At the same time, they hide an Adlerian complex with feelings of inferiority, expressed by *speaking with a voice of command* and using bombastic language to bolster their inflation—especially technical language that others don't understand —so that we have the impression that "they know everything and we know nothing." Such a person does not hesitate to emphasize our "stupidity," that we cannot understand him (*Delusion, on entering the room, everything in the room is diminished while she is tall and elevated*). This is called "inflation," being infatuated and fascinated with himself, pumped up like a balloon—*Delusion, elevated in the air; Del, he is hovering in the air like a spirit; Del, he is floating in the air*—lifted up from the earth, immersed in auto-eroticism, flying in heaven while looking down benevolently upon the masses and fostering *delusions of fancy illusions*. Fantasies and delusions—the grandiose inflation of the ego—are only devices to shield humans from the other sight of themselves.

Such a human indeed only inflates himself with wind, bouncing around like a ball. While the ego is carried off its feet, he thinks he is God among people, the one chosen by the Almighty to rule, or he identifies unconsciously with the wise old man (see Chap. 12, under "The Four Faces of the Archetypal Masculine"), who will bring guidance to everyone's life, while most humans he considers part of an ignorant animal-like crowd. To be possessed by an archetype makes him stretch and grow tall—a giant among humankind! He wants to be the savior looking for the weeds in his neighbor's garden rather than taking care of his own. "Follow me," he exclaims, "I know what I am doing," convinced he is on top of the whole worldly business. All his "minor" traits are conveniently forgotten, repressed and heaped up to form layers in the unconscious, poisoning the foundation of his life, as he does not even know that, really, *he* has become a dwarf, far removed from humanity. An archetype reaches beyond the confines of humanity, so anyone possessed by an archetype develops inhuman qualities. In his case, to love and adore himself is the beginning of a lifelong romance!

His only salvation is a "depression," a *deflation*—a truth and insight, a dose of humiliation, a pricking of the balloon—to show how little substance was really carrying his life; to show him that he was always a midget. It is not willpower this person needs, but a dose of submission to the urgent voice of his unconscious. Someone should tell him to shut up for a moment and look at himself where he is incomplete; but looking quietly at oneself is a rarity among humans. The snake that cannot shed its skin perishes. It is so with a human who identifies with his persona. There is always the risk of falling from such a height when one loses a job or position (*Ailments from: loss of position; loss of honor; loss of money*), often preceded by a warning dream of falling from a height. It is better to descend from this unnatural height without falling! We should not aim in the direction of fame and fortune, but rather grow within ourselves—in health, wisdom, empathy, and true relationships to others—not in the vast number of "friends" we have on Facebook. We must break the chain of inflation through justified introspection, with an open ear to true friends' courageous interventions.

We carry darkness and heaviness, which makes us human, but identification with an archetypal image and deity—which is imitation, conscious or unconscious—separates us from humanity. We then become a person with two dimensions, carrying the mask in front of us, unaware that there is a shadow, but preferring to identify with the psychopomp. An inflated person can never accept his shadow, so a deflation will be necessary for individuation. Otherwise, inflation will expand his unconscious, even getting out of control and possibly leading, gradually, to a breaking of the ego or into dissociation, a forceful deflation that leads to a collapse of the Self, like the pricking of a balloon. Things come into him that are entirely foreign to him, a merciless wind toppling his house of cards. The inflated person is so filled with the idea of himself—so full of wind—that in his eyes he is the greatest in his profession, convinced that other people will see him the same way. He thinks that he draws crowds where he passes, and that crowds split in admiration and deserving respect.

Unfortunately, this leads often to abuse, and even crimes. I saw a story on TV about a college student who developed a vampire interest, indulging in a habit of sucking blood. He stated that he was giving power to others, which obviously was stating that he had God power. By lowering others, he elevated himself. Overwhelmed by the syphilitic miasm, he started taking drugs, slept all day long, dropped out of classes, became aggressive, and stated after committing murder that no matter what he did, he could not get caught because he was "invincible and identified with God." Knowing something about physiognomy might have exposed his cruelty. His dull fisheyes glistening with sullen fire, the tense muscles of his face, and his tight-closed lips would have disclosed that he was not so mild and loving as he wished to appear.

A patient once confessed to me that he only read sophisticated books and magazines in order to speak the same selective language. Or he would watch TV shows and movies, memorizing the lines, studying the body language and facial expressions. But this is like saying that he cannot think his own thoughts, he can only parrot others. He modulated his voice, as well as manufactured a sexy saunter, so that women went crazy over his appearance. He became *the voice and the stroll.* This person identified with his persona to the neglect of his inner life, allowing the shadow to have a life of its own, which only became visible when the mask crumbled. But this person remained autoerotic to the nth degree. By this attitude, he only expressed enormous distance from his shadow while neglecting the Self. It is impossible to form a true relationship with someone as neurotic as that, as he had assumed the identity of an archetype, something that is beyond humankind. Such an identity is carefully constructed, replete with a new body and a new psyche. As Nietzsche claimed, "If someone obstinately and for a long time wants to **appear** as somebody, it is in the end hard for him do **be** anything else" (Hollingdale, 1977, p. 149). *(Author's emphasis added.)*

Driven by a *love of power* while secretly possessing a *lack of confidence*, an inflated person plays, or is always, the judge, captain, officer, or professor rather than the individual who gives the role its proper due at the necessary times. In identifying with ideas and ambitions belonging to the profession, they are absorbed from without, spontaneously and effortlessly. Identification with their title is very attractive and seductive, bringing much benefit to its carrier. All they want is to be worshipped as a superior being (*Del, has childish fantasies; Del, of fancy illusions; Del, he is great*). They can tell you how to conduct your life, while their own existence is a balloon changing with every breeze. They are always fishing for compliments and *weep when thanked* for their calculated largesse, conducting a life that resembles only a compensatory game for their inferior feelings. Hence it is easy to be that mask all the time, hiding the emptiness beneath a shell of decorum.

Beneath a mask of golden charm lies a thick substratum of conceit; this character invites us into his world, though never too far and only on his terms. Tasting the drug of deception, knowing a little more than the person standing next to him, evokes an exquisite relish of ruthless, private power regarding his opinions—however briefly adopted—as revealed truth, never backing down, or listening, or compromising (*intolerant of contradiction*). To add to his shortcomings, he is equally swift to give and take offense (*easily offended*) and ferociously critical of everyone except himself (*censorious of others*). He has an obsession, a belief, that somewhere, just beyond reach, is an exclusive group holding real power and influence, which he constantly aspires to find and join.

Such travesty makes us think of the packages that look big and impressive, but after removing the cotton and extra padding, the content is minuscule—yet a big price is paid for it. The price is the destruction of the owner's inner life, and unfortunately, often of those in his surroundings. A persona formed by actions, clothing, words (the booming voice, harsh and arrogant, and *speaking with a voice of command*), gestures, and manners, can be praised for brilliance, but the brilliance only belongs to these additions while the subject remains unaware of his own shortcomings, hidden and covered by these externals. Of course, he does not know that he is identical to an archetype, and none but a real friend or psychoanalyst will tell him that he does not behave as a human. But the first would instantly become an enemy if they dared, and the latter is not an option for such a person. Self-admiration is his lifelong devotion, and he seizes every opportunity to advertise himself.

Boldly trumpeting his own praises, some of them will stick, especially with ignorant people.

Although not evident, life is not smooth and easy for this individual who is manacled to a profession and weighted down by some grandiloquent title and position. It requires constant effort to maintain his veneer of strength, which seems to wash off with the smallest contradiction or misfortune. A ripple in his life becomes a gale, and afterwards there remains a kind of seasickness for some time when he tries to steady his vessel. A return to his excessive persona—to the veneer covering the internal turmoil—is desired, as it is his choice and conviction as well as his comfort. Such a human is prone to look at those who fared better than him. (If he instead would look at those who are worse off, who fared worse in life, he might console himself by that multitude.) It is even more difficult for this individual if he is endowed with a tubercular disposition, a dissatisfaction with himself, driving him from one enterprise to another and from one land to another, with moody impatience and unrealized dreams and desires that often leave him stranded with excessive cravings and disappointed hopes.

I knew a person who was a maritime captain, very familiar with life on the sea (the only form of life for him) from an early age on, who even with intimate friends and family guarded this persona to the extreme. Any conversation during an informal reunion that did not involve ships, building ships, countries he visited, orders he barked, etc., would be met by his immediate side-tracking to bring the topic back to his beloved boats—boring his entourage to death. Otherwise he had nothing to say! He could blow up like a bag by a slight breath of his power of technical language, which in reality was totally insignificant, shrouding his eyes in a blinding fog and deceiving him about the value of true existence, since all it carried was a heap of self-importance. His poor friends and family ended up depleted as if he had been conversing at a higher altitude where the air was thin. Of course, to him, lack of appreciation for his one-track conversation was only because listeners were not worthy enough to be in his presence. He did not recognize that he lived a life of blind ambition through his ego inflation. What should have been a dialogue was really a monologue, talking to an invisible audience. The truth was that he was not "interested" in you, from the Latin *inter*, or "between/among," and *esse*, "to be"; to be among each other. His mask grew continually, owing to the constant, shallow interpretation of every word and every action in life he produced. No doubt, always talking about himself was his means to conceal himself.

He was always talking *at* others, rather than *with* others. Surrounded by others, he was never among others; he was only with himself, filled with himself, speaking in grandiloquent technical terminology, locked up behind the bars of a prison of narcissism. His pseudo ego was subject to constant pressure from within to uphold that image! "I am a successful person, I am the greatest captain the company ever knew, the ruler after God; I built many ships from scratch; the Government listens to me," etc., an endless build-up of an ego that, contrary to his belief, was really minimal in variety of colors and facets. This is called a professional deformation, identifying with his function. TCM could have warned him, also, that overusing his voice with such excessiveness and passion would damage his lungs (the strength of the voice reflects the Lung Qi), and in such a neurotic state as he was, it is always the main activity (voice and lungs) that is threatened. He died from lung cancer although he did not smoke. His worry about the future (also linked to the Lung element in TCM), about coming into a life of retirement and losing this carefully built important ego, no doubt contributed as well.

Sometimes I marvel at such a person who through a "splendid" persona is hermetically sealed inside his secrets. Nothing seemed to penetrate his fragile inner world; he was able to live out his delusions until his death. Unpunished? Is he a winner? Not really! Ultimately he paid the price with a life of isolation, lack of Eros, an ill-equipped feeling function, and then a real disease that finally conquered his delusions—ending an existence that was nothing but a tightly held, organized torturous course of life—always on guard for someone who might at any moment prick his balloon of self-inflation. What he failed to know and never discovered, is that the loss of illusions and discovery of his real identity, his strengths and weaknesses, though painful at first, could have been ultimately exhilarating, leading to a life with peaks of real joy and ecstasy. But he preferred to look at his life with only one eye open—a jaundiced one, while the other eye remained blind. This is a person whose soul is dead before the body is. And where he thought that upon his death his life would be prolonged by the breath of mortal fame, there awaited him a second death, when eventually time robbed him of that too. Life continued without the "master after God."

How does such persona formation happen? Some convince and excuse themselves with stories of parental abuse, a teacher that mistreated them, or a long list of causes that account for their attitude. But if they have siblings living under the same roof, some of them do not exhibit the same annoying traits. They have a different attitude and make a different choice in life. It was their choice alone to allow themselves to be poisoned by circumstances. Concentrating *too much* on developing their superior function and identifying too exclusively with their occupation and title produces a lopsided personality, so the persona in these people becomes an iron mask which does not allow for further growth! One of the main reasons to develop such a mask is to conceal one's inferiorities, especially those of the fourth function, the function contaminated with unruly affects and emotions (see Chap. 8). They remain the doctor, or president of the United States, even when at home with family, and even after retirement. They confuse "what they do" with "who they are." *As much as such a person looks "strong" on the outside, he is fragile on the inside* (*lack of character*)*!* Typically for the *Lycopodium* person, when contradicted or challenged, he explodes in anger (*intolerance to contradiction*), as he does not tolerate views which threaten his protective psychic armor or unmask his irrational motives, while raising his voice (*dictatorial, speaking with an air of command*). Rather than the strong man he wants to project to the outside world, his sudden mood changes, irritation, and temper tantrums resemble more the state of feelings of a mere child. His successful life at work, where he is admired by others as a "born leader" (although this is motivated by the *love of power*), becomes a horrible appearance at home where his persona changes into a demon, as acknowledged by his children and wife (*contemptuous, hard for subordinates and agreeable, pleasant to superiors or people he has to fear*) with periods of explosive anger and moodiness (*violent anger; anger from contradiction*).

It is a measure of how little such a person has explored his psyche. For a man especially, his archaic anima, which remains comatose and invisible, entombed in his unconscious, leads to an undeveloped personality. Don't expect this person to have insight into his behavior that drives a wedge between him and his family and friends. He regards hate, suspicion, and lust to rule as conditions of his life, factors he is determined to keep, to secure his coveted throne. This easily leads to paranoid delusions (*China, Lachesis*) which his pseudo ego will deal with by retreating further into this one-sided mask. He confuses his individuality with his social life, feeling great and powerful, safely guarded by knowing he belongs. He identifies with a certain category, and so adopts behavior appropriate to that category. Alas, by doing so he remains isolated, removed from real humankind. He never is genuine in his conversations, laughter, and social behavior. You laugh when he laughs because you know it is expected, not because his laughter is infectious and spontaneous. The followers among his company will sit, stone silent, wiggling uncomfortably in their seats. The true individuals will never allow this a second time, putting such an individual on their blacklist of acquaintances.

How does this identification with the persona appear in dreams? Such a person is stuck and there is no distinction in the dream between his collective clothes and what lies underneath, as if his skin cannot breathe. In dreams the skin might appear thick, to be losing its elasticity, calcified, indurated, and full of scabs, or *the clothes stick to his skin.* Actual skin diseases may even coincide with identification with the persona.

B. Excessive Persona (*Veratrum-a, Platina,* and *Silicea*)

An excessive, thick mask serves to hide weaknesses of the person. In dreams it will be he *who has too many clothes* on: he takes one jacket off and another one appears and so on. The naked selfhood cannot be reached; he does not dare to take his clothes off and be naked! He is stuck in heavy armor, *unable to take his clothes off, or is overdressed in overly decorated, gaudy uniforms or dresses, or dreams of having very tough skin.* These characters are in no way easy patients, as their character armor is the molded expression of a narcissistic defense (*Lachesis, Veratrum-a,* and *Platina,* who speak in a grandiloquent manner), or a timid and fearful defense (*Silicea*), chronically embedded in their psychic structure, exhibiting constant resistance to anything that is hidden and repressed in the unconscious. For instance, *Platina* is so certain of her place in the world that she can't imagine being troubled by a little matter like blocking traffic when stepping out of a taxi and rearranging her outfit! Isn't everyone struck by her magnificent appearance, momentarily paralyzed, while time stands still?

Here is an example from the practice of how an early formation of persona (a malformed or excessive persona) in childhood can continue to wreak havoc in adulthood and lead to pathology. See if you know the remedy before I give the solution!

A patient complained to me that she found the demands of simple life with her children too hard. There was resentment, bitterness, and jealousy coming up, and what was noticeable in these resentments was that many of them were triggered by the everyday ordinary experiences of life—the sacrifices she needed to make for the children (bringing them to school and feeding them), and for her husband. Although he had a great job, he did not earn enough in her view, especially to provide a live-in maid to help with other things most people struggle with (this is an archetypal representation, a collective trait, belonging to humankind). She felt that life had chosen her as the only victim to suffer these common struggles.

Upon investigating her childhood, it was discovered that she was an only child, born into a wealthy and important family, and at school she was treated with great respect and a soft-gloved approach because of her well-known family. She was called "princess" by her parents—her father's darling, the Princess and the pea, too good for this world (*Delusion, she does not belong to this world*)—and she easily identified herself with the fantasy figure of a princess, her royalty acknowledged by everyone. This did not change when she married a powerful broker on Wall Street, as she could accompany him to banquets and outings and was treated with the reverence she expected. But everything changed when her children were born. "I became a commoner," she said to me in consultation, as she could no longer accompany her husband.

The ego adaptation (of a princess) only worked while the family situation stayed the same. But now, even with her limited qualifications, she still expected to be considered of royal origin, whereas to others she was just part of the common world and should not expect privileges because of her origin.

But ordinary life with common people was not acceptable to her. When she took up tennis, she refused to play with the beginners (where she belonged) but insisted on playing with the advanced players! She continued to identify with this consciously chosen persona. Her made-up princess persona, for everyone to see, was courteous, with an air of royalty, polite but gently condescending, mirroring her narcissistic ego. But the *egotism*, *haughtiness*, disdain, and *contempt* that would have destroyed her eventually were harbored in her shadow side, entombed in a deep cave. Invisible to her, the ego had become identified with the persona image (*Delusion, does not belong to her own family; Delusion, humility and lowness of others while she is great*). She finally developed *numbness in the face at the region of the right os zygomaticus, alternating with periods of depression*, for which she consulted me. This alternation happened always when her husband left town for business for an extended period (*fear, something would happen, that her husband would not return*). Developing such a neurosis was her way of returning to her place of importance: what physician would not pay attention to such a severe physical state! Because of parental misguided love and benign narcissism, such formation of an excessive persona can start, is unconsciously accepted in childhood, and will cause much confusion in adult life.

The remedy is obvious: *Platina!* It is interesting that after the remedy *she had a dream of being naked*. Such a dream shows that one accepts herself as she is, not as society wants her to be or as she wants to be perceived. She was able to strip herself of self-deception, to see herself naked without the princess garment of concealment but as a real person, a huge step on the individuation road. In the dream she appeared naked and not nearly as ashamed of her nakedness as she used to be, which hopefully is the beginning of recognition of her true Self, a moral unmasking of herself. She no longer was hiding her inner reality but was able, step-by-step under repeated doses of her simillimum, to wear an outfit (mask) that was proper to her exterior circumstances.

C. Inadequate Persona (*Bufo*, *Bar-c*, *Anac*, *Hura*, and *Staph*)

Inadequate persona, the opposite of excessive persona, can be created through *hereditary* factors (*Bufo*, *Bar-c*). Because of insufficient intellectual and mental tools, this person is rather blind to the reality of the world which he considers nothing but a big playground to fulfill infantile desires. Such a person never attains a state of consciousness but lives an accidental life, never having control over his ego. It is like living but not knowing that he lives, as the ego does not decide nor choose anything. Take for instance *Bar-c*. In *Bar-c* we recognize a very insecure, "small" person, a mental/emotional dwarf with a lack of individuation, still stuck even in adulthood when he should by then possess a dominant function of consciousness. *Bar-c* is a person whose blissful ignorance of childhood never ends, one who will never face the endless suffering called adult life. He is the backward child characterized chiefly by low intelligence and a general incapacity to understand. A *Bar-c*, on the mental/emotional plane, is like a child at the theater before the curtain is raised, who happily sits there with excited expectation of things to come. For him, it is a blessing that he does not know what will come, as the curtain is never raised. Growing up, *Bar-c* needs others (mainly close family) for protection and guidance in every step of his life.

Another, more frequent occurrence of developing an inadequate persona is, *Ailments from rejection/domination* in the family (*Viola-tric*, *Hura B*, *Alumina*, *Staphysagria*), where someone else's persona is forced upon the person, erasing his persona and making it impossible to form an adequate individual persona. The person *appears naked in the dream*, unprotected and vulnerable, and can appear overly defensive or frightened, or finds herself in a dream with a transparent dress on. Inevitably, such a person can succumb to grave psychic crises, especially around the time he thinks is just part of "midlife crisis." But being naked also has another meaning, that of being comfortable in one's skin, as mentioned before.

An inadequate persona can also be formed because of *poor social training*, or from being excluded from social events (a *Lac caninum*—Cinderella syndrome). Such a person will suffer from lack of poise, and unnecessary defiance (*easily offended*), tirelessly collecting injustices which invariably fill them with anger and resentment (*cursing, swearing; malicious; rage, fury from contradiction*).

Before we explore the dark side of man, a further discussion of the conscious is necessary to understand human relationships, urges, and reactions exhibited in daily life. Therefore, we need to next explore the *four basic conscious functions*, present in every individual in variable intensity.

8

THE FOUR CONSCIOUS FUNCTIONS OF JUNG AND TWO ATTITUDE TYPES

The terrifying incomprehensibilities and ferocious spirits of the omnipotent Unknown bring only peace to the human mind when understood.

The Use and Benefit of the Conscious Functions

Wherever I travel—for work or pleasure—I am constantly besieged by couples who complain to me that their other half "does not understand me and is insensitive." Let me give you a true simple example. On a tennis vacation, a male tennis friend played a "tournament" (it really did not mean anything, just a social friendly event), and when he lost his match, he lost also his cool, berating his girlfriend that she did not watch and encourage him during his valiant battle for which he deserved a monument. The girlfriend was indeed busy talking to another female who had just arrived from her native country, so she was excited to speak in her mother tongue. My tennis friend was a strict intellectual thinking type—maintaining rigid control over his appearance (he thought)—but fell apart in front of everyone when he should have appealed to his more sensitive side. Instead he became terribly childish and tyrannical. According to his girlfriend—a truly feeling person, as "opposites attract"—his feeling side was archaic, as his affection was mainly shown when, she expressed with some irrational hostility, "He only kisses his dog!" What my tennis friend did not know—as we will discover—is that such a one-sided approach to life will lead to a lack of differentiation, to *nondifferentiation*,[1] and atrophy of the other conscious functions, building an ego identical with the thinking function, always leading to emotional and physical problems. And vice versa, his girlfriend—being a markedly different functional type, living life with a dominant conscious feeling function—was possessed by an archaic reasoning, so in fact they could only speak *past* each other.

Not surprisingly, he suffered from the allopathic diagnosis irritable bowel syndrome (IBS), which resulted for years in seven diarrhea attacks daily. This IBS "dis-ease" is in effect the symbolic action and revenge of his inferior feeling function, creating an atmosphere where everyone has to walk on eggshells around him (*easily offended*) as he is touchy in any situation when an appeal is made upon his un-adapted childish inferior feeling function. It is astonishing how we can be annoyed and often deeply hurt by every perceived injury to our honor and ambition, and to every slight disdain or disrespect, which only results in destroying our peace of mind and happiness as these gestures or words that depress us are trifling and insignificant. Really, such sensitivity—analogous to an exposed nerve, a very sore spot—is nothing but an expression of a tyranny that will destroy everything except itself! As both parties seemed to be miles apart, I could not resist explaining to them the four conscious functions, which I did carefully after a clear introduction to Jung's psychological types. I knew that the slightest allusion and criticism to his inferior function would leave the man bewildered and emotional—if not hostile. My explanation soon restored peace, as he—a thinking type—liked the logic of it, and the female—the feeling one—felt understood as she was not immersed in rigid, dogmatic opinions. We remained friends and I cured him of his IBS through repetitive, increasing potency doses of LM *Sulphur*. They were married a year later as the kissing now extended not only to the dog, at least not on the wedding day, when the priest announced, "Now you can kiss the bride," which fortunately he did!

You must not presume that I am hunting to find patients on my vacation or anywhere, but this small incident (and many others) showed me the value of some basic psychological terminology. If only it was more universally known to the public! Why don't we teach our teenagers the value of basic Jungian teaching? What a difference it could make in their lives! And certainly, this knowledge is of uttermost importance in the homeopathic practice. As every practitioner has a dominant conscious function (see further), he has the natural tendency to approach each patient in his ruling mode. If he is a thinking person, he is convinced that he does the greatest benefit to the patient by explaining to him what homeopathy stands for, what principles it is based on, and how rich its history is. If the patient is also a thinking type, he might be impressed and excited, but on the other hand, a feeling type will immediately feel out of place—bored and disappointed—as her approach to worldly affairs and problems will be her feeling function, something that is most often lacking in the male thinking homeopath. You should not push such a patient to her thinking function, or you (the homeopath) will never get anywhere in understanding this patient's situation! Start to bring this patient out of her defensive shell through her feeling function, then either sensation or intuition, and only then, at the end, through her thinking function to clarify some of her blind spots. It is of the utmost importance that the treating homeopath initially set his prejudices aside and assume the persona of the patient's dominant conscious function, even if it is your nondifferentiated function—not an easy task, but a necessary exercise. Then the feeling patient will feel that her homeopath understands her, and understanding always takes precedence over theoretical explanations. As a result, the exchange of information between patient and homeopath undoubtedly will flow more fluently and harmoniously, a necessary transaction to get the "totality of symptoms" for the prescription of the simillimum. Let's explore the four different conscious functions.

Four Conscious Functions: The Gates to Wholeness

There are four functions of the conscious, the four gates to the garden of wholeness, making up the essence of consciousness. They are constitutionally present in every individual: the *perceiving* functions are **sensation and intuition**, or we can say hands-opposite-hunch, as they perceive information. Sometimes called *non-rational* functions, as they simply gather information, they do not primarily *decide*, but *experience* first. The *judging* functions are **thinking and feeling**, or we can say head-opposite-heart, as they process information received from sensation or intuition. Certain judgments must be made to organize and decide according to certain criteria, and they are therefore called *rational* functions.

When it comes to dream analysis, the four conscious functions take on another meaning, as we always have to look at the structure of the dream to see how many persons are present and what age and sex they are (see Chap. 3, "The Structure or Schema of Dreams"). Let's investigate these functions further.

The Judging Functions: Thinking and Feeling

Thinking is an *objective* judgment—organizing and deciding according to rules of analysis and logic. It tells you what a thing is as it *identifies* it. When we say to ourselves that at least three legs on a stool will support our body, we perform an act of thinking. These are objective facts—this is so, and that is that. It is logical, and a drive towards orderliness and meaning. Thinking proceeds with some deliberation and pause, evaluating the situation and looking at the pros and cons. It is a reasoning process (the use of reason and Logos) and it aims to carry through from the beginning to the end (obsessive compulsives on the other hand get stuck on the same thought and cannot go further). Thinking is probing, searching, challenging, discovering, and affirming. It involves a restless curiosity, which does not always sit well with others who have a dissenting opinion, especially with those who "*speak with a voice of command*" (*Lycopodium, Mercury*), where Logos and unbalanced reasoning become a piercing and dissecting spear, ruthlessly wounding any opposition. The thinking type is convinced that any problem can be resolved with logic and "where there is a will, there is a way," while feelings are only an obstruction and nuisance, overlooking the evidence that the heart, opposite of the head—to quote Pascal—"discovers reasons that the mind does not quite understand." This is called the "genius" of the heart, that which has courage as an investigator and discoverer, looking with daring honesty for love with wisdom that supersedes any reason. The one-sided thinking person, using this conscious thinking function as the only tool to go through life, is often someone who thinks he knows everything, but really, he knows nothing. Such lopsided use of this function only leads to a life of misery, of lawyerly disputes without end, pompous and narcissistic behavior and estrangement of others, nothing resembling the heart and soul of a dignified individual. Instead of dominating the world, which he thinks he is entitled to, the world—except for the simple souls—turns against him, which he now perceives as an injustice against such a great "leader" of people as him.

But in reality he is not a shepherd of man; he is a self-absorbed bore, easily thrown off his throne by the smallest remark against his opinion (*easily offended; intolerant of contradiction*), not knowing that he failed to transfuse his life with true light. When talking with grandiosity, big words, and dagger-like vehemence, such a person loses connection with the collective human in himself, often using "biblical" language that goes over the head of the ordinary collective human. When thinking, writing, and acting, this type is under the spell of an influx of his inferior feeling, personified by his anima (see Chap. 11). For him, applying his mind with the use of, let's say, the sensory senses, is using his mind in a rather stupid way, while intuition for him is not considered "real"! Is this person the captain and master of his soul? Nothing could be further from the truth! The more he identifies with his superior thinking function to the neglect of all the other conscious functions, the more he will suffer from the criticism of others (*easily offended; intolerant to contradiction*). His is nothing other than the child-like stupidity of those who always want to have the last word. The surface of his skin is like an open sore that flinches from a caustic agent—the insult—which is always magnified in the broken mind of this person. Therefore, he must find an outlet, be it anger (*Lyc*), withdrawal (*Nat-m*), violence (*Nux-v*), internal unrest (*Arg-n, Lachesis*), and sometimes hysteria (*Ign*), to soothe the irritated wound. These are all attempts to liberate himself, to communicate and explain himself, to allow the painful irritant to dissolve as in a volcanic eruption. The other response could be disintegration of his personality, a much worse fate.

To have no knowledge of the existence of other functions leads to inflation, often enabled by one's surrounding company, who thinks wrongly that such a person is full of wisdom and guidance. Sure, this thinking type *is not void* of emotions: it is not that he has absence of emotions, but the question is, how does he deal with them, how does he handle them? What is his reaction when the need for emotions is called upon? He has a simple answer. He sends his emotions to the cellar of his house, never to be visited, as they would only disturb his cool, reasonable thinking. For him, emotions are very powerful and frightful—mostly uncontrollable—which he represses, for he fears them more than his greatest enemy. Because his emotions expose the soft and weak spots in his life, he can't express them at the appropriate time. The trouble is, the thinking person not only has emotions, but the emotions *have him!* He is often sentimental, which has nothing to do with a good feeling function. In most men, the fourth inferior function (that which is least differentiated), or feeling (again, in most cases—see further), possesses them with extraordinary power, gripping them like the stronghold of a snake. "Emotion" comes from the Latin *ex*, or "out," and *movere*, "to move": "to move out or away" from what he usually is, or presents to others! When in a rare moment a tear is evoked, the thinking type is rather shocked and asks himself, "Why am I crying? Was it an argument I had, or did something go wrong in my day?" But leading such a one-sided, Logos-oriented life, being a "logic-chopping" type of person, will never provide answers to understanding and living life, let alone answering Aristotle's basic question, "How should a human live?" Homeopathic thinking prototypes are *Lycopodium*, *Sulphur*, and *Silicea*, who use their intelligence, encyclopedic memory, and attention to detail (*conscientious about trifles*) to obtain what they want, although with different results.

The conscious sensation function (explained later in this chapter) is also misused and not understood in homeopathy, when patients are asked, "What do you feel (emotionally)," which is the essence of the "vital sensation" method. But sensation and feeling are two terms with totally different meanings. Homeopaths would do well to refer to the French term *sensation* for the English use of "sensation," and the French term *sentiment* for the English use of "feeling" (or "sentiment"). ***Feeling*** tells you *what a thing is worth to you*, so it organizes and decides value and individual worth, a rational function. Feeling has to do with the expression of the personal or subjective value which we give to that which we perceive. When we say, for instance, "I do not like this car," or "I do like it," we give a personal value, a cool assessment, to what we perceive—agreeable or disagreeable, good or bad, acceptable or rejected, pleasant or unpleasant, likeable or not, enjoyable or not, etc. Feeling has different faces: *Lachesis*, who is a passionate feeling type, can tell you with ice cold eyes and cutting voice, "I hate you," and *mean* it, as it is as a reflection of her misplaced passion for others (anger in this circumstance), as the opposite feeling is love. Feeling can also be diplomatic, or just feigned niceness to obtain the desired goal, as the animus creeps in to create this pseudo feeling. Feeling operates (as a function: liking, desiring, evaluating; its contents, hopes, anger, etc.) with immediate spontaneity, responding directly to a situation before we analyze it, as liking and disliking are not under our control, are unadulterated. Why should one's taste or choice be ostracized? Most people want to choose the nourishment which suits their body and soul. Feeling is also associated with *empathy*. A person like *Phosphorus* with a strong feeling function can look at the face of someone, and without words spoken, realize what the other person is experiencing: pain or pleasure, hurt or anger. This is different from intuition, which does not have strong subjective responses.

So **feeling** is a *subjective* value judgment. We cannot judge objectively (thinking) and subjectively at the same time: thinking and feeling are *mutually exclusive* in simultaneity. When we put the accent on one, we automatically put aside the other. Imagine you are a crime detective, and you come upon the scene of the crime where an acquaintance has been murdered. You need to set aside your feeling function, as it will interfere with the thinking function that needs to take the dominant seat to resolve the crime. To the feeling type, thinking is rather cruel and cold. There is also a vague form of "feelings," when they happen chaotically and uncontrolled (in a miasmatic-syphilitic way) known as *moods*. Moods are also value reactions, but they are not fully conscious; they have an autonomous character, which can also lead to compulsive thoughts or delusions. Moods penetrate the whole field of "being" that we are: we *are* a certain joy, sadness, despair—they immerse the whole of our existence. "I am not myself"—something only a human can say of himself, because only a human can say it *to* himself. As Sartre said, "I am always simultaneously more or less than I am" (Barret, 1958, p. 246).

We are at the same time able to transcend this immediate situation, but it can also cause fragility and anguish in general. So, moods, obsessive thoughts, and uncontrolled opinions are the unconscious side of feeling, the germs from which feeling is made. As much as we might think that feeling (used in the wrong sense as expressing emotions) is irrational, feeling (as we now understand it), and thinking, are both called *rational*. They both work with evaluations and judgments, assessing the valuations: "true/false; pleasant/unpleasant; good/bad; just/unjust," reacting with an appropriate human judgment. Through the feeling function we appreciate a situation, a feeling, a moment in time, a connection with Nature, etc. Let's explore now sensation and intuition, the perceiving functions.

The Perceiving Functions: Sensation and Intuition

The perceiving functions, *sensation* and *intuition*, were called by Jung *irrational*, as they circumvent reason and use only mere *perceptions*, facts perceptually recorded, not proceeding from logical steps. Our senses tell us *something is*, not *what* it is (for that we need thinking!), so the **sensation** type finds a situation in which he believes. **Sensation**—the perception of reality and principle of facts—perceives things as they are, and not otherwise. *It is the sense of reality coming to the person through the five senses,* the primary source of information! It is this perceiving function that notices *details*! A sensation type (*Calc-c* is the prototype) sees an astounding mass of details in any object, a master at noticing trifles. It is like an index at once revealing its contents to the person. "How is it constructed? What does it look like? How does it function?" Sensation types like to take things apart, to see what makes them tick. They are the patient builders, great mechanics, and the children who immerse themselves in LEGOs and puzzles. They become good accountants, computer programmers, builders, architects, and military personnel, as well as mountaineers, as certain fixed rules need to be followed. They are comfortable among known facts but lose their sense of security when change happens. Sensation is often used unconsciously as a tool of experiencing pleasure: the pleasure of tasting delicious foods, looking at beautiful scenery, smelling wonderful aromas, hearing sounds of birds, touching the silky texture of clothing, etc. Of course there is also the opposite for the "hypersensitives," a first physical level of syphilitic defense: they experience sensations as overpowering and uncomfortable—unpleasant to say the least, if not obstructive (for instance, *hearing, acute, to noise, causing nausea;* and *smell, acute,* [to the scent of] *flowers*). Sensation will gather all details with infinite patience. In trying to resolve a crime, the witnesses that are most reliable—many people get convicted based on eyewitness accounts that turn out to be totally wrong, illustrating the individual relativity of sensation—are the *extraverted sensation* types. It is as if they have a camera in their head that allows them to relate quickly and accurately to outer objects. The sensation type does not look beyond what he has observed with his five senses; there is no sixth sense, something that would register a general atmosphere. So, he could appear as a "soulless" individual, as can be seen in engineers. Obviously, anything approaching his opposing function—intuition—is considered pure nonsense, but there is a danger that such inferior introverted intuition might lead to persecution delusions.

Intuition is a sort of right guess or hunch about possibilities out there in the future—being in touch with the germs of the unknown through mediation with the unconscious. We intuit what is not visible yet, as intuition gives outlook and insight; "smelling things out" before acting. Our sensation tells us that something exists, and our thinking names it, but it takes a lot of intuition to tell us what is hidden. To say "I smell a rat" is instinctive intuition! *Intuition tells you that there might be something wrong.* You don't know for a fact that something smelly is going on, but you know that there is something not kosher: "It smells bad; I have a hunch about this; Something is in the air; It seems to me that there is something fishy; My gut is telling me something; Something does not feel right; I have a sneaking suspicion; I get a weird vibe!" Intuition is a form of perception that gives us an answer directly from the unconscious—not from the senses—and some people can consciously develop intuition. Intuition, turning inward, becomes prophecy. It certainly is a good weapon (like most well-differentiated conscious functions) in the hands of a crime detective. When the suspect gives a statement that makes no sense, the intuitive detective will think there must be an ulterior motive: "I smell a rat!"

An intuitive person can convince people of the most remote possibility, a potential which might happen, or might not. Furthermore, he can create fabulous schemes and thinks for a while they are possible before he jumps to another one. Like an exuberant *Phosphorus*, the intuitive does not stop to pay attention to all these swallowed thoughts, does not wait for realization. She is always ahead of herself, never settling down with the problem, not dwelling on a single subject nor living in the here-and-now, as she wants to be removed from the body, which is like a prison and source of illness to her (especially stomach and abdominal disorders). The present is a different country where everyone else is living; the intuitive lives instead in a wonderful future of promising possibilities, always inspired by potentialities—dreading above all the repetition and boredom of a steady job. Movement is her life—discovering new avenues, new friends, new adventures, and uncharted territory—not chewing on any one problem or recent discovery for long! For the intuitive, only things that are *not yet* are real. Once they become real, she is off to the next creation, a new prospect, not dwelling further over the last thing, afraid of being caught in this single subject. No wonder some of these intuitive people are called subjects of unfulfilled promise, as they can be good, excited beginners and bad finishers (*undertakes many things, succeeds in nothing*). The tubercular person comes to mind, who dreads being locked up in an office every day, killed by the monotony of such an existence, longing for ever-beckoning adventures and possibilities, and therefore, is often the personality that does not stick around long enough to reap what she has sown.

Intuition does not care for elaborate details as sensation does, but takes a comprehensive grasp of the *whole*, even when it is not completely visible. Professions that are keen to develop this function are publishers ("I am sure this genre of book will be successful next year") and stockbrokers, who seem to possess a fine nose to predict what stocks are going to do well, year after year, and build up an enviable reputation in guiding people through the ups and downs of the financial market. It is as if intuition has erased the barrier between the unconscious and conscious mind, creating a free flow between the two. Intuition is the perceiving function that sees things in the broad context. For example: while traveling in Africa on a reservation, the sensation type will note every detail like the flowers, the trees, rivers, numerous different kinds of animals, the color of the sky, sounds of birds, etc. The intuitive type partially shuts his eyes and will simply register the general atmosphere of peaceful feeling and total silence (as I encountered in a remote reservation in South Africa, a silence so deep an outburst of activity startled me), being one with Nature—trancelike—where details are obliterated to the mind, *as if in a dream*. The intuitive finds himself mesmerized by the experience and asks himself, what are the implications of what I am seeing or intuiting? When he looks at Nature, he imagines where it came from, and speculates also about the future: what will happen to it from all the pollution and destruction occurring? It is interesting to note that the *third eye* appearing in a dream is the symbol for intuition, which gives the eye magic power to understand unconscious activities.

To illustrate the four functions, we can look at a trial process. Our jury system allows lawyers to quiz potential jurors about their thoughts regarding certain general aspects of the case, called the *voir-dire* process, from the French verbs *voir*, "to see," and *dire*, "to say." In other words, all lawyers want to "see what jurors have to say," when answering pertinent questions posed by them. Most trial lawyers, prosecutors and defense attorneys alike, would benefit from understanding these four conscious functions to discover each juror's dominant conscious function, which will play a great role in the outcome of the trial. Let's say the defendant enters the court: the thinking juror obviously will be the one logically analyzing the facts and will take his conclusion from the evidence presented. Nothing else will change his mind! The sensation type will be mesmerized by the defendant's color of dress, notice her blue eyes, the penciled lining of her eyebrows, the ring she is wearing, her mannerisms; in other words, a mass of details will preoccupy this juror and looking at the facts becomes secondary. The feeling juror might think, upon seeing the defendant, that she resembles his divorced wife, and might think "guilty" before he even hears the facts, or a female juror might find herself having been in the same situation as the defendant (like domestic abuse), and no matter what the facts are, her empathy and feeling will cause her to conclude "innocent." The intuitive juror's first thought might be, "I have a hunch that this person is innocent" no matter the facts presented! And she will defend her opinion like a lioness protects her offspring.

No wonder that twelve jurors deliberating a defendant's fate in closed chambers for the first time rarely reach a unanimous verdict, unless of course it is not at all a circumstantial case. It is the excessive identification of his ego with his dominant function that will initially pull the juror to a certain conclusion. Alas! Selecting jurors for a trial can be like a game of Russian roulette. A juror with a dominant thinking function cannot be expected to be ruled by compassion. As for the prosecutor, justice means finding justice for the victim and the victim's family—facts will be facts. But, especially when there is a clear guilty case, it is the defense's duty to find jurors with compassion, feeling people, which is *their* version of finding justice for their client.

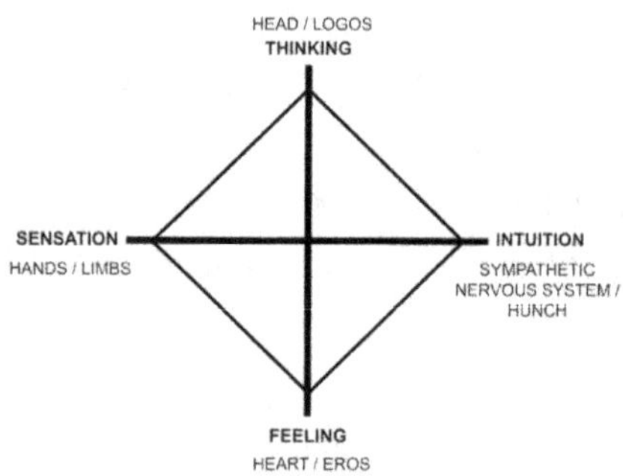

Jung's Four Conscious Functions

So how much can we work on, or hope for, to be able to use and differentiate our different conscious functions?

The Degree of Differentiation of the Four Functions

The important question is, how many of these four conscious functions can we differentiate in our lifetime? Are we the very rare individual who can honestly say, "I use all my conscious functions *almost* equally and certainly properly, as all are somewhat active!" Or are we, as most, stuck in one, our *dominant* conscious function? Are the brave and humble among us able to activate at least more than one (which would help greatly on our individuation journey)? When one more of the conscious functions becomes activated, this has the effect of changing the basic structure of our psyche, as such a change produces an alteration in the balance between the conscious and unconscious. Would it not be nice, and preferable, to be able to raise all four functions to consciousness in an equal, differentiated high degree, thus creating the ideal and perfect human being, ready to respond perfectly to any situation?

The answer is known to anyone but a fool or megalomaniac, that no such perfect individual exists. Only through hard inner work, an *approximation* can hopefully be achieved by a few. When we see a uniformly developed equal state of all four functions, it is a hallmark of a primitive mentality, and can be found more in people living close to Nature such as farmers and hunters, who have to use all their functions more or less to obtain their goals. The farmer plans when and what seeds to grow (thinking), what is most profitable (sensation), has a hunch for the upcoming weather (intuition), and must have a balanced relationship with his family and animals (feeling) to be successful. An adequate distribution of his functions is important for him to avoid going bankrupt in one season! But in general, we can state that it is just as important for all to think, intuit, perceive, and feel to be as "human" as possible, an ability given to few.

Alas, most people remain stuck in a one-sided conscious function—called the *dominant* or *superior* one—and rely mostly or entirely on this trusted function to navigate through life in *any* circumstance. To have a hint of his dominant conscious function, just ask a person, "In life, how do you act/react most of the time, almost *automatically*, when confronted with daily events and situations?" The superior function has lightning speed, is easily accessible and highly reactive. It is the eagle in the sky, always preying on what is below (and inferior), ready to seize it and bring it into his realm. It seems we would be foolish not to use our greatest gift and sell ourselves in order to live and create, but when this function becomes one-sided, when we *identify* with this superior function, it becomes much too autonomous—hindering further development of the Self—separating the individual from himself. Once we have tuned life according to our dominant conscious function, the remainder of our life is nothing but hunkering down and defending this created fortress, even when it leads to mishaps, neuroses, miscommunications, standoffs, and upheavals. It is really a pity that we limit ourselves to a tiny lot of land from which we dare not step beyond. What will be left of one whose dominant function loses strength when getting older, when one physical or mental asset after another begins to vanish? What of the other conscious functions; any hope of raising their power?

The best we can hope for—and it is a difficult task to achieve for anyone—is to differentiate one or two more conscious functions, called the *auxiliary* ones, making one, or (rarely) two more of these functions conscious. Most of the time we are capable only of bringing to relative consciousness *one* auxiliary function. For the thinking person, that is either sensation (most likely) or intuition, and for the feeling person, either intuition (most likely) or sensation. For the sensation individual, either feeling (most likely) or thinking, and for the intuitive one, either feeling (most likely) or thinking. This auxiliary function serves as a guide to temper or balance the dominant superior function, but at the same time is never as responsive to our will as the dominant function. To assimilate such an auxiliary function, and to prove its strength, requires that life actions and habits rely on this function at least for a *certain amount of time.*

Jung refers to the archaic conscious function (the opposite of the dominant one, remaining mainly in the unconscious) as an "inferior" function, in quotation marks, for it is not really inferior (well knowing that we will experience it constantly in life), but is rather the one function responsible for the unexpected turns and twists, the shocking and surprising appearance of moods, which are inaccessible to man's will and relating to aspects of this inferior or primitive developed conscious function. It acts like a trickster, only becoming conscious when we are "beside ourselves," expressing its tremendous, heavily loaded charge of emotion, leading to moods and reactions that express their infantile nature, revealing at once the owner's concealed lack of perfection. The average person does not know what he does or says in life due to the strength of this inferior function, as it is infected with the personal and collective unconscious, with the emotions and feelings of its owner, clinging to him.

When we fail to extend consciousness, we lose an amount of freedom, as the tide seems to go against the ego, undermining it at inopportune moments. "I did not mean this," we say, or, "I did not do this," though our words and deeds were visible to anyone. Where we are inferior, we are connected to the ordinary collective man, or mankind in general—as Nietzsche expressed, and entitled a book, *Human, All Too Human*—while the differentiated functions help us be more independent. In the fourth undifferentiated function we are walking a tightrope, a dangerous place to be, full of risks and tensions and, in many cases, resulting in mishaps, falls, and death.

For most male persons, the unconscious ("the hair in the soup" or Achilles heel) is personified by the feeling function—Eros and anima[2]—and as we have seen before, often represents a dubious entity whose infantile and undeveloped nature brings them frequently into a state where others recognize not only the fabricated persona they present to the world but who they *really are.*

In order to discover one's inferior function, it is further helpful to ask the following questions: "Where is your greatest suffering? Where, and in what circumstances and relationships, does life always seem to give you hard knocks that create a living hell? When are you beside yourself? When do you get upset easily? What disturbs you most in others? What aspect can you not stand in others?"

In general, we feel inferior in circumstances where we are *easily offended, lose self-control* and *self-confidence*, or are easily influenced by others, as everything that is commonly known by us, and by others about us, seems to have evaporated momentarily. At these times, the inferior function has changed us into another, "unknown" personality, briefly dominating the scene. Few indeed are those who can control with iron will a sensitive temperament capable of strong emotions. No doubt, only a small number can guide their ship through the mysterious waves of human emotions—through all the simplest, and the mightiest, feelings life knows.

As Traditional Chinese Medicine pointed out 5,000 years ago, the inferior function, associated with femininity, is found in a human's dark side or the yin. Even the two somewhat *differentiated* or *auxiliary functions* of any individual are still partially rooted in the unconscious, and few are those who can free them significantly from the darkness of their unconscious, therefore remaining more under the influence of yin than yang. These four functions are like the four gates of a fortress, where one gate—the fourth function, closest to the unconscious—is barely defended, the weakest spot, allowing the enemy (the dark elements of the unconscious) to come in. But integration and acknowledgement of the fourth function leads to better organization of the psychic equilibrium/defense by enlarging/fortifying the consciousness. Yet no one can close this gate forever, as this fourth function, even when somewhat differentiated, will remain mostly in the unconscious—though any degree of differentiation is better than none. Surprisingly, we might develop a new attitude for a more exciting, complete life by any recognition of the fourth function. But we must remain humble, realizing that it is the last function we are able to pull a little from the dark after the two auxiliary functions are somewhat assimilated.

In *dreams*, the fourth undifferentiated function presents in men as "the unknown woman," projected into a non-ego, or can appear as a young child or an animal, a dwarf, a mad man, the ugliest person, or a complete fool. Contrary to man's belief, it is exactly this inferior function that provides the renewal of life. *Only rarely do we see animals, unknown persons, and children as symbols of* ***well-differentiated*** *functions. Well-differentiated functions appear in dreams as personifications; either the dreamer, or others known to him!* This is an important message for the dreamer to recognize this inferior function as his true savior, whose intervention propels him to be a more complete person, the greatest treasure he can receive.

The third and rather archaic function, the other auxiliary "unconscious" one, is also feminine and is pictured in dreams together with the archaic inferior function, as daughter and mother respectively.

We can understand the violent battle erupting during integration of these dark elements, and it is no surprise that the dreamer (patient) will react with disgust and denial when the filth of the unconscious is put right in front of him—often a moment where the patient will turn away from the remedy intake and therapy, as the dream message is disturbing, violating his artificially created peaceful existence. Of course the patient's conscious at this point (led by the dominant conscious function) states "Homeopathy does not work for me," and tries to steer away from this "nonsense," an opportunity lost to become a more complete person by expanding ego-awareness. As mentioned before, homeopaths would do well during a consultation to temper their own dominant function, and with great care and humility switch to the patient's dominant function. For one, it is a good exercise for the homeopath to differentiate an auxiliary function. Secondly and more importantly, the patient will feel understood and will open his heart to communicate even his deepest fears and shortcomings.

"Feeling persons" don't always guarantee an amicable atmosphere, nor are they easily understood, as they are often guided by dogmatic insistence and inflexibility about values. If they do not want to be confronted with conflicts or uninteresting topics, say at a party, they turn inward and remain silent rather than contributing to the festive ambience, especially if they are introverts (*Nat-m* is such example). However, a person who has exercised this feeling function and is in balance with his attitude types (see further), is able to turn on either level of feeling—being reserved or engaged when the moment demands for it. In other words, such a person can make good use of the introvert and extravert attitudes. Otherwise, a *Lachesis* person, a feeling type, seems to sense the weak spot in others and can crush with as little as a look or a word, destroying those she believes to be her opponents. *Lachesis's* speech takes on a sort of autumnal redness of color, a combination of wit, intelligence, and fluency, but is also a drawn sword ready to kill any inferior. She uses her loquacity to overpower others (*loquacity, changing quickly from one subject to another*), and always behaves like a superior who, with wit, uses others to increase her own glory (*egotism*) and grandstanding. Words are *Lachesis's* way of ordering the jostle of life. She speaks in eloquent bursts, using her voice like an instrument, her hands and eyebrows rising and falling to accentuate each note (*gestures, ridiculous or foolish*).

As a rational function (feeling is the reason of the heart!)—making value judgments—feeling will take more time than the non-rational functions, mere collectors of perceptions. The more primitive level of feeling takes less time because it evokes mainly a reaction of a sudden yes or no, like or dislike! When we wake up in the morning there may be an immediate feeling that "we feel good," regardless of exterior circumstances like bad weather, work that needs to be done, or stressful tasks that need to be undertaken. Feeling is not what our logic would explain, but here too, it is the logic of the heart rather than the reason of the mind. And whether one likes a person or not, for instance, is not always a straight answer, a yes or no: a more reasonable, or better use of the feeling function will answer, "It depends on what you ask about that person, his characteristics and the situation presented."

We see the importance of the feeling function in being able to discriminate between positive and negative feelings and how to express them. A person might entirely have feelings of love for his spouse, but because of the inferiority of his feeling function he might not be able to express them except through some rambling—a distorted and inadequate way—embarrassing both parties. Feelings can carry a positive (pleasant, constructive) or negative (cruel, destructive) sign, but a balanced feeling function can deal with both in an appropriate way. A good feeling function recognizes and admits even negative feelings and will move us to act, reflect, and possibly find a solution to respond appropriately. It can deny a request, explain a dislike, and put long-held resentment into words.

However, there are many circumstances where the inferior

feeling function rules the life of its possessor. All too often—incomprehensible to others and the person himself—awkward situations and moods are noted. Let's discuss some of them.

Consequences of an Ill-Equipped Inferior Feeling Function

An archaic inferior feeling function makes the person lose contact with his feelings. He is unconscious of his feelings, and so becomes a person who does not know what he wants, what he likes doing, or even who he loves, and is able to fall into either a sense of worthlessness or an inflation of the ego. What would be left if the balloon was pricked? He becomes a person at risk of his own unpredictable feelings: will it be depression, irritability, despair, suicidal ideation, or indifference? A lack of moderation is created, going from disgust about things to desiring something with maniacal obsession, an unbridgeable chasm that is always present. All these feelings are a punishment for those who always lacked contact with the unconscious, out of disbelief or angst over being drawn into the unknown and incomprehensible.

The male especially is at risk in midlife and retirement age to be swept away by his inferior function into the psyche's dark side. Thankfully, homeopathy has excellent remedies to allay the fear of feeling useless and helpless, expressed by the rubrics, *indifference to everything*, and *Delusion: has lost the affection of friends and family; everything will fail; she is lost; he is unfit for this world; is despised; he is repudiated by his relatives;* and *he is lost to the world and beyond hope*, all leading to questions about the meaning of life (more about this in Chap. 14, "The Death of a Soul").

Manic depressives are another class of patients that suffer from an inadequate feeling function, as their emotions swing from one extreme to another (loss of control, a syphilitic miasmatic characteristic), expressing its distortion and disarray by creating a tool that is not available at the times it is needed by the person. Instead, their feeling function presents like a pendulum in motion, unresponsive at opportune moments as it is spending too much energy elsewhere, leading to many misunderstandings and long, accusatory discussions where, if both parties have an inferior feeling function, no one wants to be the loser! Indeed, the immobility and stubbornness of this inferior feeling function has led to many divorces! Where TCM prided itself on tranquility of the mind—a consistent course of life without excitement or depression—for modern society, a turbulent state has become the norm, not only for adults but for children as well.

Another consequence of an inferior feeling function is the *guilt* (*anxiety, of conscience*)—a syphilitic miasmatic expression —that many people put on themselves, especially when their children did not grow up to be what was expected according to the norm, supposedly because they were not "good enough" parents. And with the epidemic of autism, many mothers' first reflex upon hearing the diagnosis is to reflect on what they must have done wrong: "Did I not love this unborn baby; Did I not eat right; Was I too emotional with the turmoil in my life and did I not pay enough loving attention to my needs and the baby's during pregnancy (*reproaching oneself*)?" And if after the birth process the woman is seized by a post-partum depression, and has dreams of killing her baby, guilt increases tenfold. *Sepia* is a remedy for these circumstances, as a *Sepia* patient with her inferior feeling function is overwhelmed by so many emotions that this archaic function can't manage. Such guilt supports her ego as she is convinced that what happens is "hers" and must be set right by "her," a vicious cycle increasing the darkness of her mind. This we see in the rubrics: *indifference to everything; averse to business; despair about her miserable existence; Delusion, she is alone in a graveyard; fear of killing;* and *dwells over past disagreeable occurrences,* all expressing a dangerous emotional block.

Even victims of incest, male or female, fall prey to their inferior feeling function as self-blame often occupies their thought process: "It must have been my fault" (*reproaching himself*).

An example from the practice is of a middle-aged woman who divorced her controlling, thinking husband because she was never appreciated by him for her interests in alternative medicine and psychology. When she met a nice, feeling man, she was still overcome with guilt. Her indicated remedy was *Lachesis*, and after one dose she had the following dream.

Dream

We have been inside a house or enclosed something, maybe public indoor pool. I have a third young boy; the strange thing was that I would forget his name and I have to ask others, what is his name? I don't want to ask this really (it is embarrassing of course, a mother not knowing the name of her child). This child is easy-going, never asks for anything, then he goes to the pool and I forget about him. I am not even concerned that he can fall into the pool. Then I hear somebody screaming and I rush into a room where a baby boy is lying on his bed, I see his face and on his head is some blood and he screams, almost having convulsions, and when I pick him up he is fine. This is the first time in my life that I see a face in a dream. Usually I don't.

Analysis

This is an important dream, a great or archetypal dream. The archetypal nature is seen in the image of the third boy (her child), whom she forgot the name of (unknown), which of course refers to her newborn animus, a rebirth of her animus and more properly, the Divine Child, as he was easy-going and seemed to know everything and did not need any help from a mother. Now that she finally separated from her husband, the boy refers to the inner child of the dreamer, to everything that is unfinished, just started or in need of growth, a symbol par excellence of the reborn psyche evolving to independence, reflecting the death of the suppressed infantile personality and hindered feeling function, and the rising of the adult independent personality. It can point to paving the way for a future change of personality, which is the meaning of the eternal child or the Savior. As the alchemists say, "No new life can arise without the death of the old one." Positively this points to potentialities and possibilities in the dreamer's developing personality, to whatever has great possibility to grow and be fulfilled in the dreamer's life. A work in progress! The house refers to the Self, and the pool refers to the personal unconscious. She heard someone screaming and saw the boy laying on the bed (another symbol of personal unconscious, the seat of birth), with some blood on the head and screaming—an image resembling what really happens in any new-born birthing process! Just as after giving birth, when the physician puts the baby in the mother's arms, she embraces the child and he calms down and is fine. So, this dream has an excellent lysis showing the accuracy of the remedy. It should help the patient accept the new-born aspect (her new animus). This dream will therefore not be repeated but will evolve further as a series of dreams.

Another patient, a 35-year-old female, had set forth the goal of helping her husband and two children to realize their individuation journey. Of course, this is an example of having *too much responsibility*, which inevitably will lead to the well-known burnt out *Sepia* state. After taking *Sepia* in adequate doses, she stated that she had been having "illuminations" that showed her the need to visit certain periods of her life and process them and find peace. Interestingly, after this contemplation and after having the following dream, her clarity of mind is returning, and her emotions are changing for the better. Her previous restless dreams changed in the following dream.

Dream

I am again around people, a kind of festive atmosphere, and I am looking for a laundromat to take our clothes to wash. My husband finds a huge bathtub-like washer and I am very glad to be able to wash *all* the clothes in one load. While the clothes wash, I walk around and run into a man I perceive as gay. I observe him for a few seconds and go back to the washer and I find the clothes all gone. I assume somebody put them in the dryer. A peaceful feeling is noticed as opposed to many restless dreams in the past.

Analysis

The restless dreams before showed exactly the patient's *Sepia* state: taking too much responsibility, putting many different clothes on (which are personas) to deal with the many different goals she sets forth. In this dream she washes all these clothes (like starting on a clean slate!) and hence she feels more at peace, not carrying these loads of duties she has mainly put on herself. A good progression and lysis!

The inferior feeling function's action is also easily seen in the workplace, especially if we must perform a rather unpleasant task like firing someone. We make the situation more awkward with clumsy remarks and overthought reasons that sound more cruel than empathetic. Even at home such a person will leave the task of disciplining his children to the mother because "it is her job," while at the same time he will sabotage his wife by giving in to his children's whims, so he is the saint and likeable parent who dances away from domestic responsibilities (*inability to take responsibility; aversion to responsibility; flees from his children; aversion to domestic duty*). But having to fire someone, or denying a child's request, even freeing a long-held resentment by putting it into words—all expressions of an exercised and balanced feeling function—will bring a sense of liberation and increased energy. Frequently, women in cases of deception and grief—*Sepia* and *Nat-m* are perfect examples—will react with their distorted feeling function, with the help of their strong animus, to resort to an all-or-nothing attitude, something their lawyers like because they drag on the divorce procedures. No one has more *hatred for those who have offended*, as this archaic inferior feeling is loaded with *resentment*, *anger*, and *rage*. *Nat-m* with her feeling of being *forsaken* and her initial fantasy about what love should be, takes no prisoners. *Nat-m* has a psychic armor that covers her head to foot, but there exists a flaw near her heart: a simple word (*easily offended*) can hurt her deeply, and she will never forget but will always feel the steel that wounded her. She will rush, head down, at the person she holds responsible for her wound and try to trample him underfoot. At those moments, the purring cat transforms into a raging tiger! For her, after deception, "all men are bad without any exception" and, "men only get older but remain bad." Revenge is nothing but returning the hurt that was inflicted on her, as reflecting on it for some relief if not a sense of satisfaction. And one of the first things she might do while still married is to buy things she does not need, as she can't shop without buying due to her distorted and wounded feeling function! And her combination of conceit, vulnerability, and wounded vanity always discourages others from telling her the truth.

As seen in this chapter, it is easy to get entrapped in an archaic feeling function. How to avoid those pitfalls? When it comes to the affairs of loved ones (friends, children, spouses), a feeling function is tested in the tempests. We can lend a hand and take it upon our shoulders, but *not make it part of us*; we can be concerned, but never impassioned or brooding over others' affairs, as such involvement will injure us more than them. It is already hard enough to be involved in a balanced way in our own affairs without inviting others "inside." There is always quite enough to do to restore our house (Self), without being carried away by others. Otherwise we are always busy with other people's business!

Passions or unbridled anger are a fire that benumbs and consumes our energy, and following the generation cycle in TCM, lead to hysteria, sleeplessness, and cardiovascular incidents. At the first moment of such a turbulent storm or fierce gale, abandon the subject that is beginning to weigh on you before it carries you away. Slam the door shut, because once this emotion is in your home, it has the possibility of becoming a permanent and unruly housemate. Enter a quarrel lightly, and you are apt to get out of it just as lightly, although for the common human like me, I must train myself to do so by disposition, not virtue.

An important facet of the child's formation of the dominant conscious function is an early imposition of this natural evolving function. What happens in this case?

Early Impediment of the Dominant Conscious Function

What parent is not concerned about the future of his child, with how to guide and encourage his child, so that he or she hopefully takes the right road—obviously never a sure thing. But a child can be gently steered according to constitution and temperament, as well as true capacities, desires, and the emerging natural dominant conscious function. The latter are indeed the preferred guidelines, as temperament and constitution are innate (if not deviated through unfortunate mental-emotional intrauterine experiences), while the differentiation of types is visible from very early childhood on. I observed introversion or shying away from the object—often because of anticipation anxiety—in an autistic child who, before staying in his classroom, had to go through all the other classrooms to see what and who was in them, so as not to be surprised and overwhelmed by an unknown object or person. His introversion was also confirmed by his continuously using an alter ego name when speaking to his mother. The differentiation and one-sidedness of a conscious function comes of course later (fully developed at age 18), but the ruling function becomes visible by watching what the child prefers to do—which is always what he is good at—while avoiding what he is not good at (for example, outspokenness for the *Lycopodium* thinking child). A *Calc-c* child is more of an extravert-sensation type as he is very interested in "how things are made," paying attention to details and engrossed in LEGOs. The *Phosphorus* child, extravert-intuitive, often astonished me by the surprising gifts he possessed from an early age on. For example, to be able to see colored halos around the heads of others, and other visions, expressions of intuition. Before parents push their own agenda on their children, they would do well to allow the child's initial one-sidedness to blossom, before distorting this natural developing superior function by exerting pressure on the child to operate in a function that goes against his natural gifts.

Alas! All too often, parents—either because of their own shortcomings and missed opportunities, or because the ruling tendency in the intellectual ambitious family favors a profession with a steady and preferably high income—are convinced they are doing their children a favor by steering them towards security and conformity, rather than looking at the really important factors previously mentioned. "Trust me," they say, "take that city job, it is a steady job; they can hardly fire you and it has a good retirement plan, so you are set for life." It is like condemning someone to prison for life before they start living! Another parent might say, dictated by his own superior conscious function, "Why do you want to become a starving artist? At least then try to become a graphic artist, that's where the money is!" Of course, such a parent claims to his child, "I love you, it is for your best," but it is just the opposite. Such parents do not love their child, as they are cutting him off from his spontaneous natural wishes. They do not accept their child as he is, but want him to be something else, which implies therefore that he is unacceptable in their eyes! The child is forced to choose safety above growth; his expected performance (and salary) according to the parents' wishes is all that matters. It's believed that is what well-meaning parents should do. Don't they have the best in mind for their child? No! Although everything seems acceptable—in the parents' eyes no crime has been committed, life goes on as always, and yes, the child is not dead, not literally—unfortunately he must carry on according to his parents' desires, creating a pseudo Self if he wants to be loved and worthy, so he is not only rejected by his parents but also by himself. He receives the message that he is not permitted to follow the lead of his dominant function or he will be abandoned or punished for being "disobedient" and "defiant." This child is condemned to a handicap of possessing only one limb and zero self-esteem! Such a person becomes *help-less* and *self-less* and the feedback effect on the Self is that he is incapable, cannot master anything, and does not trust himself.

An important step to self-realization is to follow one's vocation—from the Latin *vocare,* or "to call"—to do what one is called to do! It should be a true vocation, not one imposed by custom, expectations, or stereotypical behavior, like "we should be married and have children." Wasting talents and abilities is like sailing to the wrong port, one we would hope is temporary but where we still run the risk of being anchored forever in a place that leads to a loss of spiritual life. Not everyone is an *Aurum* personality with a born instinct that he is supposed to do something great in this world, which for *Aurum* is *not* a variety of schizophrenia and grandiose aspirations that never can be fulfilled because of lack of talent and intelligence. Of course *Aurum's* road is still paved with many stones, even insecurities (*Del, he is not doing his duty; Del, he is not appreciated*), a significant burden often leading to and culminating in syphilitic reactions (*loathing of life; suicide, jumping from a height*).

From young age on, and certainly from age 18 when the natural dominant function should be fully developed, when this development has been impeded, it oftentimes means that a function which as a rule should have occupied the fourth place has been pushed to the foreground so that it takes the place of the dominant one, that of our original predisposing function. If we are forced in childhood to an adaptation that goes against our nature, it will lead to neuroses, compulsions, difficulties, and dissatisfactions in life, as the absolutism of this unnatural superior function has shut down and atrophied all the other functions, delegating them to the unconscious. Then we become an adult with a hole in the heart, always feeling that something is missing and feeling inadequate in whatever challenge is thrown at us. We "never feel right in our skin." Directed by parental traits, we always do the work of somebody else. There is confusion, awkwardness, and above all a lack of confidence inevitably leading to low self-worth, anxieties, fears of failure with *Delusions, we will never succeed in anything*, and the rest of a multitude of neuroses. In such cases the *actual ego potential* will remain unused and is delegated to the shadow side —the positive side of the shadow, the alter ego (see Chap. 10). No wonder we stumble in life when *our shadow carries a personality that is more powerful and superior than the ego consciousness.* When we reach the age of 40, this inferior function, imposed as dominant, has become a tyrant and ruler, which often leads to melancholy in the thinking type and dogmatic, animus behavior in the feeling type, because the original dominant function was not accepted and welcomed as our inborn natural relationship with the world. Often it is called a "midlife crisis," but it is a sign to incorporate our dark images from the unconscious, our animus or anima, as we will see further (Chap. 11). The challenge for everyone is to maintain a modicum of youthful exuberance and satisfaction, but for those who spent the first half of their life in their imposed nondominant function, approaching 40 and reaching the pinnacle of apparent "success," they start thinking, "Now what? How do I deal with the rest of my life?" And not uncommonly, some do apparently "stupid" things: a physician leaves his profession and opens a pet store; a lawyer becomes an artist; and the CEO of a corporation visits ashrams in India, leaving behind his opulent lifestyle to immerse himself in yoga and meditation. What these people are really looking for, and hope to find, is a new life by applying their inferior function, the spark to new life, one of the most genuine things they have ever done.

Sometimes reality can be more incredible than fiction. What if parents decide their child's profession at age 1? This story went as follows. At age 1, a couple's child was in danger of dying and both parents prayed to God and promised that if He would save their child, the child would become a priest. As we know, a child until age 5 is close to the parents as his ego is predominantly formed through mystical participation, while such a young child is also close to the archetypal images of the collective unconscious—the protective Hero Father and the nourishing Earth Mother type. That this child was already inundated with the ghost of a priest at a young age was seen at age 3, when he was telling other children what was good and what was bad, already playing the role of a saintly priest. To force a child into premature development is to drive the child more into his inner world, and in this case, to let the created persona of a "priest" deal with the expectations of the outer world. Confusion and not knowing where he fit in were direct consequences for the rest of his life. Although his parents divorced, the young man started religious studies at a young age only to find out that he was bored. So, at age 17 he tried the other road and became a physician, dealing only with radiology. But even here he was caught in a position that gave him no satisfaction, and at a later age he worked in the stock market, and later, for a pharmaceutical company. He felt guilty towards his father especially (the one in the family with the deciding voice) that he did not become a priest, even though exercising the thinking function had brought nothing but dissatisfaction, as his anima was more developed than his animus and Logos. As an adult he was still entangled in the situation created by his parents' holy promise, his destiny assigned him at an age when none of the four conscious functions was dominant, creating confusion and bewilderment when it came to choices in his life.

The Self must seek its own path and should not be predetermined as in this case by the preconception of parents. No doubt he was more a feeling type—not at all haughty and cloaked in the garment of a prestigious physician, but a person who possessed much Eros or function of relationship—yet the jobs he chose were not at all relationship-oriented, as he did not see patients as a radiologist. No wonder he traveled between Logos and Eros (*will, sensation as if he had two wills* and *will, weakness of will*), lost in a desert looking for water, the living spirit, and for a profession that would satisfy his feeling function. As an adult he developed Graves's disease with all its symptoms. Here we see that serious pathology can develop, its beginning created at age 1 by well-meaning parents who nevertheless shackled their infant to a "sacred oath," from which he still suffers as the "duty complex" has him! This can be called a benign form of *Ailments from domination*, and the patient remains caught in chains that were none of his doing. A dream that terrified him showed where he was in his life (not what he needed to do, as a dream rarely tells that).

Dream

I dream I am locked up in a coffin or cramped space and I am overcome with a fear greater than if I would be dead.

Analysis

This dream is self-explanatory. He is still caught and paralyzed in the unconscious from which he needs to escape. The coffin also indicates that he needs to die first in order to be reborn, so he can choose this time his own path to individuation, without being trapped by the sense of parental duty. The parent's voice of absolutism will have to die first, before he can discover the spark of creative energy within him; the voice of a ghost needs to be killed, a gift of death that will become life again.

None of these four conscious functions operate by themselves. They operate in tandem with two *attitude* types, *introversion* or *extraversion*, and combined will form the eight different psychological types: the extraverted thinking type, the introverted thinking type, the extraverted feeling type, and the introverted feeling type, and so on, a total of 32 (8x4) possible combinations of functions. It is more difficult than one may think to come to a correct conclusion about the psychological type of an individual, although we can say that it is mainly the dominant function of a person that determines his psychological type.

The Attitude Types

The four functions act differently if they are introvert or extravert, which will influence the entire psychological process, and thus form with the four conscious functions the eight different psychological types (see further). Introversion and extraversion are not at all our choosing, nor is one preferable over the other. Even the most extraverted person is just as much imprisoned in his own centrifugal Self as the introvert in his centripetal one. The extravert is primarily oriented to the object and objective factors, the introvert towards the subject and subjective factors. This is obvious when an extreme extravert faces a new situation: "Let's do it," is his battle cry, "I can't wait! Let's dive into it! Success is assured!" The introvert will at first recoil and withdraw—looking first for all the reasons *not* to engage in this new challenge, certainly not before he has thought about all the negatives (mainly) and plusses. We see clearly that these attitudes direct the individual's libido—the totality of energy flow—flowing to the object (extravert) or to the subject (introvert). It is easier to see (as it is often right in your face at that moment) when a person is in an introvert or extravert state, than knowing what conscious function is actively dominant. What needs to be avoided in anyone is *one-sidedness* of the two attitudes.

Is one of these attitude types preferable above the other? What would the extreme extravert and introvert think of each other? Would they be friends? Good companions, as opposites attract? They most likely would show disdain for each other, pretending that each missed the true meaning of life. Who is right? Both are! The extravert misses the richness and guidance of the inner life, the introvert fails to participate in the outer life! Although an extravert will accuse an introvert of morbid introspection and morose behavior, he confuses this with the more positive introversion. **Introspection** comes from the Latin *spectare*, or "to look at, to see." This can be passive entertaining of old morbid feelings, like *Nat-m* exhibits in her *reminiscing and enjoying about old grief*, a non-constructive state of mind. **Introversion** comes from the Latin *versare*, or "to turn, to change," turning to the hidden side, the unconscious, to change or integrate it—a positive step. Although we naturally possess one of these reactions more than the other (introversion or extraversion), we must understand that there is a place for both attitudes depending on the circumstances.

Certain periods in life tend also to go in one of these directions: puberty is a hurricane, an extreme extraverted yang state, while menopause is a time of reflection and dormancy, or yin. The person who is always in the extraverted mode might look like a spineless fool, a risk taker who never thinks anything through, who tries again and again against better judgment, leading to the next catastrophe in life! He is a nervous racehorse galloping in the world, while losing his way back home to the womb or connection with the unconscious and the Divine Mother. Sadly, in order to be successful in his many enterprises, his thinking function has become so dominant that he is unable to use his feeling function, even with those who are closest to him in the most ordinary circumstances.

The dominant and permanent introvert becomes the hermit —isolated from humankind, never exposing himself to the joys in life except those from the voice of his inner life, a cocoon that he is reluctant to leave—a syphilitic miasmatic state. For him, the cave—representing the darkness and seclusion of the unconscious—provides shelter and warmth while the exterior offers nothing but insecurity, coldness, and wickedness. He shuns the bright light of the exterior world, keeping a small flickering light in his tomb, and avoids social relationships (*social meeting aggravates*).

For mankind, trying to be more complete is differentiating three of the four functions to the greatest degree of consciousness possible, and practicing both attitudes whenever the opportunity presents itself. And then remains the biggest obstacle: getting to know the inferior or primitive function so that it becomes our greatest ally, rather than the trickster and demon. For all of us, this is a life-long Herculean task in which plenty of victims have fallen on the battlefield. Even for famous and apparently successful people, the struggle often left them injured. For instance, introverted feeling persons understand others very well, yet they themselves often experience being misunderstood. Their motto: "Still waters run deep!" Example: Sister Theresa. Extraverted feeling people know exactly what they like and dislike and can express their feelings in public freely. Their empathetic understanding of others' feelings and their ability to make others feel valued and important have the encouraging effect of creating harmonious interactions. An example was Martin Luther King.

The homeopath has deeper knowledge of the inborn constitutions and the influence of the family miasmatic background, to recognize where his patient stands—how much and on what function and attitude he has to work while removing obstacles created by high-feeling toned complexes or "ailments from"—so that the patient can be freed from inherent and acquired obstacles through judicious dosing of the simillimum.

With the information in this book, the homeopath can now also understand that when he is able to explore the patient's dream world, another important tool is added to his quest to heal the patient and transform him into the person he *wants to be* rather than the person he *is.*

General Appearance of the Eight Different Psychological Types

The two attitude types combined with the four conscious functions form the eight psychological types:

- the extraverted thinking type
- the extraverted feeling type
- the extraverted intuitive type
- the extraverted sensation type
- the introverted thinking type
- the introverted feeling type

- the introverted intuitive type
- and the introverted sensation type

Each of these types has a nemesis, or a compensatory function: the extraverted thinking type has an introverted feeling; the extraverted intuitive has an introverted sensation; the extraverted feeling type has an introverted thinking; the extraverted sensation type has an introverted intuition, while the introverted types have similar compensations. For instance, the introverted thinking type has an extraverted feeling. While *no one* is a single pure type uniquely present in society, and most are somewhat a *mixture* of these different types, it is not uncommon that many have a tendency to approach and orient the world one-sided with their trusted and familiar dominant function, with many mishaps as a consequence. We can only hope that the auxiliary functions of each type described are strong enough to temper a one-sided conscious function and exert a balancing influence.

Just as dreams show a compensation action with the conscious exaggerated attitude, the overemphasized conscious function is inevitably followed by the opposite function that will start a compensatory action visible to everyone. The mask is clearly pulled off its owner, exposing his weaknesses to everyone. He becomes the Emperor without clothes, the immature child, often vulnerable or foolish, depending on if he recognizes this compensatory state or not. If not recognized and attended to, especially when we get older, nothing but tensions and calamities will occur. Therefore, part of our individuation journey is discovering the functional hierarchy most natural to each unique individual in order to go more smoothly through life, a journey that is a slowly evolving process. As any basic idea, the theory of the four functions is not a dogma but has great value for mankind to understand himself and others.

For an in-depth analysis of these eight types, I highly

recommend and refer the reader to Jung's *Psychological Types* (Jung, 1990, CW Vol. 6, pp. 346-407 or paras. 584-671). I describe in short in the following paragraphs the main characteristics of these types, linked to the homeopathic prototype, elaborated by homeopathic remedy pictures and their fitting rubrics, and by the four temperaments and the TCM corresponding findings 5,000 years ago.

The Extraverted Thinking Type with Inferior Introverted Feeling (*Nux-v; Lyc*)

As much as this type thinks he is an original thinker, his eyes always on the object, he only follows what are generally accepted patterns and habits. And of course, he has an answer for every argument that does not coincide with his opinion. Ruled by Logos with nearly an absence of feeling (as his nemesis is inferior introverted feeling), the unconscious—the other half of his life—is never visited or acknowledged. Thus, for him thinking often takes a destructive form, leading away from emotional psychic reality and focused more on material aspirations and desires. This also means that his Eros—the function of relationship and cultivating friendships—remains archaic, creating problems with others for which he will take no responsibility. Others not belonging to this, his class, he considers losers, uninspired, lazy, and should not be walking in the same circles with him. Worse, this is the type who is a tyrant to his wife and children (*contemptuous and hard for subordinates, pleasant to people he has to fear or to superiors*) as they are merely subjects hindering his road to "success"—which is power (*love of power*)—and are only useful to serve him, while his responsibilities to them are non-existent (*lack of domestic responsibility; flies from his own children; want of amativeness in men*). He gets angry when contradicted (*intolerant of contradiction*): if he says so and so, he means so and so, no further discussion needed!

While his excessive mask reaches a peak high in the sky, an enormous block of ice sits below the surface, consisting of a multitude of untrained feelings he is totally unaware of but that rear their ugly head when he faces a situation requiring feelings. No doubt, in such a situation, besides outbursts of infantile moods such as *delirious raging*, *dictatorial behavior*, and *speaking with a voice of command*, when pushed into a corner *projection* becomes his favorite reaction. He is the one with "all the right answers" when it comes to living, a dogmatic opinion which does not allow any deviation if you want to be in his grace or belong to his elite of thinkers. Unknown to himself, he is the one losing all flexibility in life, something for which he will be punished in the second half of his life, when the question of the meaning of life is posed. He is dominated by his animus which leaves no place for real philanthropy like that in an *Aurum* personality, but his strict opinions are always phrased with "ought" and "should," as he believes his judgments should be universally accepted by the rest of the world. This type is the first one to push his children to operate with their archaic function, which is *his* dominant function: this Logos-oriented person pushes his viewpoint of life on anyone, most calamitously his offspring. He does not look for divine riches, and certainly not the one most valuable: to love others.

The world of politics, justice, government positions, teaching, and medicine is full of these individuals, who consider others who deviate from the general formula in those professions as "free spirits, unorthodox, out-of-the-loop dreamers, crackpots, charlatans, irrational lunatics." The extraverted thinking type (with inferior introverted feeling) might be good CEOs for the company they work for but create friction among the workers who feel used and exploited for the greater good of the investors or stockholders. The danger in this idealist—driven by ruthless ambition and the desire to save the world and discover groundbreaking therapeutic techniques for mankind—

is that he resorts to falsifications, twisting his research results and evidence, as has happened in the allopathic medical world. Think of the total mastectomies advocated for years for breast cancer, or the falsification of data regarding hormonal therapy for menopause, the hiding of side effects of medications, and controversies about vaccines. This is also the *Nux-v* person, always terribly overworked and never finding time for vacation. *Nux-vomica* identifies with a mask or persona with only one facet, as it is entirely formed by the one thing important in his life: ruthless ambition (*ambition increased*)! No wonder his temperament is as gentle as a sack of gravel! Even when he stares silently at the other person, one can see the rage rising in him, coating his throat with bile. This limited mask is the whole ego; there is nothing behind the mask. The person *is* the mask! This sets the tone for *Nux-vomica's* approach to the world, which is driven by his cyber delusion. *Nux-v* has many delusions (44 of them!), but the central idea is expressed by different delusions with the same meaning (one of the criteria for calling it a cyber delusion). We can therefore accept that the *Delusion, someone is in bed with him*—intolerance and hatred for competition—is the prime motivation for his limited attitude towards the world. The pursuit of goods has become an end itself, and in such a person, tending to his livelihood overshadows his life. When he deals with business, he knows how to get ahead, how to manipulate others. But when it comes to the question of living, he is weak and even less than half-awake!

The more he focuses on a materialistic pathway to happiness, the less happy he tends to be and the less happy he makes others. His "being," how important he is in his eyes and in others, his "happiness," is based on what and how much he *has*. But anyone who seeks happiness in acquisitions is doomed to disappointment (*Ailments from disappointment; anxiety about business*), as hedonic pleasures have limited staying power. Therefore, *Nux-v* indeed has the delusion that he realizes an authentic life, but in order to truly be authentic, *Nux-v* must learn to set aside pleasure-seeking well-being—the shallow, short-lived pleasure he gets from acquiring things—in favor of a deeper, more meaningful state in which gratification is not usually immediate. This way, he will not blame others or get defensive (from his conscious rationalism and counter-position in his unconscious) when he meets with less success then he had hoped for (*anger about his mistakes; anger so he could have stabbed someone; being beside himself; reproaches others; rudeness*).

Too late in life, *Nux-v* learns what he must do to be healthy: avoid excessive violent and unpleasant emotions (*anger with red face; exaggerated anxiety*), avoid mental overstrain, and take daily exercise in the open air (*businessman, worn out*). Without proper daily exercise, no one can remain healthy. Aristotle said aptly, "Life begins in movement," as this assures the ceaseless motion of each individual part in man: the heart, the lungs, the intestines, the glands, the arteries and capillaries. All are moved by our Vital Force to keep us healthy and alive and prevent internal tumult; internal motion is supported by external motion. Burnout—emotional exhaustion, physical fatigue, and cognitive weariness—will set in if our job is too stressful or intense or, as in the case of *Nux-v*, when he has been experiencing its fervor too long and excessively. The destructive power of burnout is unforgiving. It leads to stomach ulcers, recurrent myocardial infarction and apoplexy, increase of coronary atherosclerosis, and yes, death. Sleep deprivation and physical exhaustion are at the root of his demise (*sleeplessness from cares of business*)! This is the price he pays for his "religious" dogmatism regarding ambition, which is nothing but an intellectual superstition. Feelings in this extravert thinking type are not absent, but as they are introverted, they do not flow to the object. A woman could live her entire life with this thinking extravert and never hear him say, "I love you!" His real "love" is autoerotic, he loves everything about himself. This inferior infantile feeling is also the argument and justification for him to drop bombs and destroy buildings when another country does not blindly follow his policies, as he is a sort of imperialist (*anger from contradiction; destructiveness*). And often when such a person is dying—even when he only had interest before to gain more outwardly (power and riches), not inwardly—as a result of a sudden eruption of inferior function, he converts to a religion for salvation (*very religious; despair about religious salvation*). Besides *Nux-v*, *Lycopodium*, *Causticum*, and some *Sulphur* people, men are found chiefly in this type. They belong to the Liver type in TCM, dominated by emotions such as frustration, anger, and suppressed anger and have a choleric temperament.

The Extraverted Feeling Type with Inferior Introverted Thinking (*Puls; Pall*)

Eros takes a front seat in this type, as this person is overly concerned with relationships to others, to the point that approval of others is a guideline for his life (*longing for good opinion of others; Delusion, she is not appreciated; Del, he is forsaken by friends and family*). If appreciation is not forthcoming, self-worth and confidence are at a lifetime low and can only be restored somewhat by continuous sustained praise, difficult to come by for anyone. *Palladium* and *Pulsatilla* come to mind! An inferior introverted thinking is their compensation: they are afraid of offending others if they voice an opinion that might be contrary to someone's feelings (*Delusion, he has offended others*), or differs from the general universal feeling about the object. If a Picasso painting is generally considered "a work of art and value," then the extraverted feeling type will agree, even if deep down he is horrified by the abstraction of the work. Going to church every Sunday, occasionally visiting the opera, and dressing according to the present fashions provide comfort to this type. This comes at the cost of individuality, as mixing with the masses is a "positive" refuge and provides the stamp of being a "decent and good person," admired and loved by everyone—the thing she wants the most.

Unknowingly, she (most of these types are women) is nothing but a great actor, as she loves a certain painting or book not because it truly speaks to her heart, but because it appeals to the masses—in other words to her archaic mind. Don't expect this type to be a philosopher. Asking deep questions about life is something she considers melancholic and overthinking, to be avoided, so her thought process remains infantile, primitive, and crackpot like. Such a woman is also guided in her choice of husband by "he is decent, the right age, is a good provider, and wants children," leading to reasonable unions providing she does not visit her archaic introverted thinking function. Not that she cannot think, but she does not allow her thinking to disturb her distorted feelings, or rather those opinions generally accepted by the masses (*credulous*). After all, the latter are *the* guidelines in life. She fears the destructive effect of negative thoughts about the vicissitudes of life, as she equates them to black magic (*exaggerated anxiety; anxiety on going to sleep*).

Obviously, life is full of ups and downs, and this type only responds to them by presenting a multiple personality, so easily is she overwhelmed by moods (*moods, changeable, variable*). It is not rare that she lands in a continual struggle to gain approval of others, as these mood swings evoke doubt in others. How can we take such a person seriously? She hops from one opinion to another if the situation is even minimally changed and changes objective values following her different feeling states (*hysteria, changing symptoms*). When control of the superior function fails (extraverted feeling), negative critical thinking about others comes out, as this coarse function is not differentiated enough to let her mind wander over questions about the meaning of life. Such a quest she almost never pursued. Her fragile ego with a slavish infantile thinking function (*childish behavior; desires to be carried, fondled and caressed*) has the appearance of being in danger of constant dissociation or depreciation of her person (*lack of self-confidence, sense of depreciation*), a voice that whispers for a few moments that her "life amounts to nothing." She flees instantaneously from such dark thoughts by meeting people, phoning a good friend, or keeping herself busy with a banal task that defies thinking (*company, desire for; aversion to solitude, company ameliorates; Del, doing business*), as it is the oil that keeps her car lubricated. This type belongs to the Earth type in TCM, with a predominance of worries about the past and present.

The Extraverted Sensation Type with Inferior Introverted Intuition (*Calc-c*)

Calc-c is the prototype of this character. Rationalism is the religion he adheres to, but unknowingly he is at the mercy of sensation. He will use his five senses to know that something *is*: that something is real, and these concrete facts bring him comfort and peace of mind. Such an extravert sensation type rests secure on facts, solid rocks on which he stands, as he always has both feet planted on earth. Food banquets and parties are high on his list as he remains the child forever, which in many people's eyes make him a pleasant, jolly fellow, easy to like, but not interested in penetrating the soul of others. He has a desire for crude, immediate satisfaction perceived through the senses only—anything that can enhance his sensations. Extravert means that the stimuli must come from the outside, while those from the inside are not trustworthy. His main enemy, and compensation function, is the introverted intuition function, a crazy world full of mysteries and extrasensory perceptions with no place for reflection. He wanders along at about the same speed mud oozes down a hill and with about as much purpose. It is interesting to note that this leads to negative intuitions about himself projected onto others (*Delusion, there are conspiracies against him; Delusion, confusion, others will observe him*), and delusions of reference, which are gross misjudgments of any small circumstance, gestures or words, or perceived situations (*Delusion, he is persecuted*). When someone with delusions of reference meets with a mishap, he immediately jumps to the conclusion that he has been deliberately injured, insulted, or treated maliciously. *Calc-carb's* inferior intuitive side leads to the creation of unknown primitive possibilities, which leads to a deficiency of energy and increased worry for the unknown (*Del, of having anything happen; Del, about to sink into annihilation; Del, of incurable disease; Del, being sick,* and *despair of recovery*). If he is not overcome by his egocentric inferior intuition, jealousy and anxieties about his health (*anxiety, mania to read medical books*)—leading to brutality and coarse behavior (*jealousy, brutal, driving to strike his wife*)—he can be a good mechanic, accountant, mountaineer, or artist, due to his eye for detail (*conscientious about trifles*).

We have only to think how calcium carbonate makes nice coral reefs and provides a home for thousands of fish. Speak of inertia! The idea of inertness comes often sooner than later to *Calc-c*, as it is part of his innate character. In other words, it can set in *before* depression starts. Inertia is one of the greatest enemies of conscious choice. *Calc-c* is a person who tends to receive things from the outside, not being very productive on his own or paying attention to what comes from the inside. He is a good poised listener (can be an excellent psychotherapist), but his talent lies in receiving ideas, not in producing new ones. *Calcarea* always expects everything from an outside source, even in religion: God is the almighty protector (*religious affections, in children; religious affections, alternating with metaphysical concerns* [*black type, only remedy*]; *religious affections in puberty*) from whom he expects everything; it does not occur to him to put forth effort. Faith allays *Calc-carb's* deepest fears and mitigates unbearable losses (*religious affections; wants to read the Bible all day long*). He is always searching for the magic helper as found in fables and the dream world that he likes so much. He has many friends simply because he needs many hands to feel secure, so he has a hard time saying "no." He loves to say "yes" to everything and everyone, resulting in a paralytic mind unable to make decisions (*irresolution*), which makes him increasingly dependent on others. He belongs to the Earth element in TCM, dominated by worries about the past and future, leading to gastrointestinal illnesses and diabetes.

The Extraverted Intuitive Type with Inferior Introverted Sensation (*Phos*)

In view of her compensation repressed function, introvert sensation, this intuitive type—although oriented by the object and only concerned with externals—will be overwhelmed by the hard, unaltered facts of life as reality is her greatest nemesis. To her, there is nothing more disconcerting than stable conditions, which is like being fenced in, locked up in a prison from which she needs to escape at all cost. Unfortunately, it is also the person trapped in this function who forgets to live in the *now*, always being caught in obsessions about the future. She is constantly pursuing the future, bored with anything that is past. The question always lurks: "What possibilities do I have? Is there anything new in the making? Is there anything more exciting tomorrow? Can I think of another animating trip in this world?" We can recognize some of the *Phosphorus* personalities in this type, who with their changeable tubercular character can be good beginners, but often become distracted, bad finishers. This type belongs to the Fire element in TCM, and therefore a new career, or a new topic might stir up an enormous fire in her soul, only to be abandoned a few weeks later, without leaving the slightest trace in her mind of its existence (*capricious; undertakes things opposed to her intentions*). What at first appeared as the "promised land" has changed into a prison, from which she wants to break out. Stability is not part of this type's make-up. She is fired up and guided by new adventures or speculative prepositions, not sound judgments, and is often called naïve, adventurous, foolish, and biased, but no reason or feeling or argument can convince her of the foolishness of these new possibilities, so great is the power of her extraverted intuition (*desire, for numerous various things; exaltation of fancies; excitable; discontented; exhilaration; fancies preventing sleep*). Sensation and thinking, which she so desperately needs to bring her life in balance, remain in the unconscious, not able to temper the power of her extraverted intuition (*chaotic, confused behavior*).

She is the one to consult about something that is not known yet, or when stuck in a situation where the other conscious functions cannot find a way out, as she might have a fine nose for an investment or an uncharacteristic solution since her extrasensory perceptions are her forte (*clairvoyance*). Since her nemesis is introverted sensation, it is not rare that such a *Phosphorus* person overestimates her strengths and misjudges her limitations, leading to failures in her speculations and burnout in her health (*aggravates from mental and physical exertion; prostration of mind, brain fag*). She resembles Icarus who wants to fly high in the sky but forgets that the wax will melt under the heat of the sun (*Delusions, floating in the air*). Always led by too much expectancy and visions directed at external objects—which makes it looks like she is using sensation—her adventurous forays are a hit or miss, although this will not necessarily stop her from looking at the next hidden, partly unknown treasure to be pursued. "Possibilities, possibilities" is the name of the game (*desire for numerous various things*) to which everything else needs to be sacrificed, and as much empathy as she has for others, in submitting to the authority of her intuitive quests she can forget to be considerate of others (*indifferent to others; to loved ones; escapes from her family and children*). There is always a readiness to fall in love due to her innate sympathy for others (*desires for sympathy and compassion*). She can be a mixture of saint and sinner, and as a result, she more than once changes husbands and can be credited for several marriages.

She has an inordinate passion for pleasure and travel which is the secret of remaining young, with a strong conviction of having a long palmar crease, promising a long and turbulent life. While she is always interested in having her fortune told (*likes to be mesmerized*), hearing possible misfortunes are messages immediately swept away from her exuberant existence like a fly caught in the force of a gale. She is a cheerful person who emits cheerfulness without design or even consciousness, spreading it all over the place. The contrast with another person is like comparing a rock along the roadside with a jewel. She might fall in love with her "soul mate," only because she finds in him the right social connections to advance, but does not hesitate to leave him for new, more exciting prospects. In her make-up there is no split between the "inside" (character, intellect) and the "outside" (looks). She is charming and possesses an intoxicating, beguiling quality to many men she encounters. She can inspire and convey affection with such ease that few ever notice being charmed. Male or female, old and young, rich and poor, she envelops them all. She loves to laugh and to listen with deep sincerity and rapt curiosity.

Although this type is mainly found in women, men among this type are found in the speculators, risk takers, stockbrokers, financial advisors, motivational speakers, and entrepreneurs in the new dot-com companies. Driven by their strong intuition and unbridled enthusiasm, easily kindling excitement in others, their ego becomes one with all prospects and they embody their vision, at least temporarily. Tomorrow might be another thing! But fate will tell, and they accept it. We can imagine how a sensation type would react to this incertitude! For him, only people who wait for the fruit on the tree they planted can benefit greatly, while the extravert intuitive is already off racing to another unknown place to plant a seed for a new tree, often leaving him without rewards (*impertinence; inconstancy*). And as much as he is convinced that he is not a prisoner of rational judgment, by repressing real sensations he can fall victim to compulsions in which a man marries a woman who possesses his archaic soul or anima, a totally unsuitable woman, and vice versa for a woman. The repressed sensation function can take its vengeance with phobias and absurd bodily sensations (*Delusion, sees faces when he turns his eyes; Del, sees something coming out of the corners; Del, fingers are thumbs; fear of impending disease; fear of death; fear of imaginary things*).

The Introverted Thinking Type with Inferior Extraverted Feeling (*Sulph*)

Here we meet the ragged philosopher, the *Sulphur* type, with his love for religious and philosophical conversations (*religious delusions; naïve but very intelligent; ability for philosophy; dwells on religious speculations*) as his thinking is directed inwards. He can be an original thinker and philosopher, but tends to become too erudite, so to many he becomes incomprehensible and pedantic to a fault, as he is mainly concerned with his ideas (*ideas abundant, clearness of mind*). He can spin many beautiful, convoluted theories (*theorizing; thoughts intrude and crowd around each other*). Of course his nemesis and compensatory function is extraverted feeling, so he is prone to misjudgments and callously disregards feelings of others when their opinion does not fit in with his magical, spun theory based on objectivity and inner contemplation (*egotism, self-*

esteem; intolerant of contradiction). He also expects his theory to fall into the midst of society and to thrive and be accepted by everyone without criticism, although he himself is *censorious* and will retort with the sharpest tongue against the slightest criticism of his ideas, to the extent that criticism becomes contempt. This type can be a male chauvinist, which until recently was relatively unproblematic in Western society. Often, he thinks that women should be educated not for work but just to be interesting to men and to have something to fall back on if their husbands should die young or turn out to be unreliable.

Another area of insensitivity for *Sulphur* is sexuality: his selfishness and self-centeredness are at their height when he claims that the sex in his relationship is great, having no clue that his partner is climbing the walls (*A/F sexual excesses*). With a tendency to hypoglycemic headaches with annoying irritability in the morning (*aggravation 11 a.m.*), he usually shovels food into his wide-open mouth. When his wife makes pancakes for them both, he has wolfed down his half before she finishes cooking them. As his wife is about to sit down and join him, he gets up to leave because he has finished eating. This is a typical display of *Sulphur* insensitivity; his wife hopes that sharing a meal might be a little more of a social event, but he does not notice, he has other things on his mind. As intelligent as *Sulphur* is, he could increase his love for humankind, if he would consider that the highest form of human intelligence is the ability to observe without judging others (*censorial*), which would keep his provocative thoughts in a positive light rather than becoming destructive, mingled with bitterness, volatility and disdain (*fanaticism; abusive; ardent*). Insensitivity (not in his own eyes, but in others') can be his hallmark. This introverted thinking type never hesitates to pursue his creative passions and recognition for fame, justice, and other mind-boggling pursuits while his partner will be left to deal with the colorless practical necessities of life—children, house-related obligations, taxes, etc.

With single-minded determination, he excels in his capacity for enjoying intellectual pleasures when healthy and balanced (*easy comprehension and active concentration; ability for philosophy*), which are available to him on many levels, from the simplest *jesting* (although *he cannot take a joke)* and conversation to the highest achievements of the mind. His witty conversations signal intelligence and creativity. Independence of spirit is a hallmark of the *Sulphur* person as he writes and speaks with little respect for authority, detesting the hollow conformism that he finds in society in general. Being notoriously disdainful of authority, during his studies *Sulphur* conspicuously avoids attaching himself to any single mentor just to preserve his independence. He may become almost identical to this type (that is, his ego may come to identify with it) in his older days when he becomes a hermit (*discontented with everything; company, aversion to the presence of other people, ameliorated when alone; cannot bear anybody*). What accompanies him in his self-imposed solitude is what a man is by himself. Having become an introvert, he easily reaps secret joy from his solitary life. He simply prefers traveling through his own interior universe (*independent; indifference to the welfare of others*). He has become the ultimate individualist, so his wish for solitude evolves naturally and inevitably. When entirely alone, he is entertained by his own thoughts, no longer having to rely on the diversity of various people, boring conversations, or fleeting amusements.

A life of retirement and solitude for *Sulphur* has a beneficial influence on his peace of mind, for he escapes living in the sight of others, no longer forced to politely heed the annoying casual opinions and conversations unbearable to him during his productive life (*impatience; irritable when spoken to*). Relationships to things and people have become secondary, and he cares less how his theorizing links up with the real world. Love of solitude, for *Sulphur*, is the result of experience and reflection, both of which have increased with the years. And even if his life's work goes virtually unnoticed during his lifetime (Schopenhauer comes to mind), he is not one to think that the world is right and that he has been wrong. He is convinced until his dying day of the supreme value of his work, certain that it will have an everlasting and beneficial effect on mankind. He was never in a holding pattern, between a sick person and a healthy, happy immortal being among the common people. He was always that *Sulphur* who entertained everywhere with his wonderful eloquence, at least in his mind. Even at the end of his life, when the curtain falls, he gladly looks back on what he has done and bows for the last time, undaunted by what others may say and who might look upon him as an unapproachable, antisocial, and arrogant individual. While he loves teaching to demonstrate his erudition, he can become cumbersome and stray from the "line" as he is less concerned with the content of what he teaches than the way he presents his material. In TCM he belongs to the choleric Liver type, with frustration, anger, and strong drive as main emotions.

The Introverted Feeling Type with Inferior Extraverted Thinking (*Nat-m*)

A perfect example of this type is *Nat-m*, especially in its later stage after many *Ailments from grief and deception*. This deception is also felt as *a loss of honor*, and for a *Nat-m* person, loss of honor brings shame greater and more threatening than any other kind. The loss of face, the overwhelming humiliation, and the derision of others are like daggers in her heart. There is no statute of limitations on the hurt and anger that follows a partner's affair. Her life is full of gaps of unimproved feeling, for example hatred that should have been over for years (*hatred to those who have offended*). Because of *old disappointments*, the

Nat-m person is extremely sensitive to the slightest perceived grievance (*easily offended, takes everything in bad part; Ailments from being scorned*). Note the mention here of *old disappointments*: this sets the tone for *Nat-m*. As salt preserves everything, the *Nat-m* person seems to preserve all her feelings (*thoughts persistent, haunted by unpleasant subject* and *tormenting thoughts*), in a permanent relationship with the grudges she holds. As much as she is depressed and aggravated by the many slights and deceptions that befall her, she remains reluctant to bury her pain and move on (*disagreeable thoughts; dwells, recalls disagreeable memories*).

Even when small effective doses of *Nat-m* are introduced, such a patient still rebels against the threat to her protective psychic armor, the fortress she has constructed for such a long time. She holds on to her hard, protective wall, notwithstanding the great forfeiture of joie de vivre this entails. Anger, *suppressed* and *with silent grief*, will often surface. The proud grief that remained silent is often the killer of the soul. Here we see the nervous temperament of *Nat-m*, not the choleric or sanguine temperament, because most of the pain is held in. Anger is, of course, a cover for fear, the latter much more damaging to the ego; therefore, the displacement is ideal when confronted with the *fear of men* or the fear of what men can do to her (*deception causing grief and mortification*). *Nat-m* is an introvert feeling type, but, as we see, it brews a storm for which the offending party will pay with damnation (*hatred to those who have offended; hatred and revenge; aversion to men*). It does not help that the offending party steels himself to apologize; even if he was fully justified in his original behavior, *Nat-m* will hear nothing of an apology! Hate is the eternal negation. Considered from the context of the emotions, it is a form of atrophy: it kills everything but itself. Hatred that is one-sided and not expressed can lead to destructive violence (*violent and vehement at trifles*) as well as unhappy love (*love, disappointed, from sadness with silent grief*), unsatisfied neediness, and a sense of rejection (*offended easily; takes everything in bad part*).

As she feels she has been injured in the past, she is now *easily offended* by innocent remarks. It is as though she is convinced that everyone knows about her suffering and that people are out to hurt her. Such paranoia leads, again, to isolation—which only exacerbates her suffering and her incapability to reach out to others. The cave to which she wants to withdraw is called despair, and the ground is paved with the gravestones of abandoned hope (*despair about the future; despair with the pains* [emotional]; and *despair, thinks everything is lost* [*Ignatia!*]). At this point, *Nat-m* removes herself from humanity and real life, forgetting that there is no prison into which love cannot find an entrance. She forgets that when we grieve, we don't have to turn into cold marble. The most terrible thing about a broken heart is not that one's heart can be broken—hearts are made to be broken—but that in *Nat-mur's* case, grief and deception turns her heart to stone. Establishing closeness with future partners becomes very difficult (*aversion to family members; to husband; to men; to the opposite sex*). She wears gloom as a king wears purple; she often swears never to smile again. Even more, these suppressed memory fragments (not repressed, which are deeper and entirely forgotten) remain in their primitive and childish state, and as such, they are still strong and immediate. Only when they are reintegrated into the adult consciousness (through therapy or homeopathy) can they shed their primitive aspect and be corrected. These infantile memories are like an avalanche, surprising *Nat-m* and those around her with their crude, violent nature. New delusions are now formed: *Delusion: talking with dead people; hears distant voices* and *voices of dead people; sees faces when stooping.* "Dead people" symbolize a regression to the unconscious: remaining in and withdrawing to the unconscious. The world of the living is left behind (*anthropophobia; avoids company*). Part of life is striving for a relationship, but that part is now dead. Relationships do take another form, one of nourishing *Nat-m's* soul through connection with a narrower segment of the world, that of her fellow sufferers, motivated not by injustice but more by *grief causing hatred.*

Nat-m measures time by throbs of pain, deceits and betrayals, and the recall of bitter moments (*dwells over past on past disagreeable events; recalls disagreeable memories*). The remembrance of her suffering is necessary to *Nat-m* as evidence of her continued existence. There is only a small light in the cave (there is always yang in the yin), and that small light is the symbol for the remaining connection she has: her kinship with those who have suffered similar fates. Her emotions are contained within, which tends to separate her from other people. Because her feeling function is held so intensely within, in the final stage of her *Nat-mur* state, she comes across as being as cold as the wastes of the North Pole, remote and difficult to approach. *Nat-mur's* only safety is to build a wall around herself (living in a cocoon) so that nobody can get near her, shielding herself from outside contact and never trusting anyone with her real thoughts and feelings. Because the inferiority of her extraverted thinking is visible in a certain intellectual *monomania*, the same few negative thoughts need to be repeated in her mind as they are the delusions that make life worthwhile. She does not realize that this inferior thinking can become unyielding and tyrannical (*thoughts persistent; haunted by unpleasant subjects*). *Nat-m* people seem shy and inarticulate, and they find communication difficult. At times this makes her appear paranoid and hysterical. Only homeopathic doses of *Nat-m* can break through the illusory wall that hems such a patient in; few from the outside world will ever be able to find the key to the quasi-invisible door to her world or reach the precious little oasis of reality in the desert of her soul. The walls of her sheltered, tight circle of security crumble when *Nat-m* can finally open her soul to the psychotherapist—whom, incidentally, at first she does not consider to be a real person, but more a fixture there to listen to her—to unload on as she rids herself of her garbage and the skeletons in her closet. Upon leaving the office, though, she goes back to her prison cell of self-isolation, which is now dutifully restored with brick and mortar to hide the temporary opening. In the end, her heart is as closed as a fist, at least towards most people (*company, aversion to presence of other people* and *desire for solitude*). In TCM she belongs to the Water type with a multitude of fears and anxieties.

The Introverted Sensation Type with Inferior Extraverted Intuition (*China*)

Sensation by itself is of course dependent on the object considered. But also, being introverted, this type puts his own spin on the object, "the way he sees it" according to subjective perception, *making many plans at night.* If several painters of this type would all paint the same landscape, the outcome would always be different, not because they have different abilities but because they have different moods painting it, altering colors and forms according to their introverted personal state. Contrary to the extraverted sensation type, subjectivity triumphs over objectivity in this case, and the landscape is used to give expression to their inner personal psychic mood (*introspection*)! It is called artistic license. The sensation coming from the object to the artist was just the first step in perception, but was then "colored" according to what the artist felt subjectively, as he is *unobserving*, and *absorbed and buried in thoughts*, often leading to *mental exertion* and *using wrong words*. Otherwise, to the introverted sensation type, such a painting—although he can recognize the object—seems nothing like the landscape he sees, and he would find it defective and grossly, inaccurately represented. ("How could others see it this way?!") These are people, due to an increase of the unconscious, that seem entirely detached from external reality (*Delusions of fancy illusions; acute senses are blunted*), in almost a dreamy *Helleborus* state, in which one does not hear though hearing is intact, and in which one does not see though vision is perfectly all right (*Delusion, sees people on closing the eyes*). His *persistent ideas*, even a *rush of thoughts* (2), come mainly *during the night in bed* (2, *China only*), creating *sleeplessness before midnight from activity of thoughts* (2) as he spends much energy also upon fantasies of the future (*making many plans at night,* 2), and upon negative paranoid intuitions. Using inner interpretations of how he sees external reality make him appear bizarre, paranoid (*Del, he is persecuted; Del, he is hindered at work*), tending towards devaluating things, and suspicious. He can become an individual misunderstood by others, in as much as he does not understand himself (*chaotic, confused behavior*). As Jung said, "Such a type can easily make one question why one exists at all" (Jung, 1971, para. 650). Possessed by an abnormal sensitivity leading in *China* to an alternation of predominating melancholy with periodic fits of unrestrained liveliness, this type is prone to delusions of reference (*Delusion, he is hindered at work; he thinks he is very unfortunate and constantly harassed by enemies; fixed idea that he is unhappy*). He also puts his own spin on what he hears, as he is very *excitable after hearing horrible things*. His nemesis is extraverted archaic intuition, resulting not in a hunch for objective real possibilities, but rather a flair for the hidden and sordid in his surroundings, forcing compulsive ideas (OCD) of the most perverse kind (*fear of killing; gestures, grasping or reaching at something; foolish persistent thoughts at night*), leading to alcoholism (*dipsomania*) and *discontentment* as well as *discouragement* and *suicidal disposition although he lacks the courage.* With her wounded soul and *suspicious* nature, *China* will test people to see on which side they are. Each question of the homeopath is initially perceived as a threat, even as an insult, from which the patient needs to protect herself (*suspicious; Delusion, of vexations and offences*). For such a patient, this will only lead to a road of *despair with the pains; lamenting;* and *Delusions, of being forsaken. China*, with her strong emotional antennae, rather likes intense and deep, probing conversations, not superficial chit-chat. Abstract art, creative writing, painting, and poems are positive tools to escape her troubles, but often isolate her even more as she appears eccentric.

The Introverted Intuitive Type with Inferior Extraverted Sensation (*Lach*)

The introverted intuitive type is an individual bound to the unconscious with visions and perceptions of images (archetypes) belonging to the collective unconscious, often products of an inaccessible nature, releasing a torrent of strange contents disconnected from the natural occurring sensation characteristics. Every detail of the visions is explored with great interest by this type, as if the person uses his senses to see in detail these inner images, until the whole vision fades. She is truly the intuitive who remains detached from these images as if they do not belong to her (inferior extraverted sensation). This lack of guidance by objective stimuli (*senses dull, blunted; senses vanishing off*) and restless changeability (*restlessness, driving about; delirium, changing subjects rapidly*) are common to the introvert intuitive type: internal perception has become equal to "sensation," a useful tool for a creative artist but not helpful at first for an ordinary individual. Of course, they are the great *clairvoyants* prophesying future realities, who through powerful feelings of foreboding can foresee events which then happen (*prophesying; presentiment; trance*). They are like human seismographs that have bodily sensations ahead of important or emotional events, not unlike twins who say that they feel each other's pain even when they are hundreds of miles apart. They can be the creative artist and poet, who has *excitement and liveliness in the evening, a kind of fanciful imagination; he sits up late at night at work, with great activity; he is impelled to productive work in the evening*. But in general this introverted type, possessed by the details of his inner experience (*increased activity of fancy; scenes and occurrences throng to him in an unusual amount*), has little desire to express himself (*talks only when alone*), as his discourse is of a fragmentary character—projecting aloofness, lack of sympathy and warmth to others—making him misunderstood and unappreciated in general (*impatient; desires positive answers when this is not practicable; contentious so that he quarrels with everything about him; raging about trifles*). Who but a patient and inner-oriented friend will have the composure to listen to him! But what is unfamiliar tends to be inadmissible and is therefore not accepted, and these types are regarded as persons who are suffering from inflation, having left earth and are hovering in the sky (*Delusion, floating in the air; Delusion, body is lighter than air*). Through his intuitive function, this type taps into the unconscious, even to the extent that he feels guided by a godlike figure through whom his inspiration comes. Sometimes delusions of grandeur, of omnipotence, and of being possessed are the result: *Delusion, he is charmed and cannot break the spell; Delusion, he is under a powerful influence* and *Delusion, in the hands of a strong power*. The *Lachesis* person does not even wake up while unloading the mass of accumulated ideas; he might use dreams to digest the unprocessed conscious material and create another "master work." What this type tries to express—although often with minimal success—are his inner perceptions in an understandable language, somewhat resembling the difficulty the homeopath encounters in the consultation room trying to translate the language of the patient into the rubrics and observations of the provings. But this individual, if remaining infatuated and intoxicated by inner visions, has a hard life in front of him, dictated by a fate of his own making and shortcomings, convinced he possesses remarkable talents (*Delusion, he is under superhuman control; Del, of fancy illusions; Del, in the hands of a strong power*). Depending on the progression of the *Lachesis* state, the vacuum created in the ego continues to grow, while the well-functioning sectors of the ego become narrower and narrower. And yet, he can teach us to turn inward at appropriate times, to be one with silence and introspection, to listen to the voice of the unconscious (*meditation*). We must learn from the actions of this individual—propelled by the perception of a treasure of inner visions—rather than being captured by the verbosity and gifts of gab of an everyday society. The former is an education far superior than what is thought.

The previous chapters have been devoted to an understanding of the ego, the persona, and the four conscious functions according to Jung. It is time now to explore the most hidden part of humankind: the unconscious giants, for most buried in a tomb, growing minute by minute.

SECTION THREE

Elements of the Personal and Collective Unconscious

9

THE PERSONAL AND COLLECTIVE UNCONSCIOUS: THE BURIED GIANTS AND UNEXPECTED POWERFUL OCCUPANTS

"He who has learned aright about the signs that come in sleep will find that they have an important influence over all things."
— Hippocrates

It's What You Do in the Dark that Will Put You in the Light: The Agonizing Battle Between the Conscious and Subconscious Mind

Looking at history, follow the dictum: *Si vis pacem, para bellum* (If you want peace, prepare for war). Man believes that he needs just one more war to end war, while really any war reduces the individual to worthlessness. Although Horace in his *Satires* claims, "A wise man in times of peace prepares for war," peace is on man's lips, but war is in his heart. Wars demonstrate the impotence of human restraint and arrangements in the force of overwhelming passion. Consequently—as shown in this world —our attitude is centered upon finding means to protect ourselves and knowing how to proceed to conquer the enemy, while deliberating to go fight them on their territory or to secretly undermine their government.

Instead of a war acting outward, less known is the one acting inside and against us, often more destructive because of its hidden venom (representing our Trojan horse). While our attention is focused on the above musings, we pay no attention to the internal war within us—a horrible discord—one that brings more havoc to our daily life than the ubiquitous battle rattle in the world. The enemy, whose presence requires constant vigilance, is located within, what Rousseau called *une âme déchiréé*, "a torn or shattered heart," a solid base for a permanent state of war.

We need to have an exclusive interest in our inner Self, a discovery of our internal life. The war within should give us the opportunity to progress as humans, to stir our passion, to prod us to develop our capacities to the fullest. Above all, we must go *down*, go "inside." Our conscious is concentrated on the outward aspect, but the underworld within shows us how it is *in us*, down there. The war inside often inflicts on the Self many, sometimes ineffaceable, wounds—even decay of the soul—reducing our capacities in life if we are not able to expel them from our spirit, finally disrupting the whole of our future personality. I truly believe in pacifism because I consider it a sound philosophical doctrine that should rule humanity. But pacifism is ruled by reasons which have very little to do with human action, as emotions are the moving forces among humans, waking up the most basic animal instincts leading to automatic reactions.

In fighting the war within, it does not suffice to become a soldier, as a soldier *is told what to do*, which does not necessarily contribute to building up an improved Self. In order to succeed, one must become a *warrior*, as a warrior *knows what to do* when listening to his inner voice and ripping off his mask. For a soldier—before the battle is joined—plans are everything, but once the battle begins, plans are often worthless as the enemy's reaction cannot be predicted. Planning, for the soldier, is just guesswork. A warrior on the other hand will be guided by his moral code and a flexible attitude according to how the battle unfolds, so he can avoid simple mistakes leading to deadly endings. A warrior is born with a natural insouciance and strong nerve born of implicit moral reserves, so even in great danger he is calm and apparently indifferent, never lacking the courage needed to face great danger and vicissitudes of battle. The person in discovery of his underworld, his dark world, should be warned that he must travel through a country possessed by numerous powerful and warlike savages of gigantic stature, fierce and autocratic, treacherous, cruel, and hostile. The warrior has therefore to possess a determined and resolute character to accomplish this mandatory excursion, dispelling every notion of fear, not daunted by the battle but drawn to it, eager to discover what he will to advance his conscious life.

The war we face within—the descent into the unconscious —is no mere expedition to explore newly regained territory. It is always a military expedition into at first a hostile and repugnant territory, until it has been conquered and integrated piece by piece. Among the less successful fighters, we find some with a highly-strung temperament and more animalistic responses resulting in obvious nervousness, often leading to a reaction like a powerful tiger caught in a trap, angry and afraid. We should contemplate and study our own becoming, to discover the gravity of the struggle for self-birth that we have to wage on ourselves and our fate, a road rife with fluctuations and hollow victories beside moments of real joy and all-too-quickly-fading, boisterous conquests. Our internal war is not a single battle, but rather a series of momentary engagements, none of which determine our legacy. But with each conflict—providing it is no Pyrrhus victory, one tantamount to defeat—steps to enlightenment of the Self are achieved. Rather than viewing such steps forward with astonishment and delight—temporarily reaping a beautiful harvest of pride and joy, celebrated by a quickly erected monument—we must now be more resolved to not fall into the next trap set forth by the fickleness of ever-changing life events and the autonomous power of the unconscious seeking a tighter rein over the Self.

When diving into the unconscious, will our mind become unhinged and shattered, creating a neurosis, or worse, a fugue dissociation or a real one? Exploration does not need to lead to this dangerous loss of control if we collect with a cool mind the information obtained and process it in a positive way. Is this a journey into a bottomless abyss, or is it an exploration in the utopian "land of milk and honey"? The choice is ours: the unconscious either becomes the visible or invisible front—a choice with great consequences. This integration of dark hidden elements leads to an eruption of freedom, independence, power, and divinity. The elucidation process resembles the sensation we feel after climbing a misty mountain, when upon reaching the summit the mist suddenly clears and a magnificent view is visible for many miles in all directions. Enhanced visibility of the mind results in ever-extending enlightenment and freedom; invisibility guarantees imprisonment in the dark forces. How to counter the strategy of error?

It should be clear to anyone: the way is the strategy of truth, courage, and willingness to expose the dark aspects of the grounds within that confuse and conquer the Self to create a pseudo Self. We need not only be honest in this war on perpetuated lies and delusions roaming in our unconscious, but to be wise. Otherwise the Self will be a monument to the strategy of error. Most don't believe in this internal war, and consequently think misfortunes in life are caused by fate rather than by a lack of introspection and correct choices in life. We can be like fishermen and every day go out upon the sea and throw our net into the water, but if glued to an unbalanced persona we catch nothing, for there is always a wind blowing from the land and rough waves rising up to meet us.

The unconscious needs to be like a waterfall, perpetually moving to try to create homeostasis as integration takes place, rather than resembling a frozen sheet, hanging motionless in the air after the Ice King has kissed it, resulting in stagnation. Such stagnation is cruel to those who sleep in her arms; it can cause a being to change into nothingness. If we would only devote more time to the phenomena of internal emotional chaos and force ourselves to look in at the boiling crater of our own threatening volcano! The reason we need to take on this enterprise is that we do not know what we are going to discover—darkness or enlightenment. As we descend, we do not know what lies ahead. We are entering a heart of darkness—a desert-like landscape—strewn with sand dunes, thorns, fata morganas, and a few oases. If we are mentally committed, we will bring out our fullest talents. Alas! All too often we get entangled in a Gordian knot, an intractable problem that will recur and recreate us, forming a Self that is out of reach and more important, unknowable. Here is a dream of a woman that reflects the descent into the unconscious with a favorable result, although this plunge from the conscious to the unconscious appears dangerous at first.

Dream

I am together with three other unknown people—as far as I see, one woman and two men. We are climbing down a rocky hill, on a very small island. The rocks are not safe—often when one person has gone down a bit a rock falls, down into the sea. I let the others go first—but see that it becomes more and more difficult to go down and I feel sort of frightened (I worry if I can go down at all). In the end, there are no rocks left to go and one has to swim and take one of the little floating elements (I can't remember from what they are made of) to get around the corner, where something new starts which I cannot see yet. I manage and float and it feels good.

Analysis

Despite the perilous descent towards the unconscious (water) she brings up the courage to descend from this small island (conscious) on a slippery, rocky path (reflecting the obstacles in life to overcome). Although frightened, she persists and comes to the water (unconscious) where she finds a floating device to bring her to "something new" which she cannot see yet (she needs to dive, to go under the water to discover what she can find in the unconscious), but she is relaxed and feels good. It is a good lysis of this dream. The woman in the dream is her shadow, and the two unknown men represent her non-fused animus (in reality, she was a subservient person to her husband).

Are we aware of the inner war within ourselves? Can we make a choice?

War or Peace Within?

Most of us seem to be in a semi-*Helleborus* state: our vision is intact, yet we cannot see clearly into the "intelligible" world, the guiding and forceful component of life, the conscious. As Plato mentions in *The Republic*, "Man needs also light or illumination ... to obtain the power of knowing the Self" (Plato, 1955).

When will the sands of time shift? Noble and ignoble misfortunes make their owner sift through the debris of the Self's malfunction. Doing so can be wicked and dangerous, at moments inviting a measure of dread. Who is this Self that consciousness is unable or unwilling to acknowledge? Plato's *Phaedrus* expresses this battle between conscious and unconscious very well, in his allegory of the charioteer and the white and dark horse pulling the chariot (Plato, 2015). It is the continuous struggle in the ordinary collective man, between the light/conscious (white horse) and the dark hidden nature, between will and the dark animal instincts (black horse looking for its natural master, the shadow), between reason and desire, modesty and temperance. In *Phaedrus*, the horses are ill tempered, hardly yielding to whip and spur. This is a battle where the charioteer (the Self) is continually engaged on his journey to self-realization, while struggling with his horses, seeking a haven where he can live his life in the greatest happiness attainable. Should we annihilate the inferior dark steed? No! This goes against Nature, as good inevitably invites bad; they are always intertwined. Should we not, rather, *conquer* and *tame* the dark horse?

In his *Principles of Philosophy*, Descartes stated "*Cogito, ergo sum*": "I think, therefore I am" (Descartes, 1988). For some philosophers, however, "being" comes before "thinking." For example, Albert Camus (journalist, writer, and existentialist philosopher) reversed it to: "I am nothing, therefore I am free." But is it enough to sail our ship through life? We think we lead when we are in fact being led by our unconscious. Our conscious seeks one goal, while the unconscious imperceptibly draws us towards another. Light is always necessary to life; we hope more than a sunbeam crosses the pane to illuminate the dimness of our life.

Profound acceptance, rather than struggling like a trapped bird—immersed in some degree of depersonalization or detachment from the Self—is the key to glue the two worlds together to form a better Self by integrating the newly discovered elements of this vast hidden world. And rather than the end, it becomes the beginning of something in ourselves, unknown to that point, a miracle of what our world can be. This individuation process is usually a slow process with ups and downs, often resembling an elevator with many stops in a 50-level hotel, where the slow-moving lift makes little sound beyond a rumble. When the door opens to the consciousness—an apprenticeship in elucidation—there is a sudden expansion of the world, analogous to the sudden encounter with sunlight and fresh air when coming out of a cave, when you are met by an inexpressible fullness of immense luminosity. But first we must go down into our dark world!

When to start this investigation? Do we wait till we experience a loss of identity? Do we risk becoming a stranger to ourselves? Do we look in the distance and find ourselves to be a vague silhouette, an object lost in the fog? Do we take a deep breath, and take a step back in order to jump better into a world where we don't know what we will encounter—tempests, storms, or dormant calm water—reflecting the recollections of past deeds? Upon descending into the dark tomb, invisible traps are placed here and there, waiting for us as we look for the truth in ourselves. We should hope we are awake in that old dusty room, when bathed in sweat, exhausted, and fully aware of the gravity, although familiarity surrounds us: the cobwebs we spun every day for years are left unbroken, because treading lightly in the unconscious was our savior. This room contains undisclosed memories of catastrophes, like the smell of sulfur after an explosion, ancient things that never gave up the secretive attitude fiercely guarded by impassivity. We may be stupefied by the view of these well-guarded secrets, and often at that instant feel unforgettable moments of fear whistling through our spinal cord.

That this process of individuation and the formation of a new Self is always a struggle is experienced in the following dream.

Dream of a 50-year-old man

I am walking in a street and I heard from friends that there was a party in a new apartment building. I am walking by myself to this building that was still not finished. When I stand in front of the building, I see that it was built in two parts as the middle of this building was still open, a level that was completely open and unfinished. The party was supposed to be in this space. I find it dangerous to have a party in such a place, but I enter the building anyway, but I never arrive at that level where the party takes place. I arrive in another place in this building, a place where no one had lived so far, as I see all kinds of building material on that floor. I never hear any music, nor do I see anyone else. I walk a little around and I hear noises and see several rough types (6-8 men) looking for me. I hide because I can see they have no good intentions. I become very fearful, and as I am in the back of the building I try to sneak up to the front. At this point I realize I have breathing problems. When I am at the entrance there are two portals, one in white and one in red, and above each portal hangs a digital clock counting the time. I try to run away but don't know where to. Then I wake up.

Analysis

Obviously the indicated remedy *started the process of individuation* as he sees a building (the Self) of which two parts (conscious and unconscious) are separated from an unfinished space, an emptiness, where a party should take place: it shows the gap between lower and higher parts of the Self, no time for celebration yet as it feels dangerous. The place where he arrived was part of the Self, going upwards to consciousness, but this is a place where a lot of material is present, though no job has been initiated. All the tools are there, but labor to reach higher consciousness must start. When he is there, he can't hear the music nor has he met anyone else (indeed there is still this gap where the party needs to take place). He is isolated (still in the unconscious but moving upwards). Then "rough males" appear, looking for him: the different suppressed facets of his shadow, the instinctual side of him too (drugs, alcohol). He was hiding in the back (unconscious) and slowly makes his way to the front (conscious) of the building and arrives at the portal (the border between conscious and unconscious). While he is doing this, he gets breathing problems (breath=energy/libido/soul strength), so apparently this is a difficult task for the dreamer to work his way up towards consciousness, integrating the suppressed side of his shadow. There are two portals or entries, one in white (symbol for consciousness/purity) and one in red (dark passions/unconscious/danger/blood/ violence, etc.) and each has a clock in progress counting the seconds passing. This indicates time to act, to make his choice of which portal to enter; to become more elucidated or stay in the dark, the danger zone. There is no lysis in this dream yet, but at least there is movement!

In conscious life, prudence and common sense seem to be the guiding forces to avoid madness and fateful choices. But it is undaunted courage, a whiff of lunacy, and the desire to seek truth that are needed for the descent into Dante's underworld. How to obtain this new improved Self?

A New Existence Waiting to be Born

Upon being asked the question, "Are you ready to visit the skeletons in your closet? Because sooner or later you must do it." "Oh yes," we say, "Show me the way!" With a burning desire to discover the dark side of our inner house, coupled to the request to become more whole, this idea is stuck in our head and spun frenetically, shredding our mesh of thoughts like the strands of a cobweb. But upon the first plunge, our heart tightens, and we immediately regret our previous, naive enthusiasm. Indeed, the rapture fades instantly upon experiencing the horrid sensation of annihilation, immobility, and loss of power when submerged in the turgid and wearying waters. In order to have courage, we need to have a certain amount of energy and willpower to overcome numerous terrifying discoveries. The collective human should spend many hours dangling a fishing line into the mysterious unfathomed depths—the unconscious —waiting for a bite, to be rewarded with a nourishing fish, the expansion of consciousness.

When will we respond to the ongoing invitation to delve into the unconscious instead of fleeing, repressing, and avoiding its urgent message? The sea (collective unconscious) can be a place of purification and renewal, as well as salvation, when we dive into the deep wreck of ourselves; when we glimpse the dark elements to be illuminated—also known as integration—and find a well-chosen moment here and there to acknowledge them, and to bring them into the light (like selecting tracks for an exciting playlist). Following the conscious choice to do so, the unconscious can either be nothing but quicksand, an abyss of darkness and the inside of a tomb, or becomes a cave with great treasure awaiting us, a field blossoming with helpful ideas and insights.

Some guidance from the unconscious is seen in the following dream belonging to a 64-year-old *Phosphorus* woman with a strong will, or animus. She had the dream on her birthday, which fell on a day just before spring, one day after a small dispute with her husband. Using her animus, she responded critically to a suggestion of her husband, but afterwards was insightful enough to realize that something in her reactions (personality) had to change, which she desired.

Dream

I have a very small plot in my garden, a square-like plot. Nearby I planted some lily of the valley, but to my despair none of the seeds took, except one on this nearby small square, where it was transported by the wind and grew into a strong plant and was just about to bloom. It was a very fragrant and beautiful plant to look at, and then shortly afterwards, it totally disappeared, eaten by ants. Then I saw a little spider on the place where the flowers would have bloomed. I became angry and wanted to kill it.

Analysis

Planting something in a garden refers to new potentialities to be achieved, changes that we want to happen. As she had this dream on her birthday, it referred to a "rebirth," the formation of a more complete Self. This desire for rebirth was confirmed by the kind of flower she was planting: a lily of the valley flower is a very fragrant (full of life) white flower—called the whitest flower on earth—blooming in the spring when everything comes to life after the winter, a rebirth of plants and light, helped also by the Wind (seasonal climate according to TCM) to spread the seeds around. White stands for innocence, purity—referring to the pure intent of the dreamer to investigate her unconscious in order to improve the Self. The little square represents the Self—the perfect Self, portrayed as in a mandala with its four gates, representing Jung's four conscious functions. Ants—a kind of insect—always stand for something "bugging" us, small irritations, stinging remarks and anxieties. Spiders often stand for the dependent emotions and conflicts we feel, "caught in a web," connected with family or trapped by an emotion, a basic survival instinct, initiating an action from the animus. Will I be eaten/destroyed by this relationship? The spider's level of sensory and feeling perception is extreme and important for its survival. The dreamer's reaction is anger, wanting to kill this spider, who prevented her from forming a new Self. A spider (as well as ants) hides or lives underground mainly (symbol of the unconscious) to wait for the right moment to kill its prey. Her anger also reflects her disappointment that this beautiful flower (the new Self) was not allowed to bloom yet. But at least an attempt was made (by investigation of the personal unconscious), which is positive—a message from this dream to continue the journey to self-actualization. The time to plant or the location was not right, as this dream occurred just before the real onset of spring.

Mishaps and misfortunes induced upon us by our wrong choices are unfortunately not the firm admonition which should bear fruit to guide the rest of our life. Do we remain blind, unable to know our whole universe, our Self? Will we miss the enlightenment that would steer our life to a happier road? Alas, for most, walking the path of self-realization is abhorred, as if it carries contagious disease. Is there no alternative between remaining quiet or landing in a raging storm?

The Discourse of the Other

Although ultimately the goal is illumination or help in reaching higher consciousness without succumbing to inflation, descending into the unconscious is a harrowing and suffocating experience, resembling a plunge into a prodigious storm of thunder and lightning accompanied by a deluge. As a mystical principle says, "The descent (*in the unconscious*) is for the sake of the ascent (*reaching consciousness*)," and, "The way to ascend unto God, is to descend into one's Self" (*author's additions in italics*). Usually the journey to heaven—the top of the pyramid of consciousness—is very far away, but hell (dark unconscious) can be reached in a day. And daily life in general, for most, illustrates how very close hell can be, as the condition of being asleep, or unaware, seems to be the condition of the average person. In order to become more complete, we must fall from our high mountains, down into the valleys.

For only the second time in my life (the first time was when I moved from Europe to the United States), I decided to consult the *I Ching* to resolve the sphinx-like question: "How to put ourselves on the right ladder rung to start the path to self-actualization?"

I threw the three coins six times with some trepidation, not being at all sure I would receive a clear answer. I drew hexagram #3, titled, "Difficulty at the Beginning." It said:

> This hexagram indicates the way in which heaven and earth bring forth individual beings. (*In other words, the reunion of the conscious and unconscious—author's note.*) The superior man . . . arranging and organizing the inchoate profusion of such times . . . to pause and take thought . . . to persevere and constantly keep the goal in sight. (Wilhelm, series XIX, 1977)

It would seem logical that we will be attracted to the mysterious in ourselves, but as soon as we work up our courage and start this discovery voyage and the descent to the unconscious, we are caught up in a whirlwind of mixed emotions, lifted up in the air and slammed down in the next moment, confused and bewildered, asking the unconscious, "Am I really the person you forcefully tell me I am?" That is the real power, when two opposites meet! As we descend into the unconscious, we do not know what to expect. Is the sea dormant or will it wake up? When we hear the roar of the storm, our heart beats like a bird's wings flapping in panic, and we become as powerless to slow down as the wind is to stop itself. Our heart reacts like a bird trapped inside the hall of a temple, looking for a way out. Heart rate goes up and down, like a cork on water, without ever settling down to where it is supposed to be. Metabolism is revved up. It is as if our heart tries to punch its way through our chest, and as if in a moment of collapse, we sink into a final depth, a surrender to the fear experienced when undergoing the voyage in the unconscious. The unconscious comes to the foreground like a raging chaotic river, and if we do not have an eye inward upon it, we will never discover that the greatest enemy threatening us is from within, not from without. We need to get our hands dirty in order to have a foundation to build upon; we need to accept the ugliness in ourselves to create a new, better Self. We need to walk the plank and make this mandatory dive.

Who, then, wants to continue the journey? Climbing Mount Everest seems to be an easier task, as descending into the unconscious is like being confronted with mountains of darkness, trapped in the prison of a body, or dropped in a jungle amidst hungry lions! Is it not more convenient—yes, pleasurable—to avoid the battle of life and continue to live dancing in the clouds (*Delusions of fancy illusions; Delusion, body is lighter than air*)? It appears that we all have a touch of disintegration and a mild form of schizophrenia. Is it not more expedient to claim that this dark world in us does not exist, and that our life resembles paradise filled with laughter, joy, love, and abundance, rather than being drawn into the hellish world of Lucifer with jealousy, hate, envy, and lust for power? As the latter world exists in all mankind—a part of the collective unconscious—we use our powerful personas to disguise ourselves daily, like a chameleon who changes appearance and color while doing little prancing steps. But then overconfidence, pride, and haughtiness take over, capsizing our vessel as it's overtaken by the sudden typhoon created by our ignorance and blindness for real life.

When will we be able to avoid the dread of nothingness, often apparent at the end of life when, looking back, one sees that an unbalanced Self was formed? When will we take our machete to hack a new path through the jungle of the unconscious (even if this new path is just a few feet away)? When will we realize the marauding force from the unconscious playing havoc in our conscious? Why do we not listen to our inner voice, as if we have plugs in our ears? As Socrates proclaimed, "An unexamined life is not worth living!" How to proceed?

Adapt Your Conscious Mind to the Suggestions of the Unconscious

The unconscious never sleeps but just waits for an opportune moment to take over the conscious or ego temporarily, imitating a kind of schizophrenia. We need to go up and down, going from the unconscious to the conscious, to bring dark elements up to the light. Often the birth and beginning of more consciousness can invite either feelings of inferiority or megalomania—not necessarily the blessings that we hope for. Courage is the best slayer of the old Self. In order to grow, we need to dare ask the unanswerable questions: "Who am I really? Do I live life as an ordinary man with vices and virtues? Do I live unconsciously with this mixture of characteristics, or do I reside continuously in the sky? Do I want to stay on this island of consciousness, without going down to take even a slight dip in the sea?"

We often live our life like water flowing down a hill, going more or less in one direction until we splash into something (an accident, disease, a shattering event, a divorce, a mishap, a faux pas, or a wrong choice with bad consequences) that hopefully forces us to find a new course, one that streams upwards towards enlightenment. Alas! When such misfortune befalls us, we curse a certain fate which created situations that are "not of our doing," and when they are recurrent, we blame someone else for tricking us and landing us in hot water. For most of us, it remains a fallacy to attribute every unfortunate outcome to deliberate intent by others (ideas of persecution), entropy, conspiracy, and unfortunate fate, while neglecting the possibility of personal incompetence, and bad priorities and choices. When complaining about fortune, we seize the first opportunity to vent our spleen about injustices!

One such character is *Nat-m*, the stubborn feeling introvert, who most often has an inner monologue that proceeds uninterrupted for a long time (*dwells on past disagreeable occurrences, recalls disagreeable memories*). This becomes stale and vicious, and feelings of insignificance and inadequacy may never go away, as her thinking is like riding a stationary bike of dread, *hatred*, and bitterness. With a tendency to alienate herself and blow things out of proportion (*easily offended; oversensitive*), her ill-equipped feeling function always finds a way to justify her thoughts and actions. Although mulling over sad thoughts (*sad thoughts persistent; haunted by unpleasant subjects*), she often puts all her energy into striving for something positive out of life—becoming a crusader—since striving provides the entire grammar of her further life. Yet the mood of malaise and doom permeates most of her existence, creating temporary insanity, trapping her like a fly caught in a jar. She retains a nearly obsessive pleasure of looking under a bandage at a wound (*dwells on past disagreeable occurrences*).

Often, we seem to be just chessmen moved by an unseen power. And most of us have at times felt like an *Arsenicum* person, suddenly called upon to bear an intolerable burden (*despair of recovery; fear of cancer*). At that point, we wish to be an actor appearing in a Greek tragedy or a French vaudeville, merely pretending we are suffering, or making merry, but real life is different. The world might be a stage, but we are mostly badly cast. We resemble puppets of a monstrous show, and for many, days that break in beauty end in dark storms. Too many people think that everything happening to them in this world is an accident, when really, most of the time, there is no such thing as an accident. We may blame God, the devil, a spouse, boss, neighbor, and possibly the rest of the universe to account for our destiny and misery. In actuality, except for the unexpected turns of fate like unemployment, economic crises, wars and actual accidents, we can state, "Fate is most likely the sum total of our stupidity and wrong choices, the total of human sagacity and folly, of pathos and heroism, perverse judgments and waking fantasies, hubris and squander, inattention and loss of faith." Fate is largely self-made, as it usually contains an element of freedom of choice and responsibility! Providence is not an excuse for inertia!

It's easy to see that when good fortune comes to us, we can be consumed by it with ever-lasting longing, as if it is God's given right to us. Just when we think there will be no end to a series of great fate, it will desert us when we least expect it, creating upheaval in our life followed by bitter reproach towards fickle fate. We forget the true nature of fate and fortune. It has not betrayed us, but only lulled us into compliance and increasing expectations, when showering us with a cornucopia of alluring happenstances. Fate has not abandoned us, only followed its nature and showed us both faces. We should remember we are the two-faced animal, flip-flopping in life to the side most convenient and profitable to us. We must accept fate's rules, with its continuous change, not curse it as cruel, and shed no tears when switched from unexpected happiness to the depths of despair. Accept that one day you are the pigeon, and the next day you are the statue.

We must assume that life is a mixture of spangles and tatters! As we make decisions, and sometimes decisions are made for us, we shed our life that might have been. Really, it is difficult to know when we look back at our life what we should give ourselves credit for (or blame) and what we can attribute to luck. When we dare to look honestly at our life, it appears to be filled with so many contradictions, with so many twists and turns, that it seems incomprehensible that they could be produced by the same individual. But even the man full of wisdom and deliberation cannot state that virtues (from the Latin *virtus*, meaning "principle") can fill the role of fortune! Who is at the helm of such fickleness? It is here that knowledge of the four conscious functions and the inhabitants of the unconscious (anima, animus, shadow) becomes primordial, and needs to be followed by a balanced application and appearance of the governors of our life. Real life is full of inconsistencies, and despite what fate offers us, striving to achieve baby steps to self-realization is the principal aim of wisdom. Every stage of life is subject to changes because constancy and foresight are rare finds among humans, so life seems to be more like kaleidoscopic shifts of rise and fall. Fortune comes like the day; sometimes filled with sunshine, sometimes hidden in gloom. We must learn to accept whatever comes along without regret, and not take either gratification or disappointment too seriously.

We need to use that rusty key for the creaking gate to the unconscious, where a roaring, merciless tempest reigns, a shrieking whistling storm in the black forest of our depths. We must descend to establish order. By shrinking a world at one end, we grow at the other end, changing our perspective on life. This can also be expressed in many dreams, extending over years, if the patient is not able to liberate himself from the suffocating grip of the unheard, although delivered, unconscious message. I remember a patient who was raped by her father. As a child she dreamed of buildings—the Self—collapsing, and by miracle escaping from the wreckage. She ran and ran until she was some distance away, and when she reached a place of safety, started to inventory her body, touching every part she could reach, counting fingers and toes, the way a mother does to a newborn, to see if all were there. And then she saw that blood leaked from a wound she could not see. In other recurrent dreams her face had fallen in little pieces, and she gathered up all she could to find a surgeon (magical helper) who could put them back together into a person she was able to recognize (looking for rebirth).

If integration of unconscious elements into consciousness does not happen—mixing the powers above with the powers below—or if one exhibits belligerence towards this mission that Carl Jung called "the individuation process" (Jung, 1990, CW Vol. 9, Part I, para. 83), becoming an individual rather than an obscure person in the masses will not happen. Too many people identify all their life with one aspect of themselves: skin-deep beauty, a marvelous singing voice, an ability to excel in a sport, being the star quarterback of the college team. But when that is gone, where do they end up if failure to grow never occurred? The integration, step-by-step, of our dark hidden elements becomes the difference between the clarity we see in the sky (conscious) and the clouded view on earth (unconscious). This process of ascendance and transcendence is a lifelong, difficult battle, a morass or quicksand that most get sucked into.

Recognizing the dark aspect of the unconscious is not enough if appropriate action is not taken. This seems strange and illogical because we naturally assume that if we recognize obstructions on the path to individuation, we then at least make every effort possible to remove them. But complacency, and lack of courage and moral strength, is far more common in humans than the desire and drive to truly become a more complete person. What does it take to move the inert ordinary human forward and open to new ideas? One must become a child again, an unprejudiced and curious being, for new territory to be found!

Traditional Chinese Medicine is one of the only practices (besides homeopathy) that is almost theory-independent, as its principles are based on accumulated centuries of accurate observations, with noted periodicities of day and night, and occurrence of the seasons and climates with associated diseases and emotions, etc. Any physician trained in Traditional Chinese Medicine knows the theory of the Five Elements, and that the Water element (symbol for the unconscious world) is the most versatile and powerful of all the elements. Water can wash away Earth; it can put out Fire; it can wear down a piece of Metal and sweep it away; and Wood can't survive without being nurtured by Water (the Water-Wood generating cycle). We must therefore understand that water changes shape and flows around things and finds secret paths no one in his conscious mind has thought about. Water reflects the power of, or is analogous to, the psychic force of the unconscious, that can release some "water" between the conscious and unconscious in order that psychic growth takes place. We must glean the movement of the universe or macro-cosmos around us (in which we are a micro-cosmos) and time our actions so that we are not fighting the currents but moving with them. This is different from the mechanized, reductionist, non-holistic and non-whole-view-embracing science that allopathy is.

What then is holding us back from proceeding on this journey? Where do we look to fill in the gaps in self-knowledge that will permit us to answer the age-old question, "Who am I?" What constitutes a good or fully functioning person? It seems that the need to know is blocked by the defensive fear of knowing. To strengthen ourselves and expand our consciousness, we must be like a tree sending its roots into the ground. For self-realization to take place, for a better change when meeting a fork in the road of life, suffering itself is needed, and much transformation. So often a traumatic event, a serious disease or set back in life, prompts the patient to pay attention to introspection and investigation of his unconscious—the voice of his dreams. The following is such a case.

Conscious situation: A 30-year-old man suddenly found out he had a brain tumor. It was a benign tumor, a meningioma with a large cyst attached to it. The brain was really pushed out by the cyst behind the tumor and the surgeon needed to drain the cyst first before operating on the brain. He removed the tumor completely and the operation was deemed a success: end of story. Or was it? For allopathy, besides a follow-up later, nothing else was needed. It is here that the shortcomings of allopathy are exposed. First thing advised by his homeopath, right after the man heard the diagnosis, was to take *Ignatia* 1M acutely to dampen the shock of "hearing bad news" to avoid formation of another tumor (metastasis), which is a common occurrence. (One should read Dr. Hamer's theory of The German New Medicine where a *new* tumor is discovered, not a spreading of the original one, away from the brain and in a *different embryologic leaf*, e.g., in pelvic bone.) But after *Ignatia*, necessary for the homeopath to discover and ask—since it is an acute finding—is, "What event preceded the formation of this tumor?" (In accordance with Aphorism 5 of the *Organon*.) And secondly, after the operation, or before: "Did the patient have any dreams indicating the more precise and hidden conflict he was going through?" (A situation Dr. Hamer called a "conflict-active phase.")

Upon questioning, this patient indeed had a "hanging conflict," one unresolved. He had started a new job with a lot of enthusiasm but recently was unsure that it really was his vocation, and now he feared he may never find his real calling. I asked him for dreams after the surgery to see if they could give information that I could not receive from his conscious. He had the following dreams.

Dream one

I am walking at the seashore, on the seaboard with a rucksack. On the seaboard are many other travelers, young people. They invite me to sit with them and we start to talk. I have to communicate with gestures and short sentences as we do not speak the same language. There is one among them who claims that he can fly, and he demonstrates it for us. Then I put my sleeping bag on the ground to sleep with them and the same young men start to ask me questions which I do not understand at all. They also give me food to put in my rucksack, but the quantities are too big, so I am holding this food in my hands, not knowing what to do with it.

Analysis

The patient is on the border of conscious and unconscious (seaboard) where he meets other young people who speak another language. "Several people" indicates a collective problem, but interestingly enough, these young people have already investigated their journey to the unconscious as they "speak the collective language of the unconscious," which our patient does not understand. One of them even shows him how he can fly, which is an encouragement to free the patient from his monotheism and to integrate unconscious elements to reach conscious heights (insights). They invite him to descend into the unconscious (sleep with them on the seaboard) and ask him further questions he does not understand (the patient has not at all investigated his unconscious, and therefore does not understand these collective questions). Why is he so far removed from his unconscious? Is it because he is identifying with an archetype (called inflation), as these young men are still students—in other words, still in their learning phase of life, open to learn more, but this patient does not speak their language? Further dreams could confirm this. Then they offer him food (=psychic energy) to be able to make the journey to self-realization by investigating his unconscious, but the amount offered is too big at the time, so he just holds it in his hands, puzzled as to what to do with it. Here, he already had a dream that was a guide to encourage him towards investigating his unconscious since he seems too far removed from it. This is a totally new concept for this young patient, that the unconscious would guide him in what to do in his further conscious life.

Dream two

I walk in a street of an old South American city with a lot of old cars and a lot of commotion. I enter a house where I come into a common corridor leading to many doors. I enter a room with a lot of disarray; it is dark, with much old furniture and many items on cupboards. A half-dressed old man talks to me in Spanish, but I understand only half of it. What I do understand is that he wants to heal me with a certain potion to drink. He shows me a cup which I have to warm up first with a strange system with a USB-like connection. As I struggle with this, he continues to give me instructions which I do not understand. Suddenly this old man disappears, and I at first stay in the room. Then I leave the room and come into the previous corridor; I return through the same door and now I find in the same room an old woman who asks me why I came into her room. I tell her "I am looking for the old man," to which she reacts in a very excited manner, stating that there was never a man in this room and that I am crazy. As I try to leave the room to look for the old man, she follows me and literally impedes me from going, as she jumps on my back to pull me into the room again. When I wake up, I am confused.

Analysis

The patient is walking in an old foreign city (the unknown Self, with new opportunities or chances) and then enters an old, dark house (the unconscious) full of garbage and old things (the shadow side). There he meets a half-dressed man (the wise old man) who promises to cure him if he drinks a certain tea potion (medicine or remedy). Usually the wise old man is called upon in dreams when the dreamer is in a difficult situation, when the dreamer really needs his guidance. (In the past, this archetype was found in the form of the medicine man, who was worshipped, feared, and venerated as much as the strict medical physician later in history.) But the patient is not able to understand this man, so the wise old man leaves after seeing that his instructions are in vain. What this means is that the patient thinks he does not need, or cannot accept, advice from a person, not even from the wise old man (one of the four personifications of an animus figure, see Chap. 12). This might point to an identification (which is an imitation) with this archetype, or that he needs someone or something else to resolve his problem. When the patient tries to follow the old man, he comes into the same corridor as before (the Self with many entries or doors) and he chooses to go through the same door and room and finds to his surprise the Divine Woman, a personification of the anima figure. This old anima figure compensates for the lack of experience in his conscious life. At first, she told him there was never a man in that room, but when the patient wants to leave, she jumps on his back, stopping him from leaving. What she is really saying: "If you want to go further on this journey through the unconscious, you need me, your anima figure; there is no use in continuing your trip if you don't take your female side along." It would have been better if the woman in his dreams was a young woman, as it would signify the birth of a newly forming anima. Dreaming of an old anima means that this man is too young in his own consciousness, that he lacks experience, so the anima is very old to compensate for this conscious individual. This dream tells clearly that he needs to set aside his dominant, unbalanced, conscious thinking function and possible identification with an archetype (the One-That-Knows-All-The-Answers or God or the wise old man). And he needs to exercise his atrophied and unused conscious feeling function, or his immature anima (or his weak inferior conscious function), in order to find solutions for the dilemma or conflict he is facing in life. There is no lysis as he wakes up confused.

The next day the following dream appeared.

Dream three

I am in an old school. I think I am a student, but first there is no teacher present. I am older than most of the other students. I have some words and fights with some of the younger ones as we don't agree with each other. At some point it looks like I will be the teacher but then someone enters the class who (definitely) looks like the teacher. All the students sit down but I am not at all interested in the lesson.

Analysis

A school is where we learn the lessons for life. Interesting enough, he is in a classroom with much younger students. This means that, although he is older, he is still an apprentice, an inexperienced youth, a young student at life, not an accomplished and developed individual yet. But then he imagines he might be the teacher (which is the wise old man), but this refers to an inflation of the dreamer, imagining that he is already further than he really is in his life experience. This is yet another warning from the unconscious when compared to his first dream where he also met students. Then the real wise old man enters the class. He always enters in the moment he is needed. This saves the dreamer, because if the dreamer would be swallowed by the archetype of the wise old man this could lead to psychosis. As the younger students want to learn, the dreamer, because of his inflation, is not at all interested in the lesson presented.

In a **following dream**, soon after the previous one, this inflation is repeated as he has "a little book with me in which I scribbled some lines, nothing of importance. I tell the others 'I am a writer,' and they believe me. I tell them too that I want to publish a book but that it is not ready yet. I tell them literally that 'first one has to write a book before one can publish it.'"

This clearly relates to fairy tales and aspirations which have not been achieved, as instead of a book he has only a small book with some scribbles in it. The inflation is not dissolved yet, and this is a repeated message to investigate his unconscious. Hopefully further dreams, after the simillimum and possibly psychoanalysis, might show an attempt to journey into his hidden side. There is no lysis in these dreams; rather these dreams are part of the same series or same chapter of the book of life. A new chapter is not started yet.

In the **next dream**, the same night, he dreamt that he was fighting against soldiers and tried to deceive them into believing that he was an ordinary person. Possibly in subsequent dreams he will be killed, as this always signals the start to a new and improved personality. The more he identifies with his excessive persona (teacher and writer in this case)—called inflation—the further he is removed from his unconscious, and the much-needed investigation of his shadow side. For the moment he is still lost and has not even begun to write the story of his life—his true achievements and aspirations—as he is identified with an excessive persona.

This patient needs a new consciousness; he needs a series of transformations of his consciousness, a death followed by a rebirth, often personified in dreams by a phoenix rising from its ashes, or by the hero who is swallowed by the whale (Jonah) and then either kills the beast from within or gets ejected, or by a snake shedding its skin, or by a tadpole transforming into a frog or a caterpillar into a butterfly. Such rebirth can only start when he achieves detachment from his inflation of the wise old man, otherwise he pays the penalty as he did with the formation of a meningioma, an over-built sycotic expression, analogous to the inflation. These dreams will further help the homeopath not only to understand the real conflict but also to serve as guidance to find the simillimum, as the patient might start a series of dreams ending in lysis. Only then is a radical change of attitude and character possible: the inhibited person becomes free, the fear-ridden more courageous, and the unscrupulous more conscientious. Every incorporation of a neurotic symptom will accompany a character change of the ego, even for those childhood justified phobias and traumas that were completely transformed and preserved into a character structure. Most people remain unaware or ignorant of the fact—meaning, do not see something that's not exactly obvious—that the control of life is steered by a vast continent called the unconscious or subconscious, as it lies under the radar of consciousness. Yet it plays a primary, important role in the stability of the psyche, just like the foundation of a house is built upwards from the basement and not from the attic downwards.

That the unconscious is often the motor behind conscious behavior was easily seen in a 5-year-old *Calcarea-c* boy. His mother left on a seminar for seven days, but his father took good care of him. During this time, when out with his father, an unknown dog ran up to him. He froze in sheer panic (*Ailments from fright; fear for dogs*) and urinated in his pants. The next day he seemed normal and no remedy was given. When his mother came back a few days later, he showed first aggressive, disobedient, and naughty behavior towards her (sign of an *obstinate Calc-c*), to "punish" his mother. He also came down with a 104°F fever and sleeplessness, coming up to his parents' bed every night. As one can see, *Stramonium*, the remedy that wants light (consciousness) and a great remedy for *separation anxiety*, should have been given immediately after the acute incident with the dog (*fear of dogs*). Both events, the fear of the dog and the fear of abandonment and separation, were pushed into the subconscious (suppressed does not mean disappeared) but remained strong enough to create and guide unruly conscious behavior. Previously, a homeopath had given *Calc-c* 10M (his constitution) and *Aconite*, but both failed to cure the fever. Here is the report I received of what happened after *Stramonium*:

> For S. I found enough rubrics where *Stramonium* was represented in fever yesterday that fit his state. He had no striking reaction to *Bell* 1M (and I never bothered to go to 10M after finding *Stram* in the rubrics). His fever was down 5 degrees in an hour and a quarter, to 99°F, but no evident response in mood or energy or otherwise (you wrote in *Discovering Life* that a *Stramonium* fever is less inflammatory than *Belladonna* fever, and he was no redder in the face than in the body, nor had the *Belladonna* keynote "bursting headache" at this point). I gave him what I had of *Stram*—one dose of 200C from a 4 oz. bottle. Ten minutes later he was asleep and slept the whole night to the relief of us all. Fever was down this morning, and he is almost free of it tonight at bedtime. He was in a good mood and had energy to move about in the second half of the day, so curative in the right direction. But you were right, it was evident to me today that he needs a higher potency than the 200C, to address the state at its core, and a higher potency probably would have relieved him sooner of his fever, too. I am grateful you helped us out, now I know how to continue at least.

Another remarkable fact after the first dose of *Stramonium*

200C was that the boy, of course not knowing the remedy, came the next day to his father telling him he had a dream in which *a light brown dog came to him and put his paw in his hand*, evoking a feeling of trust and love. The next remedy given, not unusual to calm down the awakened psoric miasm after such an acute fever incident, and especially in view of *A/F embarrassment*, was one dose of *Sulphur* 30C, ½ tsp. from the dilution cup, which stabilized him again to the more independent boy he was before, easily saying goodbye to his father to see his friends.

Another example from the clinic showed how from childhood on, a terrifying event can put an indelible stamp on the unconscious leading to neurotic and incomprehensible behavior. This was the case of a 7-year-old girl who could only barely talk to her mother about what happened three years after the incident, a traumatic event that occurred in school when she had to go to the toilet. Being afraid she would lock herself in the toilet and not be able to open it to get out, she left the door ajar. Three boys came in and opened the door, which shocked her to the core. We can use the following rubrics: *A/F mortification; A/F shock; Delusion, she has done wrong; Del, she is a criminal.*

From then on, she had excessive reactions to anyone approaching the toilet, even at home, screaming and jumping up nervously. She was also very *sensitive to reproach*. Understandable at such an age, she was afraid she would be blamed if she ever told her parents about the incident. Other rubrics to this case were the following: *A/F embarrassment; A/F fright; A/F mortification; A/F shame; confidence, want of; Delusion, life is unfair to her; forsaken feeling; foolish behavior; childish behavior; gestures, makes ridiculous; grief, deception from; hiding himself; inactivity; irresolution; reproaching oneself; shameful; somnambulism; taciturn; undertaking, lacks willpower to undertake anything; weeping from admonition; yielding disposition in children; face, discoloration, pale; extremities, awkwardness; sleep, falling asleep late*. Computer result: *Ign* 88; *Nat-m* 67; *Op* 66; *Puls* 66; *Lyc* 65; *Sulph* 61; *Lach* 58; *Phos* 54.

When I saw her in the clinic three years after this incident, *Ignatia* was still the remedy needed!

Response to *Ignatia* 1M, 2 drops from 8 oz RSB:

> Parent's Report: Since the dose of *Ignatia* 1M yesterday morning the exaggerated insecure behavior has disappeared. I gave her the dose of 1/4 tsp. directly from an 8 oz bottle. She was very taciturn the whole day yesterday, still pale after school but more composed. Very even in her temperament, even a smile or lightness of her being was not easy to arouse. She fell asleep earlier than normal and quickly. This morning I still thought she seemed a little "heavy," burdened, and thought the dose had landed possibly a little too hard on her. She got home from school two hours ago, and now the positive change can be seen in increased lightness overall, more spontaneous talking, talking freely and expressing herself with balanced confidence. She was less pale but still slightly dark under her eyes. No doubt she is better; talks, smiles, and laughs, and has overcome the state of inertia and is again in her normal creative mode. I can hear her right now humming a song to herself, a safe sign that she is in her good mood! She always does that when she enjoys herself and what she is doing!

It was clear that this child was able to finally shake the shackles off and become a free person again.

For most people, the unconscious is the invisible enemy, which is always more dangerous than a visible one. What path to follow?

The Truth Will Set You Free

If we allow one conscious function to dominate, especially the thinking function (see Chap. 8), which recognizes only intellectual enlightenment or "elucidation" without further trying to exercise and bring into the light of consciousness the other conscious functions as well as the unconscious elements (shadow, anima, and animus)—the integration of the latter is called "illumination"—we steer a boat whose rudder is fixed. Thus, it is impossible for the helmsman to change course according to the winds, the "spirit or God-like essence" that determines the vessel's direction. This leads to a conscious life turning more barren and meager while the unconscious swallows up more and more land, becoming a threatening and compelling force. We will wake up one day to find out that we have only lived half our life, when our journey comes to a crashing halt on a cliff or undesired land. It is inevitable. Wholeness, reaching the summit of consciousness—the only desirable goal in a human's life—can never be achieved this way, and remains a never-ending quest, merely the object of wishful thinking! Our first goal should be to create a degree of widening consciousness and to illuminate one's Self by recognizing the individual and collective unconscious, realizing that the long arduous journey to self-realization is not an automatic course without ups and downs. It requires a steady helmsman, one who can use the rudder to change course when encountering obstacles created not only by inescapable instances of fate but also by the autonomous activity of the unconscious, testing our will and desire to approach that wholeness with grit and determination.

Unfortunately, awareness and increasing consciousness do not come automatically with age. Once while traveling, I got to know a woman in her 60s who demonstrated all the emotional make up of a *Pulsatilla* person: she was not married until age

40, wandering around the world as an innocent child, *yielding*, *needy*, talking constantly to everyone, even about nothing. To her, everything was "fantastic and beautiful" (often only to her), and when she became sick with diarrhea, rather than face the truth and seek help, she said, "I am not hungry, I am going to do some crosswords in my bedroom." But she did have an interest in dreams, as her archaic feeling function was often called upon. So, one day she told me with great childish enthusiasm the following dream.

Dream

I walk with an old man upon a road next to a canyon. At some point we come to a line of demarcation and we stop. I look in his eyes and without words spoken, I throw myself suddenly into the ravine. Halfway down, I get wings and I fly gently to the bottom of this canyon. How wonderful that felt!

Analysis

Upon asking her what her favorite fairy tale was, she told me it was the story of Peter Pan. This did not come as a surprise to me, for she acted like a person who did not want to grow up, clinging to her husband every moment. This dream revealed quite a bit. It sounds like a fairy tale, where she receives wings so she can be that little butterfly girl (in reality, she looked frail, petite, and vulnerable), fulfilling her journeys in unexpected ways. In the dream she is accompanied by the wise old man, an archetypal image of masculinity or animus. Apparently without words, through the power of his eyes, she receives the message to jump into the ravine or abyss (in other words the message was, "Go and explore your unconscious!"), but thanks to this childish Peter Pan miracle she can fly, so she lands at the bottom of the canyon, which represents the collective unconscious. It reflects again her closeness to the collective unconsciousness—in her case, the need to be near a "hero figure," her husband, for protection and to be able to stay in this rather infantile fantasy world even at her age. She beamed with childish joy over this dream, not understanding at all its meaning: a message to integrate the unknown elements into her consciousness—to finally grow up rather than stay in the infantile protection world with an undeveloped ego! She likely may stay there for the rest of her life and feel happy, but miss the opportunity to become the person, the individual, she could and should become—a loss mainly for herself.

Regarding the personal unconscious: what is this component of human nature, that invisible entity, misunderstood, preferred to be denied or forgotten by most as if it were something of a ghost that makes its appearance from time to time—mostly at inopportune moments? Is it just a warehouse consisting of everything that the conscious forgets or wants to dispose of, or does it also contain elements that were not formed in the conscious mind in the first place?

The Ever-Expanding Garbage Can

It is evident that everything gone from consciousness has not ceased to exist. All of us have had moments when we come into a room to fetch something but cannot remember what, until prompted by unexpected actions from the unconscious. This personal unconscious contains ingredients that were not strong enough to transcend the threshold to keep them conscious. Even more frequently, when convenient we deny things we have said: "I did not say such thing," we exclaim. Yet if we would have recorded the conversation, we would be astonished how easily we transferred these conscious contents to the unconscious. No doubt we all have these experiences, proof of the powerful and useful unconscious to save us from uncomfortable moments, as we want them pushed out of sight. As Nietzsche said, "I have done that, says my memory. I cannot have done that, says my pride, and remains inexorable. Eventually—memory yields" (Nietzsche, 1967, p. 270).

Of course, the possessor of these neuroses is often betrayed by "Freudian slips of the tongue"—curious lapses of speech or hysterical attacks of fainting, or engineering of dangerous attacks—where sudden reactions are required but the patient is overcome by unexplained hesitation. The action of a hostile unconscious and the power of autonomy of unconscious elements can be seen in stumbling, awkwardness, trivial accidents, self-injury, and in dangerous accidents (all syphilitic expressions of losing control) that have been at work for a long time.

We need to be implored to listen to our unconscious voice, and without prejudice take the opportunity to perceive its important psychological activity and unite the opposites through a middle path, so aptly described and preached in TCM 5,000 years ago and symbolized by the concept of Tao, translated as "meaning." To translate meaning into life is our objective. What will be the desired result of integrating the contents of the personal unconscious together with the elements attached to it? No doubt, a broadening of consciousness and an obliterating of our blind spots. Above all, becoming a different and more complete person should lead to compassion, empathy, and foremost humility, which seems always to be the last virtue. Empathy and compassion are virtues because they practice valuing and paying attention to others. It sounds like the best present, all around, we can accord ourselves, but this is only the case if we have a critical understanding of the process of integration of unconscious contents. Everyone is tested when thrown into a noble or ignoble misfortune, as it poses the question, "How will I react to calamity—accepting, rejecting, or trying to get something positive out of it, when fate has turned its back on me?" We must remember that it is not the existence of the problem itself (the NWS), but our attitude (compensation) towards it that gives it power for good or evil. Determination and undaunted courage can come out of grief; or degradation, meanness, and spiritual apathy can come from it. Out of riches and power may come selfishness, self-gratification, and materialism (e.g., *Nux-v*); or opportunity to serve and practice the art of giving like a balanced *Aurum—to be*, not *to have*, is the message!

Integration of unconscious elements and movement towards cure can be seen in the following dream of a male patient after a first dose of the indicated remedy.

Dream

I am a medical student and scheduled to do a cataract operation on the left eye of a woman. I am surprised that they ask this from a beginning student, and I feel some trepidation about this, as operating on an eye is an important and dangerous task. I am assisted in this operation by an older female medical student, who preps the patient, and a male technician. I go ahead in getting ready for this operation while the patient is already under anesthesia. Contrary to most of the medical students who have postponed their first operation numerous times, I seem willing to go on. I carefully watch the older student to make sure that I will be able to prep a patient if the occasion will present in the future. But then, before I can proceed, the woman wakes up. Then I wake up from the dream.

Analysis

At least this dreamer has started the investigation of the unconscious and especially of the state of his anima. The left side corresponds to yin, the unconscious, feminine, nourishing and protecting part, and the left eye signifies the sight and introspection of the unconscious. Other students have postponed their first operations, showing the collective nature of this dream, as integrating unconscious elements is a universal problem, not just belonging to the dreamer. The dreamer is still "a student" like the other characters, meaning a student of life, gaining insight but not a professional or adult yet. But at least the dreamer, under the influence of the remedy, has already started the process of investigation, willing to go on, unlike others who postponed this journey. Further doses of the *same* remedy in judicious, opportune moments will move the case forward.

This brings us to the point of investigating the garbage can mentioned before, in more detail. It is a rather easily accessible entity of the personal unconscious, with an enormous capacity and limitless libido: the shadow, or closest family member of humans! Just as many characteristics of personality can be found in the study of the four conscious functions, many other characteristics (such as jealousy, hatred, empathy, morality, responsibility, etc.) cannot be measured by them and remain secret, as they are part of the inferior function, hidden, and must be confronted in the shadow.

10

THE SWAMPLAND OF EXTENSIVE GHOSTS: THE SHADOW SIDE

"Nothing is more your own than your dreams."
— Nietzsche

The Secrets and Lies that Become Our Life

Among the symbols of the individuation process there are a few that stand out, appearing in human or animal form in the dreams of countless people who are often unaware of them—the chief ones being the *shadow*, the *anima* in man, and the *animus* in woman—archetypal figures, which the dreamer will encounter initially. These archetypes (from the Greek *arche*, or "beginning, principle") are not at all invented but can be found centuries back in the dreams of people of all mankind as well as in fairy tales. Whenever a personal figure appears, be it anima, animus, or shadow, the dreamer can be sure that the unconscious is becoming active—that the unconscious is inclined to form a connection with consciousness. Usually the shadow is the first one to appear in dreams, followed by the animus (for women) or anima (for men). As we will see, these figures have a frequent and disturbing influence on our life, and as products of the unconscious they seem to act as secret autonomous guards, with mixed qualities that we remain mostly unconscious of. Everyone has secrets, sometimes to protect others but generally to protect ourselves. Most people keep their inner conflicts hidden, even from themselves, until the unconscious psychic force makes them commit irrational deeds, even cruel ones, as they can no longer resist the enormous force of this hidden energy. For some, deception and lying is a second skin and few ever manage to pierce the armor of mystery that clads them. We all at some point have the illusion that we are following a rainbow in the sky, but eventually we encounter our living being, a blend of shadow and light, because there is no escaping engagements with our dark passions. Outwardly we can look like a kind person, while inwardly we are often egocentric, cruel, and possess cold traits cleverly concealed from everyone.

Carl Jung states, "By shadow, I understand the 'negative' side of the personality, the sum of all these hidden unpleasant qualities, but also the insufficiently developed functions and the contents of the personal unconscious" (Jung, 2009, p. 209).

Good and bad in any individual are inextricably one. The shadow is the underside of human nature, a side that is unavoidably present in every human individual, and mostly appears to us as the pettiest, meanest part of our personality, easily deflating our ego. It can also appear in dreams as a desperado, a criminal, a dwarf, or the inferior brother. As we will see further, *acceptance* of this dwarf as part of ourselves—not rejecting it—is necessary. The shadow's contents are found when we peel back the extreme façade and veneer of our persona, and lo and behold, another Self is discovered within ourselves, an alter ego. We detect what lies beneath: fragility, lies, loneliness, deception, flattery, posing, playing a role before others and even ourselves—a constant flutter around the flame of vanity. We discover untold stories of shameful secrets, the enduring pain of grief resulting from early traumas, or a secret yearning for the spotlight, power, and domination, as well as destruction, backbiting, rip-offs, sadism, tyranny, disloyalty, ignorance, triviality, contempt, treachery, detachment, coarseness, and jealousy—which swallows most of its own venom and poisons itself, creating a chronic, bleeding ulcer—and a desire for self-aggrandizement. This vast cornucopia of vices correlates with the prevailing dominant miasmatic predisposition and is comprised of the emotions that set the human heart ablaze and quicken its pulse, yet are, for the most part, never subject to closer scrutiny. Sometimes, such emotions may be a fleeting thought, like finding malicious pleasure in seeing others' suffering or misfortune (*laughing at the misfortune of others*). A human's shadow seems to be a pile of tinder, always in search of a match. At any moment, we can be driven into one of these tempests, terrifying us, more so because of the difficulty of figuring out what drove this unruliness and how it can be assuaged. How frightful, even intolerable would it be, if everything false was stripped away; how much of humanity would be left? All too often, we are unable to dispose of these ill drives and dark passions, behaving like a gardener who cultivates the shoots of vices. We may seem to be living as productively and profitably as a beautiful fruit tree, while really, we are creating only a wilderness. We must try the impossible: the truth, masked and veiled perhaps, but eternal. The dictum "Love your neighbor as yourself" should remind us that our closest, permanent neighbor is our shadow! Accepting it as part of ourselves, embracing and taming it, is part of becoming more complete.

Most among us don't even undertake the battle of freeing ourselves from dark elements, but even for those who attempt to, liberating ourselves of their influence is not always achieved. Some mud always sticks, requiring further attention for additional progress to be achieved. But at least, for them, the overall picture is not one of unrelieved, false pride.

The goal of keeping the lid on the garbage can is always to construct an alternative, alluring reality. Maybe on our gravestone, a collective epitaph should be written: "Out of shadows and phantasms into truth." Of course, it would be an acknowledgement that comes a little too late. Integration of the shadow's dark elements means succeeding in penetrating the veil woven out of delusions, illusions, and evaluations, to learn—through the process of elucidation—to see the situation as it is. For most of us, the shadow remains a cellar so filled with filth that it is nearly inconceivable that an urge for truth can be found in this horrid heap, as we are immersed in illusions and fancies. Is there ever a time when we want to be naked, or laid out in an illuminated glass case?

We often think of ancient tribes as savages and barbarians, but modern humans seem to be caught by a savage streak that was unknown to those "savages" (humans are by nature corrupt). On his trip to Brazil in 1556, the French priest Jean De Léry, who lived with one of Brazil's best-known tribes for more than a year, the Tupinambé, compared them to his French race at that time, writing:

> [They] do not in any way drink of those murky, pestilential springs, from which flow so many streams of mistrust, avarice, litigation, and squabbles, of envy and ambition, which eat away our bones, suck out our marrow, waste our bodies, and consume our spirits—in short, poison us and kill us off before our due time—nothing of all that torments them, much less dominates or obsesses them. (De Léry, 1990, p. 57)

So much for "primitive" versus "advanced" cultures! Those primitives seemed to know only truth and untruth, belief and unbelief, without modern man's uncertain gamut of finer shades. The philosopher and essayist Michel de Montaigne

(1533-1592) held the same opinion when he talked about the settled life, exempt from agitation, of the natives of Brazil:

> They die only through age, which some impute to the clearness and calmness of their air, but I rather ascribe to the calmness and clearness of their minds, void and free from all passions and cares, toiling and unpleasant labors, as a people that pass their life in a wonderful kind of simplicity and ignorance, without letters, or laws, and without kings or any religion. (de Montaigne, 2014, p. 147)

Reading these words, it seems that the beauty of the primitive, the human and natural, could still take hold of us, creating a paradise of near magical reality now lost!

It is uncanny how many different characteristics can be released from the shadow. We seem to possess an elastic capacity to maintain a degree of immorality, pushing aside the inner voice of a higher being, the wise old man. Are we aware that this other part of us—our bête noire, a crook, a traitor, counterfeiter, a criminal, leading a debauched lifestyle—is prostituting ourselves, and that it portrays the seamier side of our existence? Are we at risk to make our illusions and dark realities so vivid and persuasive that this existence becomes life itself, the new normal? Does such "realism" metastasize out of control? It becomes a continuous balancing act in our existence to even portray a modicum of normalness. Are we aware of our moral failings, or do they become part of this imperfect existence? The shadow at the reins of our chariot creates a seductive, deceptive, and paltry world, a turmoil of delusion and lust, in which we recognize untruth as a condition of our "undisturbed" life.

Those rare humans who don't happen to take part in this system of illusions and self-denial are assumed to be fools, freaks, or ignorant. To most, being naked—to be looking in the mirror with clarity—is equal to societal suicide. Such an individual is shunned and condemned for not knowing "the rules" they should follow for acceptance, to be part of the "successful" human family. Why should *they* avoid the avenues to power, acceptance, and prestige?

Conformism is the norm in humans, the adoption of uncritical attitudes, taking the early path of self-deception in the form of desired, created personas. But are we falling down the rabbit hole and mutating our life into Fantasyland? The unconscious in which the shadow resides is a world of scattered rocks in a sea. We must dare to venture down to where all the ladders start, in the rag-and-bone shop of the unconscious, in order to help the philistine in us (guided by materialism) discontinue the drab business of ordinary living. Most of us start on the lowest rung of the ladder, a needle jab in the heart of the philistine, for the last thing he wants to be reminded of is his spiritual poverty, although it is the first step to achieve a positive conquest by the spirit.

Should we finally lose patience with our erratic behavior leading to missteps, misfortunes, and even to losing our minds? Should we finally learn from the sphinx to ask the question: "Who am I really? What in us really wants truth?" We will have to take the risk, with open eyes, otherwise we will sink deeper in a self-created morass of deceit, a stain that will never disappear but only gets larger.

A Stain that Spreads and Sooner or Later Stains Us All

Most people are so inconsistent, even excited in their behavior —ruled unconsciously by the forceful shadow—that they exert themselves like exuberant horse riders gone wild and covered with sweat. Irritation in themselves arises when something touches a sore spot, which most of the time they would like desperately to hide. Sometimes we are caught by sudden mood swings that we cannot account for: everything in life seems to be going well, work is rewarding and everyone in the family is healthy. Yet there are moments so bizarre, contradictory, and overwhelming, that at first the best tool to describe them is metaphor, modes of narration that function in a less linear way. We hope, mostly in vain, that these moments of gloom and destruction will not emanate permanently from our dark underworld, before we start thinking that our chromosomes must be altered.

A life of chaos upends everything, creating ripple effects, unforeseen consequences, and moments of despair, not so much for the perpetrator (who often remains blind to breeding chaos), but for those around him. We can only hope that the imposter will survey the wreckage and draw some lessons from it before destroying the Self of so many others. Maybe we need to invent a variant of luminol, the chemical that reveals spots of blood in the dark at crime scenes—one that can illuminate all the dark spots of the human psyche—so that the persona can become more a reflection of who we really are, rather than a commodity to sail through life with, allowing a "criminal" to get away with "murder" and homicide cases gone cold in his all-too-long lifetime.

The realization of a persona destroys a deception, leading to the discovery that it was just a mere semblance of who we are. Our shadow makes us all hypocrites, as it can counterfeit any physical appearance. The shadow, a cornucopia of mostly inferior traits, governs human life with an ever-changing content and shape of incessantly passing moods (unless repetition in these moods creates the existent euphoria of the manic or the depression of the melancholic, or a pathological liar, or the birth of a psychopath).

Do we need an inquisition of our deepest secrets to take place? No! We need a thorough personal investigation of our dark side. And we need not be a prosecutor, but a fair-minded, impartial judge! Every "house" has skeletons struggling to come out. How much better and liberating for us would it be if they could be free to roam in the full light of day. Of course, we have the greatest difficulty accepting the shadow. We are constantly acting in a Greek drama, mostly one without a lysis, as the play never ends and the curtains are never drawn to salute and congratulate us in our performance, or valiantly won battle. For most, it is never-ending, as an actor finds every cause in the world to never let go of his false persona. Poverty of goods is easy to cure, but poverty of soul is almost impossible to remedy. It seems that we always find a way of pushing our stowaway—called our dark side—on board the vessel of glorified, convenient personas, preferring to live a life of eternal blindness and denial.

Unfortunately, familiarity with vices and immoral acts does not breed contempt, as it should, but rather becomes an asset for maneuvering through life's difficulties. In general, we strive to shore up our vision of ourselves, so we have no tolerance for justified criticism or the wise counsel of friends, or above all the inner voice of our unconscious. Opinions of well-meaning friends will not (or little) modify our character, but what they can bring forward is an illumination of dark elements that hitherto remained obscure to us, buried in a deep tomb. When well-meaning people point to the real us, we usually cry out that we do not recognize ourselves in the image they draw and seek refuge from it by pointing an erasing finger at their derangement. Our projected persona is even more effective if we have a charismatic personality (from the Greek word *charism*, which means "spiritual gift"). But as we can see, this is a gift that can either be used or misused, depending on one's moral strength not to succumb to temptation and corruption. Too many use this asset to follow a false agenda rather than one that is good for the well-being of others.

Our view of our own condition is always friendly, as favoritism and narcissism blind judgment. "Know thyself," the command Socrates issued to philosophers in his time, is most often subject to counterfeiting. To know ourselves, we must look *in ourselves* and *keep true to ourselves*, requiring in-depth, honest investigation. But who has the courage to tell the truth to himself? Who dares to drag his whole stock of evil into the light? It is like inviting a storm but suffering from potentially permanent seasickness. How can this voyager in distress be rescued, put in sight of the land he seeks?

Whatever effort is called upon, the difficulty is that we cannot get away from ourselves. Most of us, tragically ignorant of the extensive ghosts at work in our shadow side, replicate our old mistakes, the stupid errors and infantile reactions, when facing otherwise reasonable issues. But these giant ghosts cannot be underestimated. They continue to exert their silent work with a program bordering on autocracy, so we must be prepared for the eruptions of the unconscious. The hopeful outcome is that the shadow is not allowed to assemble fuel and flame to scorch the Self before we leave this earthy life. He who conceals his vices from others usually does so from himself as well. As physicians and homeopaths, "cross-examination" of others' lives during our consultations should impel a *self-examination* of our own life. Maybe the humble and courageous among us should ask others what they think of us. But what a surprise! Say we ask five of our best friends for that opinion, and then discover they do not talk about one person but about five different individuals. One will tell you that you are the most generous person he knows; another may say you cannot hurt a fly; the next will disclose that you tend to be harsh with your family but less contemptuous with your friends and superiors. Another will be convinced that you are always edgy in your behavior and cannot be contradicted about anything, while another will swear that you are the most attentive and patient listener he ever met.

This begets the question, "Who are we really?" Maybe none of those, maybe all! None, because after all they are mere perceptions of five other people, not an opinion belonging to you. All, because each of these opinions might have a valid basis in observation of your personality.

That leaves us with the difficulty that no one really knows himself. But limited knowledge of oneself can be built up with humility, psychic courage, and a desire to walk the road forward. It's a walk strewn with obstacles that plead with us to remain stagnant or even go backward, but no doubt this would be incongruous with our true personality and with our dreams. Alas! We don't all have the appetite to increase minimal familiarity with our true Self, therefore limiting any progress that can and should be made. All we can do is be ourselves, to grow up to be none other than ourselves, a web woven from its own complexities, from its own choices (too often perceived as fate). "Life is lived forward, but can only be understood backward," said Kierkegaard. To put it another way, midlife reckonings revise the events of the past to make the present comprehensible.

Why should we not sweep the contents of the shadow under the amnesiac rug? Not accepting and correcting the shadow—because of lack of insight, cowardice, laziness, and spiritual penury—leaves us an empty shell, a crude and fragile travesty of what we might have been in our life.

Inside the inner adobe—the thickly constructed wall of our inner city—the air can be stale, humid and hot, where for most no whiff of clean air or blue sky can penetrate to freshen the effluvium of the dark conqueror. Why then are there moments that bring frayed nerves, sleepless nights, and even nightmares; how is it that these thick walls allow an insane ruler to escape? Most prefer to keep the inner city under lock. We choose to stay in our "summer palace" to get a good night's sleep, living with our eyes closed and ears stopped. We should all be stung at some moment by a gadfly, a tormentor, just as Socrates knew how to sting the citizens who otherwise would sleep on, undisturbed for the rest of their lives. Non-investigation of the shadow, with no purging of unexamined pre-judgments, renders distress in the physical body, but even greater is the danger to our spiritual life and quest for self-realization. Is there a dominance of the unconscious over human self-awareness, or an instinctive nature (unknown to most) opposed to it?

The Shadowy Figure: A Search for Resolve or Refuge?

"Who am I? And what am I?" What is man's nature in deeds, words, and intentions? Most think they know; few are those who do! What is visible to others is a created helpful persona, projected as the Self, leaving the shadow to lurk in the unconscious. For the most part we are unconscious of our shadow, and therefore it does not really exist in our world. Hence, by rejecting our shadow we reject our inferior personality, the dwarf and fool in us. It is a warding off of the evil eye, producing an *Anacardium* figure with the *Delusion, of having a devil on one shoulder and an angel on the other* (a split personality), which is a reflection of the morality compass of mankind —"morality" coming from the Latin *mores*, associated with rules of behavior. By not acknowledging our shadow, however, we in fact weave a web in which we imprison ourselves, where we could have envisioned a much larger horizon had we integrated our shadow's darkest elements. Alas! We think that whatever we do, we always do the "good." That is, we always do that which seems to be good or useful to *us*. Oscar Wilde had a "solution" for missteps and sins: "The only way to avoid a temptation is to yield to it!" (Wilde, 1966). But character is destiny. If we do not acknowledge our past misdeeds, we are bound to repeat them. What are we to do? Maybe we should look to do good in regard to others, not harm?

What is correct belongs to the few, but hopefully their example is like lightning and thunder moving the masses.

Unfortunately, in our present political world, free rein is given to fake news and limitless immoral behavior in plain sight without consequence. Such disease is sadly contagious and perverts the youth, who see unlimited freedom and disinhibition as a mission in life, not recognizing that such a life is full of destabilization and danger, one in which the shadow, part of the dark unconscious world, can transform into an internal abyss. Is this where humankind will go adrift? It is still Augustine (theologian/philosopher, born AD 353) whispering in our ear, "The truth about the truth is that it is too dreadful to those affected."

We resemble a strange crystal, which is one moment clear and the next clouded, an expression of spurts of the incessant battle that goes on within, where moments of morality conflict with passions of greed and lust. The shadow's actions do not resemble rage or full retreat, but only attack and withdraw at inopportune times. Even when we have the best intentions, our animalistic instincts often get the better of us because they are alluring and seductive, putting the body at war with the mind. This soon goes on for a prolonged time, taking us captive in the wilderness of frivolous desires and empty ambitions. We obtain "riches" by the victory of an army tilting to soldiers of vices, unaware of the coldness of their glitter and that the price of falling for their allure is the loss of our soul, as we commit crimes continuously with apparent impunity. For many among us, life might resemble King Sisyphus's existence, who when punished by the gods had to roll a rock to the top of a mountain, only for it to tumble down when it neared the top, repeatedly. But at least he will be remembered for his labor towards his purpose.[1] We can only hope that a hard look at the hidden depths of the soul is able to start the process of integration, loosening the grip of the wrongs of our doing on our desperate soul. Such integration of dark elements will only be achieved by "blood, sweat, and tears." But what exactly about morality is so difficult to grasp?

Defining morality should be easy, right? I find it easy: integrity is doing the right thing even when no one is watching! Everyone should know what is good or bad, what is right or wrong, is it not obvious? If it would only be that straightforward to define. Moral sense consists of a certain specific emotion as well as judgment of approval towards various kinds of acts. Of course, right or wrong always has consequences which need to be taken into account, with the right action always having the best possible outcome. The difficulty is that there is always the eerie temple that houses both good and evil, a seductive ambivalence, and the power of unacknowledged prejudices, a shadowy area in which the inner lives of so many are played out. Our values may all be written down on paper, but our actual life goes on mostly as if morality does not exist. In modern times "going viral" is more important and attention rewarding than being moral. But what is important for us is our personal appropriation of morality—"appropriation" coming from the Latin *proprius*, meaning "one's own." As the English poet, essayist, and playwright T. S. Eliot (1888-1965) said, "Humankind cannot bear very much reality and it is doubtful whether they can bear the reality of being told so."

Morality is more than what is just, as it designates what is beyond the sphere of normal obligatory duty—what we cannot expect everyone to do. But rather than seek this high ground, we tend to run away from our shadow with the swiftness of a thief caught red-handed. Morally destructive patterns of callousness, manipulation, and materialism are so engrained in our routine behavior that we often do not even recognize them. No matter how many friends, neighbors, and strangers we encounter, everyone crossing our path is capable of inhumanity. Consciously and unconsciously, our shadow side is what mostly guides our life in respect to oneself and others. In subtle and not so subtle ways, this is now accepted as the norm in society. We also prepare enough fences to have no real fear of having to compete with our unconscious: ignorance, denial, projection, delusions and illusions, are among the defense mechanisms we use. Pangs of conscience are, to most people, a very endurable pain, and practice and repetition in wrongdoing rapidly diminishes them, so introspection, if exercised at all, is very brief, and at the end becomes altogether absent! Maybe finally, a spark of insight falls into the soul of a more integrated human, who then finds the road to live by it. Hopefully humanism will triumph rather than sink in the swamps of nothingness. The ground around us is littered with humans who are unconsciously riding a horse out of control, making themselves smaller than they really are. How long will we continue, bewildered? Will we ever be enlightened?

No one is perfect, and to become more tolerant of the faults of others is the first lesson in the religion of humanity. Regarding ourselves, we hope to have the impetus to strive to do better. We must give expression to who we truly are and enlighten our conscious. Put down the drawbridge which allows unconscious energies to come to the surface. Let darkness be illuminated so that we can liberate ourselves from the suffocating yoke that threatens the journey to a more fulfilled life. Here is such an example as seen in a fast sequence of dreams, under the influence of judicial doses of the simillimum. The 50-year-old female patient finally begins to explore her unconscious, changing it from a swamp (literally in her dream) to an attempt to get nearer to the door of the unconscious world.

Dream one

I'm barefooted and walk through a dark and slimy swamp. But somehow it feels as if it has to be like this.

Dream two

I'm walking by a pond which is dark and more looking like a swamp. I'm a bit disappointed; I can't really enjoy the walk.

Dream three

I'm walking down towards a pond. People (friends) are calling at me to come and see how nice it is there. I walk down, it's dark and I discover a beautiful pond with lots of wonderful plants growing all around it. Then the friends ask me to embark on a small boat, which I do willingly, and we row through plants and cascades and around rocks in a marvelous water landscape. I wonder at each turn as we wind our way gently into the area, discovering more and more beautiful landscapes and sceneries.

Analysis

Dream one: Walking barefoot is to be in contact with reality—the reality being that there is also the world of darkness, the slimy swamp. But she does not feel disgusted by this and says, "It feels like it has to be like this," accepting there is a dark side to her.

In **dream two**, she is still somewhat disappointed that the pond she thinks she will see is still a swamp, which decreases her enjoyment—being again confronted with reality.

In **dream three**, when friends call her over to the pond (reflecting a collective dream, as it involves more people), she discovers that the "swamp" has much beauty in it (the golden nuggets to be fished from the unconscious), so she does not hesitate to embark on a boat (a symbol of a great journey of transformation) with her friends, discovering more and more beauty—a very positive step to be willing to discover the unconscious. This reflects a positive direction of cure and a step forward into her self-actualization.

But what about cherishing our illusions if they make us happy? Alas! Such a veneer of joy must be continuously supported by further illusions, more bizarre, foreign, and destructive than we can imagine. These illusions are nothing but an escape from the dullness and boredom of a meaningless life, a lack of prospection, and a kind of daydreaming. That energy should rather be spent for advancement on the psychic level. We must liberate ourselves from the part of our being which already contains the seeds of decay and death—even while being alive—to come down into the path of true life; not just catching hold of our outer garment or persona, which is usually the reflection of a hidden life, but finding a newly discovered Self, a newly found substance and not the fragmented, mummified mask that has hypnotized us for most of our existence. This way we will bring light to ourselves and lift ourselves to our feet. We will then become taller, brushing off the cobwebs of our unconscious, opening the door to self-communication and dialogue with others. At that point the unconscious loses its grip, and the rising into consciousness is like a surprise balloon, finally ascending from its anchored place in the dark unconscious.

A perfect example of such cleansing is reflected by a typical *Phosphorus* woman with great desire for travel and freedom, who had three dreams in the same night. This repetition of dreams always reflects the same theme, showing more clarification and, at the same time, indicating a possible going forward in one's journey, as expressed in this patient.

Conscious situation: Her husband suffered a heart attack and now she feels trapped in the situation as she must perform more functions than before, taking care of a dog and her husband, cutting down on her own time. Here are the three dreams, experienced the same night.

Dream one

I have an apartment and look for a roommate to share. A lesbian butch shows up. I was taking a shower and before I turn the water off, I ask her if she wants to take one. She takes one and says when coming out of it, "The water was too hot."

Dream two

The roles are reversed as I now look for an apartment to share. This woman is grossly overweight. When I show up, she tells me "I want to get pregnant." I leave as I don't want to live in an apartment with a baby.

Dream three

I am on a bus driven by a male and all the passengers are female. My best friend is on the bus too and looks like me, tall and slender. We stop to visit a building on our own. Coming into the building I tell my friend that I want to take a shower and I tell her to let the driver in the bus know to wait for me.

Analysis

All dreams take place in an apartment or tourist building, reflecting the creation of a situation of a temporary Self. In the first two dreams her shadow side does not reflect at all how she really looks, but as it is her shadow (with characteristics she does not like) she takes showers, a cleansing of this shadow. Even in the third dream, where she was on a bus, she tells her shadow to tell the male driver (her animus, who is the active force) to wait for her as she is still "cleansing" her shadow, before she wants to continue on her trip with these many women, reflecting that the dream has a message for women all around. These were insightful dreams for her, as their message was clearly understood—to cleanse her shadow—to integrate the unruly passions (shower was too hot) dwelling in her unconscious. Is everyone as attentive to listen to their dreams?

Alas! For most, our first duty in life is to be as artificial as possible, to be identified with a deceiving persona. Our second duty we have not yet discovered or heard of. We detect the defects and decrepitude in others that are more clearly present in ourselves. It is far more common to see the roots of evil in others, though it is as visible as trees in ourselves. We should not spare ourselves from searching to find out if the vice of the neighbor is one that has taken deeper root in ourselves, and not remain keener in judging others' lives but lazy when it comes to correcting our own. Instead of acknowledging and exploring our shadow, we fall into a state of life in which we remain in a shell that gradually hardens and imprisons us, making progress impossible. We might say, "This is the way I am, don't try to change me," feeling that our entombment should be celebrated for its constancy! Sadly, such rigid preconceptions and convictions do not create a beautiful life. What a mistake it is, to be so deep in a dormant state that alarm bells have no more effect. The shadow has become a maleficent force whose solvent action easily finds a vehicle to plow through our conscious, creating havoc all along. There is great danger that this entity takes total autonomy and control; its wild horses of fate will run away with the light chariot of our fortune, which can even lead to an appalling end (for example, dissociation). Far too often, our praiseworthy intentions are as withes of straw in the fire of the underworld! How to stifle this ignorance and self-aggrandizement, and awaken dormant vices and virtues? What to do with the tyranny of the shadow? Will we always stand in the darkness of its slavery? Or do we consider tasting the sweetness of liberty? Why do most prefer to project their shadow, rather than use it as a tool for self-realization?

As Cicero once said, "Any man can make mistakes, but only an idiot persists!" By successfully projecting or suppressing the shadow on a day-to-day basis, we often achieve that desired grandiose persona, which grows like a genie released from his bottle. People around us who are always determined to find something desirable and wonderful in everything we do or say only stimulate our shadow, which allows our unconscious to overgrow like an impenetrable jungle. Only determined explorers—a small remnant of diligent, truth-seeking people—fail to affirm our genius that is so loudly and annoyingly pronounced.

Like a lightning-quick minded *Lachesis* or *Sulphur*, mankind can develop a humorous vein, stimulated by constant practice and, yes, by extraordinary natural gifts. But without integrating the unconscious elements, this fair ship of extravaganza and masked life will inevitably come to wreck on the shoals of spiritual poverty, even *before* earthly poverty. Confronted at that point with reality, instead of conquering and overleaping this poverty, we more often anchor our boat in the wrong port where it is tossed and thrown around by the unruly ocean that our unconscious has become—the only way left to assure ourselves of a modicum of self-control.

But can such a person, an intense pleasure-loving and power-seeking individual, wait forever? No! His persona has already grown so much—the desire to dazzle and astonish so great—that he identifies with it, wanting to wear his peacock feathers all the time, and at all cost! And of course, there is that advantage of having a big shadow: notoriety, often the forerunner of fame (ill-gained for sure), is always commercially and professionally valuable. As such, because the bar of morality is set so low, he really does not care what others *say* of him, just that people *talk* of him. Increased self-assurance creates defiance and his black soul turns cold as stone. More commonly than not, there is great concern about a speck on the outside of the platter, while the inside is never peeped at—much less probed and investigated! Suppression and projection are the rulers of a human's kingdom! And eventually the black cloud of hate, deceit, and condescendence will become more and more threatening to the Self, and if not destroying it, will only produce a freckle of what life could have been. Just as there is no season as beautiful as the brief northern summer, in an area where, three-quarters of the year, cold and darkness rule, this short reprieve from snowstorms and blizzards resembles the minor (and often self-served) "good" deeds, masking everything we want to avoid: that we are not a shepherd, a guru, or even a king, but more like the majority of mankind! So spring, when birds arrive in flocks and flowers spring to life on all sides—so beautiful and oh so brief—resembles the correct attitude and conduct of the ordinary human, all too brief a season in an entire life!

The mirror teaches us what we always should know: that we are horribly normal. The collective, ordinary man, is made of the same stuff as all; he is "us." A man who can confess his weaknesses is strong indeed! "He that is without sin among you, cast the first stone," as stated in scripture, or Shakespeare's version of the same truth, "Use every man after his desert, and who should 'scape whipping?" Human beings differ in accidentals only: in dress, manner, tone of voice, religious opinions, personal appearance, habits, interests, etc. Human nature, as history shows, can be called dreadfully universal with little chance of progress. Most people, by definition, are perfectly ordinary. Oscar Wilde phrased it in in his play *Lady Windermere's Fan*: "We are all in the gutter but some of us are able to look at the stars" (Wilde, 1966, p. 417). In other words, some of us can rise from unconscious dark instincts to enlightenment, to become self-actualized, an example of free men. Sadly, those who reach self-realization, to some degree remain mostly invisible among the masses, even if they stand out as a beacon in the darkness. We are taught more by bad examples than good ones, as they are more common and, unfortunately, create the average standards.

There is nothing easier than hiding in the shadow side (a frequently used form of escapism), being the possessor of a liar—one who can get by with fearless statements and superb irresponsibility while disdaining proof of any kind. Helped by a one-sided thinking conscious function, morality does not come into question for such a person. "What morality?" he says, "I am more adroit in presenting truth according to my wishes." Lying for him has become an art, requiring careful study and devotion. Usually it starts with exaggeration of the facts (sycosis) and evolves into lying to manipulate, rule, gain undeserved recognition and respect, and, no doubt, increased social status. A true liar's voice is so loud that no one can hear what he says! Some never invoke moral disappointments because they never create moral expressions, dispensing altogether with ethical pretense. Lawsuits, racial bias, and skirting the truth are just part of the fabric of everyday life—bumps in the road to imagined glory—as the liar's most prominent character trait is shamelessness.

Most liars think there is a distinction between stealing and cheating, the latter to get people's money for nothing, selling something that is advertised as being worth much more than it really is, making others believe they are getting a bargain. But how much difference is there between that and stealing? What guides most people's belief is that no one will find out and things will work out for the best (for them!). Considered the worst that may happen—because of lack of moral principles—is they get afflicted with temporary loose stools (*diarrhea from excitement and anticipation*). And such a debased man says, "Why should I not act this way? It brings me glory, power, and riches!" Contemptuously, he regards the honorable man who correctly follows the moral code—especially when his action is a dangerous or laborious task with no compensation of exterior riches—as a fool.

How do we view and use our shadow side? Are we to be conquered and corrupted by it, or to possess it and use it to our advancement? Hammer or nail—which? We know that humans don't possess infinite virtues, so the myriad vicissitudes of struggle will test all our powers and determination in life. And every victory leads to a new battlefield; no rest this side of the grave! Will we take discipline and honesty into service? What will we make of it? The answer is critical to governing our life: it is a choice between the suicide or liberation of the soul.

Of course some will say, "I was temporarily carried away by my passions," but such a man has no idea that he is rooted and anchored in character traits that are holding him hostage, unless he finds a way to break the chains of his personal cell by following the rules of right-living and right-believing, which is morality. Some might concede, "I fell continually into some minor misstep but that should not be a hindrance to grow and evolve." But this is ignorant of the concept that "Small drops of water hollow out a stone," as expressed by the Roman philosopher/poet Lucretius (94-55 BC). The sheer repetition of small drippings is enough to affect our moral compass until we get lost in our search for light, remaining on the path of darkness in a vast wilderness.

The investigation of the shadow side is for most an unbearable and unachievable self-confronting exercise. Therefore, we prefer to exist with a dual personality, living a life of fancies, while obscuring the source of real life and growth, the unconscious. The shadow is like a coin that rolled under a piece of furniture and remained there, lost; out of sight! As philosopher Michel de Montaigne stated in his essays, "We are, I know not how, double within ourselves!"

Having strayed from the right path, as most do, we resemble an angel stripped of his halo. And most often, we easily exercise projection as it does not require too much effort. That is, we discover the false truth in others, and do so with pleasure, but remain blind to our own ugly recollections, judgments, and evil expectations and deeds. As writer La Rochefoucauld (1613-1680) expressed in his aphorisms, "We all criticize in others what others criticize in us," and, "Failings known to us are easily forgotten" (La Rochefoucauld, 2006, pp. 45, 24). Rarely do we turn an eye inward, for it would shake our foundation.

A sad example is the current hypocrisy of the Catholic Church. As reported in numerous news articles, at least 50% of priests are gay, and yet they continue to condemn homosexuality. In addition, it remains a fact that many of the homophobic bishops and cardinals have been (and are) gay, following the well-known truth, "What you hate in yourself but cannot face, you police and punish in others." It has become clear that those in the Church hierarchy obsessed with the homosexual question often *turn out to be* gay—how naked these bejeweled emperors can appear! The reality is that celibacy is not easy. Besides risking emotional problems like depression, isolation, and living a false life, abstinence also can lead to physical disease, most noteworthy cancer (*Ailments from continence or celibacy; sexual desire suppressed*)—prostate cancer in men and cervical/breast cancer in women. When will the Church get rid of hypocrisy, dishonesty, and dysfunction—and acknowledge that indeed the clergy is not free from carrying a shadow? (This applies to all clergy, of all religions.) The solution to the problem is also a collective one: don't create a pseudo Self, stop pretending, and you will find freedom! The suppression and projection of the shadow and the accentuated exposure of the persona (called inflation) should not become a default setting to which we invariably return.

No wonder we prefer violent opposition to changes, taking a revolutionary road to integration but remaining tone-deaf and unaware, preferring to reside in the clouds and leave behind the terrific threats and powers from below, cutting ourselves off from real life. We prefer to live life with a shipwrecked mind, as a plant removed from soil. We regard working on our shadow as futile, either ignoring it or convinced that we can overcome it with willpower—even when we go through life with broken wings. Yet in the shadow everyone is like everyone else. The shadow is as real and abiding as an attachment to a house, or better, is our closest sibling or twin. Integration can be a Herculean task of digging our way out of ruins, patiently and laboriously, like a survivor of an abandoned city or a wanderer lost in a forest, attempting to mark out tracks. Being conscious of our shadow traits requires great daring and humility, especially to reveal moral knowledge, the dichotomy between good and bad. Carl Jung adequately states, "It is quite within the bounds of possibility for a man to recognize the relative evil of his nature, but it is a rare and shattering experience for him to gaze into the face of absolute evil" (Jung, 1978, CW Vol. 9, Part II, p.10).

We are afraid to see reality as it is, as it hurts too much. Sure, some of us might confess to having a "bad streak in character" to keep peace in our household. But this thought is followed by doing nothing, so our house—the Self—remains unchanged. That character observation might be real, but it has not become a reality since the thought was never followed by a connective action. A mere confession does not mean that an ugly event is not going to happen again. But to expect us to display in public our innermost motivation, our most hidden private matters, is asking the impossible, a task only for superman or a philosopher king (although we would only get confirmed by others what we deep down in our heart know ourselves). There is always that collective human trait of an utter lack of trust in others, for fear of being discovered for who we really *are*, not how we want to *appear*! But we should be thinking about what we are doing, and thinking should begin with remembrance, leading to a revolution to secure an approximation of completeness. To sustain such achievement, we at least hope to find a spouse, good friend, or physician to accept our private shortcomings with grace, so that it does not lead to a possible dangerous exposure on which others will jump, as dominance over others often rules the life of humans, especially in those that have no power over themselves.

Another way of dealing with the shadow when it escapes from the unconscious and a vice is committed, is the excuse, "Doesn't everyone make this 'mistake' (euphemism for vice)?" And this is always followed by, "No one is perfect," to mitigate the offensive act committed. We can call that a consensual validation: for such a person, the fact that millions of people show the same vice (be it jealousy, cruelty, etc.) should make it more acceptable, but the common sharing of a vice does not make it a virtue under any circumstances. Seneca's advice (Roman philosopher, 4 BC) was to interact with people who can improve us (to allow ourselves to be influenced by them), and with those we can improve. When people hide greed (*Nux-v*) and lust for power (*Lycopodium*) in their shadow, when it comes out in the open it is considered by most just an annoying trait ("That guy is a jerk"), but in reality, it is one of the diseases in that person.

The fact that such a human gets away with it is the cause of this disease festering, until finally he gets burned out (*businessman worn out*) or becomes *impotent* and *dictatorial* because of identification with such a persona. In the case of *Lycopodium*, dangerous illusions come from a hidden sense of inferiority, so to offset this characteristic, being thin-skinned, he resorts to passion, anger, denial, a hint of fury, and throwing up his hands in despair. That he is not enlightened shows in his dogmatism (*intolerant to contradiction*). His real genius is in being theatrical —self-presentation is his greatest talent. His apparent self-confidence is just an enrichment and modification by his ego's coloration, as there is no base of inner strength: when one single stone (one glorious aspect) is removed, the whole edifice collapses.

Some of us excuse dark elements of our shadow because we received harsh treatment in life by one of our parents. This might summon sympathy from others, but it does not make *us* automatically sympathetic and powerful like a hero or knight, which is only wishful alchemy for fantasy life, not real life. What we need is introspection, introversion, and humility, a place of silence and calm, so that this event does not become an eternal excuse, ruining our life and that of others. As the ancient Greek philosopher Epicurus stated, "The beginning of salvation is the knowledge of sin." It is evident that we don't know how to correct ourselves if we don't know where we are wrong. It might sound harsh, but it is the only path to follow. We must be our own prosecutor and then our judge, not an eloquent lawyer who tries to convince twelve jurors that there is "reasonable doubt" regarding our guilt. I agree with French philosopher Voltaire, who said on his deathbed when asked if he wanted to confess his wrongdoings, "Of course I regret all my sins, especially those which I did not commit," acknowledging he knew he was human. I think, at the end, the most interesting thing about a conscience is *how* it answers, not *to whom it answers*.

Centuries ago, Plato had already stated in *The Republic*:

> I want you to go on to picture the enlightenment or ignorance of our human condition somewhat as follows. Imagine an underground chamber, like a cave with an entrance open to the daylight and running a long way underground. In this chamber are men who are prisoners there … and the exit is blocked by a fire, the power of the sun .... (Plato, 1984, p. 313)

There have been innumerable interpretations of Plato's cave allegory, but following Jung's interpretation, the cave—a relative fixed symbol of the unconscious—is depicted here as a "prison" to humanity. Not that we are eager to dwell in it and explore it, at least not consciously, but far too many humans in general want to remain there, as acknowledging the imperfections of their lives—when peeking through the door to enlightenment (light/the sun=relative fixed symbol of consciousness, the dazzling radiant world of the mind)—will reveal the falsehoods, skeletons in the closet that are able to shatter all illusions and fancies we are living. "What he saw before was foolery, but now he saw more rightly" (Ibid., p. 313).

This ascent from the dark is almost suicidal, a shocking enterprise, as self-realization is as blinding and painful as an initial encounter with the direct sun. But courage should be called upon, then the long painful road to becoming more complete will be started, as succinctly expressed by Hahnemann in his exhortation, "*Aude sapere*," or "Dare to know." We live in the dark, not seeing real things but only shadows, living the life of one half-blind. Only continuous trips to the dark cave to integrate its shadowy elements, and facing the light, will bring man closer to self-realization.

Rather than turning an eye in the right direction, we must first return to the cave (the unconscious), then have the courage to turn this instrument (the eye) to the bright light of the sun (conscious), in order to become more complete, more at peace with ourselves, and to be a model educator for others. Plato expressed the importance of this in his idea of a philosopher king: "A person who is not rich in gold, but in what is necessary for a happy man, the riches of a good and wise life" (Ibid., p. 319).

Few are those that confront the moral issues caused by their conduct, which would be a more meaningful way to make amends and free themselves from long held skeletons. And alcoholism and drug addiction (*morphinism*), forms of self-poisoning (as they often become an irresistible impulse to throw away everything in life), are two syphilitic miasmatic traits that must be taken as entry points to find the patient's simillimum, so that relapses are reduced to a bare minimum or none! We need to listen, with at least tacit acceptance of the moral urging to change, or the long arc of deceit will continue, and progress will not happen. Freedom and enlightenment do not happen because we *want* to see the light. They happen because we do not find it necessary to live further in the dark as a man half-aware, fooling ourselves and others. And as we come nearer to the candle, our eyes will adjust, and allowing for the accommodation and time that it takes will become part of our journey and growth. The truth is that we must seek enlightenment from the depths of our own inner darkness. Renewal can only come from what has heretofore not been accepted and assimilated, a bottleneck that few seem to want to pass through in life, a very painful and anxiety-provoking process. Why do we put up with leading such a diminished, autoerotic life?

Invisible Personalities, Occasionally and Forcefully Perceived

"There is no light without shadow and no psychic wholeness without imperfection; to round itself out, life calls not for perfection but for completeness" (Jung, 1953, para. 208).

The truth, and integrating the dark elements of the shadow which fail to fit the ego ideal, brings relief—even if it is hard to bear, unpleasant to think about it, painful to confess and miserable to reveal, especially to ourselves let alone to those we love. The shadow is the archetype—an essential building block of the personality—closest to the personal conscious, the most easily accessible part of the personal unconscious. The shadow can therefore be considered the first exercise in the investigation of the unconscious, the novice stage, before we reach the deeper, more intimate and inaccessible parts of the personal unconscious—anima and animus and other archetypes—a puzzling encounter which requires more insightful activity.

These revelations reveal the true person in ourselves, not the well-fabricated persona—the imperfect individual, often limping and falling off the wagon—but a person we should love and care enough about to walk the dangerous, narrow isthmus that blocks our way to happiness. By paying attention and being willing to accept the cooperation of the unconscious—by looking back and encountering the shadow (=the unconscious) —some pointers will show why we stumbled in the first place. And as we come down from the sky of greatness, and land (not always softly) on earth, we are told we are normal ordinary human beings. This acknowledgment that the shadow is as powerful and big as the other world will stop us from cherishing illusions about our wonderful character.

As much as we may think we have removed the shadow—an impossible and *not* desirable goal—we are reminded, often by the shadow itself, of our moral and intellectual defects, of our cowardice, arrogance, and our criticism of even those nearest to us, in the subtlest ways (especially when we think we understand all our own problems). The horrible discord in us—this internal battle—teaches us the striking lesson that we must forgive and accept our errors; discord is the great evil of the human species, and tolerance and acceptance is its only remedy. Every personal psyche contains crude emotions and inferior potentials and many more negative elements that can be *restrained* and *retrained* but not eliminated. How to tame this shadow? Before this animal can be tamed, it must be caught! We need psychological courage for that, and courage of the heart. We could start with an attempt to be honest and demonstrate discipline, to be aware of and accept our shadow, and to apply our desire to be introspective. This way we keep the evil in full sight and can wait for the next episode to see if we use our psychic energy in a positive rather than a negative way. Not an easy task, as reason does not always have the upper hand on the shadow's passionate and overwhelming strength, and indolence is the easiest way out for most—to remain in the dark. Even admitting to some deplorable traits is not eliminating them; that is an infantile illusion. The most we can hope for is to strike an accepted balance between light and shadow: acceptance and experience of the shadow elements is crucial and creates a chance of change. Focusing mainly on our good identity will only increase the evil in our unconscious.

We must always consider the good and evil in us. "Virtue" comes from the Latin *virtus*, meaning "courage, excellence, character or strength" (the number one virtue being humility, a mentality shown in the will not to be favored at the expense of another). Yet where there is virtue there is vice, an ever-present black spot in the snow-white consciousness. As recognized in TCM centuries ago, there is no yang (light) without yin (darkness). But who does not prefer to remain floating in the white clouds of consciousness, a land of fancy illusions?

Would it surprise you that all of us have heaven and hell in us? At any moment, in everyone, there is a deep-rooted, monstrous lust for disarray, arguments, fighting, savage violence, and above all, for the gutter. Most of us deny and repress the possible thief, morphinomaniac, alcoholic, and murderer in us (the latter being a collective trait of the fearful shadow figure), so we remain blissfully ignorant. Most cannot answer the question, "Do you belong to that class of criminals?" because the question has never been asked. That well is just too deep and dark! The primitive in us never disappears, as we remain controlled by passions and emotions that should have died centuries ago. At least, we should hope that we can abandon the delusion that good can be gained by evil means, a first step to silencing the darkness in ourselves. Behind the curtain, our individuation has stagnated, as we have become nothing but ordinary men, subject to primitive instincts. No man is white or black; every man is freckled! All of us have the emotion to kill; when we strongly dislike someone, we involuntarily wish he was dead. And even if we have not killed anyone, most of us have read some obituary notices with great satisfaction. Hanna Arendt (1906-1975, brilliant essayist and philosopher), coined the phrase "the banality of evil" to explain how easily ordinary people can slip into monstrosity. Of course, there is also the lesser known "banality of good." This refers to unknown, ordinary citizens who quietly show kindness to the needy, the hungry, the displaced and dispossessed—a silent battle that occurs in everyday lives. It is only a question of choice, of morality that tilts the victory to the angel over the devil.

Although one cruelty does not deserve another, we universally seem to possess an innate trait of revenge, a strongly syphilitic trait, especially found in the homeopathic portraits of *Nat-m*, *Nit-ac*, *Lachesis*, and *Nux-vomica* (*revengeful; hatred of persons who offended him*). Revenge is nothing but a defensive return blow, which we deliver to try to put a stop to the pain before the painful event becomes an everlasting torture. But in acting out of self-preservation with overwhelming thoughts of restitution, one is only robbed, as feelings of revenge serve no useful purpose to building up an improved Self. The previously mentioned characters, however, will equate deception with (*Ailments from*) "*wounded honor*," and feel compelled to restore their respect.

We attempt to deceive ourselves by trying to appear better in our own eyes. But however hard we try, scraps from our previous masks remain on our face, and we are unable to tear them off. And so, we hobble further along, not being able to find ourselves, as we keep wearing what has become a reconstructed, shabby mask. What we don't realize nor anticipate is that we resemble a fly who negotiates the strands of the spider's web before becoming caught there, struggling. Are we staying engaged in a Greek drama of life where foolish notions play the lord, and a jumble of misunderstandings and misdeeds play the vassals? Are we caught in the torture of that annoying but persistent question, "Do we live from without or from within?" Is there a force to be found in us to put a bridge down between the two, or are we always gazing to the other side with sadness, inertia, indetermination, and unresolved emotions? Mostly, unknowingly, we are stuck in one world, as lightning-speed emotions (that may catalyze our journey inward) are quickly trampled by "solid" reasons. Homeostasis must wait! For how long? What remains only results in a glaring, miserable existence in all its colors.

As for the original question, I want to live from within, to collect any tiny grains of gold and bring them to the light, a heavy task but worth achieving, as I can then try to become responsive to the inner urge to become a more wholesome human being. And although I am a *Sulphur* personality, even at the end of my life I do not want to become a hermit, because I desire to stay engaged. For real life also needs influences from without, in order that our actual fortifier—the unconscious—can exert its justified actions for mankind, not just for me. But what a struggle it is! I have no illusions that it ever will end. But trying is better than giving up!

Unleashing the base instincts is a collective trait of human beings. Paul Gauguin, the celebrated painter, put this concept in his own words: "Nail up some indecency in plain sight over your door" (Gaugin, 1958, p. 21). His wife left him to go back to Copenhagen with their children as she loved the successful broker he was before, not the penniless artist he became. He died in Tahiti in 1903, wracked with suffering from acquired syphilis before he could benefit from the sale of his wonderful paintings.

There is a multitude of characteristics of the collective man in the unconscious of *each and every* individual. Humans have always been slaughtering each other, as they still do today; they have always been liars, cheats, envious, and greedy individuals. There is much proof of the blindness of human nature when we are carried away by our passions. We are full of weakness and error; let us mutually pardon each other our follies and misdeeds. The wicked foolishness of man is the first law of nature. As Aristotle proclaimed, "No outstanding soul is free from a mixture of follies." Everyone at some point has thoughts of committing a criminal act—Road rage, anyone? Nuclear marital dispute, anyone?—but morality, self-control, and introspection will hopefully get the upper hand in this ferocious battle. We should remember the immortal words of Confucius: "Live as you would have liked to live, when you are dying; treat your neighbor as you would want him to treat you."

The shadow is not an innocent appendix with a lot of dangerous destructive powers when activated, but is like a suction cup, unwilling to let go of the past, a resistance against the new, making man fall off the wagon time and time again. This paradox, that we can be a moral being and at other times a despicable character, is the difficulty we must overcome.

Is it worth it? Do we achieve anything? By bringing the shadow into consciousness, we reduce its power, therefore gaining a degree of freedom, and then it is up to us to make moral choices, ethical decisions, and exercise self-discipline, rather than avoiding these choices through neurosis and childish outbursts. Such testing of the shadow can occur several times a day. A simple example: you see someone in a store drop a $10 bill on the floor. Your shadow side might tell you, "Oh, you can keep this money, no one will see it." It is here that you are faced with the moral choice not to follow this little fantasy and negative thought. Besides being the basis for our individual morality, accepting and recognizing our shadow aids in building up humility, humor, and less critical and judgmental behavior towards others. After all, humility is not debasement but a corrective to self-love.

Here is a dream from a male patient (it is worth noting here that the shadow always appears in a dream as a person of the same gender).

Dream

I am in a place with many other people and I seem to be very angry with another man. Even if he is just bumping me accidentally, I retort with hitting him furiously. My reactions are tenfold what he did to me. It seems that everyone else present approves because nobody seems to be surprised about my reaction or voices a different opinion. Then I wake up in a normal state.

Analysis

The analysis is obvious: There is no acknowledgement by this patient of his shadow side, as the dreamer reacts very violently to something that clearly belongs to him. He does not recognize that he has both personalities, and the fact that everyone else around him (collective unconscious) seems to approve shows that this is not only a reflection of the personal shadow but also of the great strength and contagiousness of the collective shadow, as most people react this way and we all get infected with the contents of the collective unconscious.

As much as stepping on someone's shadow was a bad omen for primitive people who believed that it injured their soul, I cannot express enough that we should all let someone step on our shadow, giving us a kick in the butt, informing us of what we are trying to hide from others. Acknowledging and accepting its content and using it as a guide in life would make us all better persons, before we steadily increase the shadow stratum to a thick layer—an outcome that is difficult to bear.

Primitives did not want to be photographed either. In a picture of native Lakota Indian women, in the book *The Killing of Crazy Horse* by Thomas Powers, all the women can be seen averting their eyes from the camera, in the manner considered seemly by the Lakota, as they feared their soul would be taken away from them if they looked. All, that is, except one who gazed openly at the photographer. She was married to a white trapper (Grey Eyes), and was therefore influenced by modern habits (Powers, 2010, p. 136). But for most Native American Indians, having their picture taken meant they would die in three days!

We should not fear looking into a lens focused on our true Self but should welcome it, as we should welcome our shadow being stepped on! The shadow is a trickster who can deceive even the simplest, most well-meaning soul. At the same time, it can also make itself known to everyone, causing the house to collapse at inopportune moments. That this shadow has a continuous strong drive, or libido, in our conscious life is shown by the following male dream.

Dream

I am with another man in a dark alley. Although this man seems to be blind, he looks very menacing to me, so I hit him with a whip and then try to bury him in the sandy stretch beside the narrow road. As I leave him, the sand keeps on moving and I run quickly away, taken by fright.

Analysis

As seen here, the shadow often appears as an inferior personality. Most people flee from their shadow, but burying it and running away, rather than confronting it, will only come to haunt its possessor in the form of numerous neuroses and sometimes even mass hysteria. The energy from the unconscious, and particularly the shadow, is always actively working in mysterious ways. Running away will not decrease its activity. Accepting and letting this figure come into our life often turns out to be helpful in the most unexpected ways. Here is a real example that my wife witnessed on her travels.

Conscious situation: My wife was traveling somewhere in the company of ten people. She observed that one woman knew how to twist her husband (a *fille à papa*) around her little finger, always looking for rescue in the father figure. This woman was always seeking attention from all others too—like a child needing constant approval and love (*Pulsatilla* comes to mind!). Then she revealed this dream to everyone at breakfast.

Dream

I dreamt about a young girl, and in my dream, I proceeded to kill her. I was very upset when I woke up because I adore children!

Analysis

Her dream tells her to kill the child in her (her alter ego or shadow side), so that she would be more acceptable to others. The child is usually the childish aspect of the dreamer (same if it is a boy, in a man's dream), a graphic demonstration of something that has happened or of who she really is. It is a piece of primitive life. She had to sacrifice her infantile state of mind. The adult person in this dream does not know how to resolve the problem except by expressing her unacknowledged aggression, and when everything is dark the only thing to do is to become hysterical or childish. As we can see, the figures in her dream connect her with a tough, "no-nonsense" confrontational energy that she fears, for it threatens her self-image of a sweet, helpless, cared-for princess—the darling of her husband and who "adores children" (that represent herself). This often happens in a father-complex where the little girl is "daddy's girl," and growing up, infected with this complex, is able to twist her husband (and men in general) around her little finger (representing the Strong-Weak Woman) so that he can't resist giving this poor little soul everything she wants. How can the homeopath discover this dark side in practice if not through dreams?

What to Ask to Discover the Reverse of the Ego Ideal

Here is an important question for the homeopath or therapist: "How, in your first interview, can you attempt a glance at the shadow side of your patient?"

This is critical, since the shadow contains everything your patient wants to hide, the ugly, the not so good, and above all, the cyber delusion which we want to know. You can ask the patient: "Describe the personality type you find most impossible to get along with." "What do you hate, or are most repulsed by, in people?" "What makes you angry about other persons?" "What traits in others disturb you the most? "What (in this person) gets under your skin?" As the shadow represents the opposite side of the ego, it always embodies those traits that the patient dislikes most in people.

Unbeknownst to himself, most likely the patient will produce a description of his own forgotten and repressed characteristics, which he easily sees in others, not in himself. There is of course a fine line between what is truly objectively perceived about the other person and what is "thrown onto" the other (called "projection," from the Latin *pro-jicio*, or to "throw upon") to hide his own weaknesses. Projection is always the visualization of a complex. These very qualities are so unacceptable to the projector precisely because they represent his own repressed side: *we see immediately in others, what we turn a blind eye to within us.* In other words, disowning our own manure is the way to go. Or is it not?

If we think that another person is arrogant and power-driven, then replace in thought that other person with "I" and ask if we are not arrogant and power-driven. In so doing, we might discover what complex has gotten hold of us! It should be clear that we are really projecting our own negative traits if the intensity of the accompanying emotion with which we see the fault in someone else rises above a normal rational observation. When we exclaim with furor that we "can't stand this person's haughtiness," we should investigate if we ourselves do not carry even more than a whiff of this arrogance. It is like that person's face in the mirror has become ours, always shocking and painful to see! The negative qualities in others which don't bother us as much and don't raise our ire, are usually not likely to be part of our shadow. Whenever we project, the compulsive nature of the projection denies us the freedom to take or leave it—in other words, denies us the freedom of choice, as we are under the power-drive of the projection. As too often seen in crimes where someone kills their lover because he'd "rather kill than lose her," this is nothing but a projection of the murderer's own archaic anima.

This is one of the purposes of the shadow: it is the archetypal urge to blame someone, to find a *scapegoat*, to blame others to justify oneself, especially if the one blamed is of the same sex. To justify ourselves, we become a warrior, a fearsome lawyer, or more likely, a collective ordinary person who can think day and night about whose fault it was that something went wrong—even finding another fault that eats up the old one—but one thing is sure, it's always someone else's mistake. By doing so, time does not heal, and walls do not conceal, because the roots of things go so deep that only the simillimum can pull them up! Shadow projection can even be collective, leading also to prejudice and racial intolerance, precluding the possibility of Eros—the function of relationships—resulting in religious fanaticism and wars.

Through awareness of these projections we can become conscious of the unconscious processes in ourselves. This can lead to reflection, from the Latin *re-flexio*, or "*bending back*": what we have been throwing outward to someone else, is returned to ourselves, like a boomerang, so that we can reflect on it and see the real meaning and ownership of the projective contents. An Indian guru once expressed it:

> You have to gather your own manure and put it on your own plants. Most people are foolish and carefully gather their own manure and throw it away and then they go out and buy someone else's manure to put on their plants.

It should not surprise us that a repressed shadow leads to a lack of sense of humor, and inability to laugh at ourselves. That is because one becomes far too judgmental and unforgiving of other people.

When committing misdeeds, our "desiring I," whatever it was aiming for—greed, power, or lust—will find difficulty to cease its activity, and most likely will be followed by another frivolous if not inhuman action, creating a permanent state of mind, especially if crimes go unnoticed. Regret, the "conscience I," is just a brief afterthought, losing the contest, while quickly being delegated to the cellar of the unconscious. Can there be a truce and friendship between these two "I's," so that a more permanent unity of mind, one bound together, can appear? Even "knowing" that we are going to do wrong will not exclude the choice of the will, as desires, passions, and imaginations triumph all too often, setting our house (Self) on fire. So, is there such a thing as a unified mind, or is this concept merely a tool for moral education? Only true love achieves it, not auto-eroticism but a love for justice, which seems to be the hardest to grasp. It is also true love for others that will be the glue that binds together, a steadfastness to be enjoyed, stilling the mind's restlessness, leaving a lasting footprint.

But is our cellar only stocked with negativity, a hoarding place to pile all the debris of life—the ugly, the shameful, and painful—or is unexpected treasure to be found there also? Can an oasis be found in the desert of the soul? Most think (or hope) never to visit this barren country, but can we find there at least some redeeming virtue? Is the shadow just our inner arch-villain, or can it also be our redeemer? Let's find out!

Seeds of Growth in the Garden of Unrest: The Positive Side of the Shadow

The shadow—although, by definition, a negative figure—is not all bad. While possessing infantile and morally inferior contents, it surprisingly possesses certain positive repressed traits also, valuable qualities which point to a different, long-forgotten background. Meaningful and valuable contents and characteristics can be buried in the same garbage can as the rotten and vile mass of forgettable things. So, the shadow can contain valuable traits that are needed by consciousness to live a more complete life, to help reclaim a gift or passion for the person desiring to redirect his life because he has been living below his real capacity! Even those who grew up with much privilege did not always see the runway to their calling, but botched the take-off for various reasons, so reality fell short of high hopes. The school yearbooks are full of beaming pictures labeled "Most Likely to Succeed," yet some of those promising individuals were never able to meet the lofty expectation. This land of might-have-been is peopled with such gorgeous shadow shapes. We are easily sidetracked by the many pitfalls of life, and even by well-meaning parents who force their children to operate in their archaic conscious function. Worse, when the patient as a child was always told that she was stupid and will never amount to anything (an animus's voice that can recur in dreams), such undue criticism (*Ailments from domination* and *rudeness of others*) can lead to timidity and inertia, paralyzing future life.

There are vocations suited to natural musical, athletic, or artistic talents. It seems a cruel gesture of fate if those talents were suppressed by a patriarchal figure because of purely financial and materialistic reasons. Real talents are then forcefully cast away in the shadow side, where they remain non-stimulated, withering away as a tree that longed for water but never grew into its full potential. In this instance, where the shadow personality can be thought of as the unlived life—an illness from which one can die (*Lachesis* is a perfect example)—the shadow is not the dark brother but the lighter of the "two brothers," the one that needs to be acknowledged and freed from his cage to show his unknown splendor to the world. We can only hope that this liberation comes as soon as possible, and not around middle-life when the situation often creates the well-known "midlife crisis."

Negative events in childhood combined with certain constitutions create other reasons for not living up to one's potential, producing neurotic invalidism. Timidity and lack of self-confidence are often clear signs of such neurotic invalidism, but even if a person has all the intellect and beauty that Nature can provide, when one child in the family was favored because of such characteristics while the other ones were neglected as their "future could never be so bright," the favorite can suddenly be overcome by burning feelings of guilt over having received too much while her siblings were cast aside—realizing, as an adult, that she was not favored because she was loved, but rather was exploited for the parents' financial and social redemption. "Once you are a physician, a lawyer, a great actress … you will take care of us in our old days," was the real reason and mantra. We should not be surprised when this favored person, destined to be the success and pride of the family, ends up living a drab and colorless life. Such a person may cast away her pleasure-giving talents and use aggression and hatred in her self-imposed miseries, reproaching others unjustly for missed chances and illnesses that have occurred, as she is caught in a web of secret self-pity, evoking the sympathy of like-minded sufferers, which is sufficient solace to deny even metropolitan enjoyments like museums, concerts, libraries, and exhibitions (*indifference to pleasure*). For that person it is all about revenge against the parents, and therefore she refuses to live a life according to her talents, full of bitterness about the injustice against her, while working in a menial job far below her capacities, desires, and expectations, putting her in a state of neurotic invalidism.

A *Sulphur* personality can be another black type remedy in this class of the never-bloomed, but his reasons are quite different. Although blessed with a critical and intelligent mind, he can revolt against society from a young age on and becomes an ascetic hermit in whom self-deprivation and contrary behavior are self-imposed. He can neglect his appearance, live in small dirty places surrounded by his precious books, and decline to entertain people as well as refuse the occasional invitation from the few that have not run out of patience, which eventually they will.

Besides feelings of guilt (which can come even when the crime was nonexistent or not associated with a heinous crime or grievous sin), and besides distorted love from parents as mentioned before, some unfortunate souls quell their talents as they are forced to take over the role of an absent parent early in their childhood (*taking too early responsibility—Carcinosin, Sepia*), which can create hidden anger at every family member

—the absent alcoholic or drug addicted father or mother, and those she needed to take care of for whom she sacrificed her life —obliterating her growth and future potential. And most of us to some extent indulge in a degree of self-destruction under the guise of being a victim, evoking sympathy as a reward while avoiding looking inward to the shadow.

Another person, after steady progress and every indication of a great, promising future, suddenly changes track and veers off in a less fruitful direction. And there does not have to be a major incident triggering this detour. Often it is a minor issue or difficulty occurred in life, in which the person was unable to adjust himself because he wanted the world to adjust to him, thereby destroying himself at the very moment he thought he was succeeding.

Sometimes the surface of the positive side has a *general collective positive* result with a *personal negative value*, as seen in the life of Gandhi. With a view to spiritual perfection and service to the poor as well as justice for his people, Gandhi relinquished the pleasures of life, abandoned his family and lived in utter simplicity but *without* withdrawing from human society, very different from the ascetic who withdraws as a recluse.

So, the unconscious is not just a bin for receiving the conscious mind's rejects but performs a therapeutic function by showing the conscious mind what needs to be done to get rid of unease and unhappiness, and to achieve fuller satisfaction in life. The real question for humanity will be: "Will the shadow be your friend, your favorite sibling, or your enemy?" The course of your life will be greatly influenced by this choice! Accept your shadow and it will become your best friend and counselor; ignore it and there will be no other entity that is more hostile during your life, creating instances where you will be embarrassed by the tricks it can play on you. Unfortunately, many are too ignorant and lazy to think about the moral aspects of their life, so the unconscious, good or bad, is left behind in a granite tomb!

An example of a male dreamer suffering from severe destructive arthritis in ankle and wrist joints and ankylosing spondylitis showed the different aspects of the shadow, some more benign than others. He was a critical, angry, and "entitled" person, all physical and emotional syphilitic miasmatic expressions. Here is his story, as told in three dreams (reportedly "of very different natures") he had one night.

Dream one

My wife, my brother, and I, are in a car driving around when we are told there are storms of some sort arriving in the area. Next thing we know they are two zaps from the sky like lightning bolts hitting the ground on both sides of us. The ground was dry and turned into a very wavy water mass. All of a sudden, my brother, the driver, is zigging us through crazy waves, passing cars and heading for safety. I am being like a backseat driver telling him what to do but he takes charge and gets us to safety. Out of harm, he crashes the car into the garage of a house, and I feel disappointed that we crashed, but happy that he drove so well and that he was confident and in control.

Dream two

My good male friend is driving me around on what appeared to be a four-wheeler trying to scare me and makes us crash but I am not letting him take too much control and I am infuriated that he wants to harm me. I go to see his dad to let him know how sad I am that he is turning into this power-hungry creature that only cares about himself and money. I am very emotional and on the verge of tears because it really saddens me that he is like this now.

Dream three

An ugly older man in a female strip joint is pushing cylindrical objects into the women, into all their orifices and even some holes in the body that do not exist in real life. I do not want to watch as it disgusts me, but my curiosity takes the better of me and I peak once in a while and then I am too disgusted. The dream ends there.

Analysis

Three dreams in the same night usually carry the same message to the dreamer, in slightly different forms but all reflecting the importance of their communication. The first dream shows the dreamer with his anima and his shadow driving in a vehicle in a place that is going to be stormy (the unconscious). Indeed, this is an investigation into his unconscious, as a lightning bolt (sudden change and impression) turns the dry ground into a watery mass (starting point into unconscious). His brother, or shadow, is driving the car (he is in the back seat, which tells us that he is not in control of his life journey), but his brother (shadow) at least tries to avoid an accident (showing the good side of his shadow) and heads for safety. Then he crashes the vehicle in the garage (unconscious) anyway, which is disappointing to the dreamer (still showing the "accidents" in his life which are under control of his shadow) but at least he feels happy his shadow maneuvered him out of a bigger catastrophe.

The second dream shows a more malicious side of his shadow (his "good friend"). Here too the shadow is in control of his destiny (at the wheel of the vehicle) but his shadow tries to scare him (or rather warns him) on purpose and crashes the vehicle (rather than avoiding an accident as in the previous dream). The dreamer went to see his friend's dad (the wise old man) to complain that his friend was a power-hungry creature who only cares about himself. The dreamer realizes the aspect of his alter ego, or shadow, which contains the syphilitic selfish nature. It made him very emotional in this dream, realizing the ugly side of this person (himself).

The last dream expresses a dark side of his shadow again. An ugly old man (not the wise old man), probably his old shadow, is doing ugly sexual things in a female strip joint, basically raping their bodies with cylindrical objects (symbol of a penis). The dreamer does not watch as he is disgusted by this, but there is a power in him that makes him peak once in a while, showing the control his shadow (containing sexual animalistic instincts) still has, although diminished, as he is disgusted with these actions.

These dreams carry the same message: his shadow side still has too much control of his life, but in a less powerful way than before, due to the remedy he received lately.

Another warning dream, given by the unconscious as a friend, was from a woman who was a very thinking-oriented, highly opinionated individual, always looking down on "common" people. She was proud of winning daily battles in a male dominated environment, as she was operating in a very competitive, ruthless corporation. At the same time, she complained of having difficulty gaining friends outside of that world, and of a cold, unresponsive husband and children. She was resistant to any psychological intervention and refused any homeopathic remedy "that could change her personality," as her husband and children were to blame for the daily, insignificant nuisances. She was brought to me by the following dream.

Dream

I am walking on a rocky road, the wind blowing and howling, which made every step difficult, but I proceed, driven by my strong will and determination. Then I see a dark, female figure sitting at the entrance of a cave. She stops me and says, "Don't look inside or you will be blinded!" With my usual determination I proceed anyway, and an old-fashioned torch illuminated the cave. To my horror, the lady at the entrance of the cave, who has followed me, is transformed into an ugly witch with pockmarked skin, and she is stabbing little female babies to death. I wake up in horror, and at first have difficulty opening my eyes.

Analysis

The dream is self-explanatory. This woman's one-sided, male determined attitude had killed all conscious feeling function in her drive to succeed in the desired corporate world. But her path in daily life (common things) remained difficult (rocky road and howling wind). Of course, she feels "other people are responsible for that" (=projection). Then she meets the lady, her shadow, who sits at the entrance of a cave (the border between conscious and unconscious), who warns her that the investigation of the unconscious (the cave) is a dangerous undertaking with risk (of blinding her). She proceeds anyway, driven by her indomitable will (animus), and sees that this lady shows the dark side of her (shadow), someone who is ugly, vicious, and killing female babies. This signifies the beginning of possible transformations to a better anima, and feeling function, and Eros; to everything that is unfinished, just started or in need of growth. A baby is a symbol par excellence of a reborn psyche. Then she wakes up in horror from this dream that warned her she must allow her archaic anima and feeling function to grow, showing clearly how she is perceived by the rest of the world: a cold, killing, corporate machine that has repressed any femininity. It should come as no surprise that *Sepia* was the first remedy needed to start her new life, a life that found a place for her natural capacities for love and intimacy.

Is there another circumstance in which the shadow takes over and forms the personality? Psychopaths come to mind!

Big Brother Takes Over: The Shadow Reigns in Psychopaths!

By now it is evident to the reader that we all have a shadow filled with a mixture of unrealized possibilities and dark elements. As mentioned before, children initially have a small shadow, as they develop their personality under the guidance of adults (parents and teachers mainly). When they take on more adult imitations or advice, not only does the person grow, but so does his/her shadow. There is one class of children that allopathy has not figured out—not how to treat them, nor where they originate from—the psychopaths! I hear every mother of young children repulsed by the term: "These little angels, how dare you use such a name to describe their behavior!"

Even Plato admitted that humans do commit evil acts "voluntarily," but he also stated that he did not know what to do philosophically with that disturbing fact. Until recently, the diagnosis of psychopathy was seldom mentioned. Not until 2013 did the American Psychiatric Association include callous and violent behavior in its diagnostic manual, *DSM-5*. Of course, psychopaths have always been with us, recognized by homeopathy (long before allopathy did), putting these traits under mental/emotional *syphilitic miasmatic* traits. Even before 2013, allopathy (as usual) invented many names to avoid calling children psychopaths, as it carried too much of a stigma. Even now most physicians shy away from this terminology, and rather call it "callous" or "unemotional" traits, harboring a cluster of behavior problems with names that describe a myriad of characteristics: malicious, lack of remorse, destructive, oppositional, delayed empathy, reactive attachment disorder, manipulative children—all describing the most outspoken behavior the child exhibits. But in the end, these are meaningless words that do not provide any tool to the parents and the child to detach from this chaotic world. It also remains a mystery to allopathy that some of these children develop into normal adults, while others end up as murderers.

To homeopaths, psychopathy is exclusively catalogued under dominant syphilitic miasmatic or hereditary traits, not in the limited allopathic sense in which "hereditary" always means finding "the same named" *disorder* in the family. Just as every homeopaths knows, the syphilitic root, if strongly present in the family (sometimes on both sides: father and mother), can give rise to an array of diseases with *different* names, all belonging to this *same* root: suicide, murder, depression, bulimia (food does not satisfy when in the midst of plenty, but is used to hide inner pain), anorexia nervosa, autoimmune diseases, destructive diseases on the physical plane (Parkinson's, M.S., Wegener's syndrome, congenital heart diseases such as VSD, ASD, Tetralogy of Fallot, other genetic mutations, etc.), sexual perversions like incest and masochism, and conditions such as autism, Alzheimer's, ALS, psychopathy, sociopathy, visual and auditory hallucinations, schizophrenia, etc.

Going back 250 years, long before allopathy recognized or named this disorder "psychopathy," homeopathy had already recognized and treated the disorder because homeopathy does not treat the disease but rather, "*the man* with a disease." Having the anti-miasmatic theory at its disposal, homeopaths saw the peculiarity and individuality of these children (Aphorism 153 of the *Organon*). Allopathy is based on protocols and names of diseases ("the disease in a man"), and is at a loss even now as to how to treat these children, to the despair of the families who are as bewildered as their physicians by the behavior of some of these children. It is worthwhile to cite a few examples I have seen in the practice, and to compare the homeopathic versus allopathic treatment of children with psychopathy.

What is the newest allopathic approach for psychopathy? In treatment centers for troubled children, the focus is now on "taming" (what an awful word!)—not *curing* children with psychopathy. Sounds a lot like all other chronic disease treatments where the word "cure" is replaced with "control," or "remission." What is this taming about? First, this taming takes place in high-security juvenile facilities where the main idea is to acclimate the child to a world different than the chaotic world he came from. This process is called "decompression." In other words, when one of these youngsters commits an infraction (even throwing urine and feces on counselors), no punishment is instituted; the child is simply put in an isolation room and the counselor returns when the child becomes tired of this behavior. There might be no violence as an answer to this behavior, but these children learn that there are no rewards given unless they behave—like accumulating points to join "prestigious" clubs where they receive privileges and treats. For example, playing Xbox, getting candy, pizza, baseball cards, staying up a little longer, etc. To me it looks like a form of coercion, or bribery, easily perceived by these psychopathic children who can be smart manipulators to get what they want: every deed that would be considered normal in any other child "*has*" to be rewarded. Their acts are usually not impulsive but premeditated, thought out. I wonder how this would work at home once they return from the institution? And what if they don't get a reward? What about other normal acting siblings at home? Does every normal behavior need to be rewarded to prevent callous behavior from being justified? I would hope the world would not work this way, but instead that "good" (aka normal) behavior leads to rewarding careers and lives, and that this insight would endure. Interesting is that one of the allopathic hallmarks of psychopathy is an *overactive reward system*, prime for drugs, sex, or anything else that delivers a moment of excitement, including being allowed the Xbox. So, are we then already at a young age activating this system? And through this reward system, is the root of the problem (not understood by allopathy)—the syphilitic hereditary miasm—eradicated? Certainly not, and that is why care givers cannot assure parents or predict how many of these children can stay a good course for life. In fact, once released, they are not followed up with anymore and recidivism of this behavior in the mosaic of its symptoms will pervade society silently, destroying their lives and the lives of others.

I remember several of these patients in my practice. One was a young boy, who from early on—and with increased intensity when his younger sister was born (*jealousy between children when the newborn gets all the attention, driving to kill*)—was very possessive of his mother, showing inappropriate sexual behavior to her. He would go shopping with his mom, and tell her all the time, "Will you marry me? I want to take a shower with you (*jesting, erotic foolish; Del, of a wedding; Del, is going to be married*)." And even more perplexing, "Let's kill dad and my sister so I can marry you and have you all for myself (*desire to kill, thought he ought to kill somebody*)." When he had sessions with a psychotherapist, he would always ask for a certain video to be played till the therapist realized it had some sexual content in it (*lascivious, lustful*). For the homeopath looking for Aphorism 153 syphilitic symptoms, *lewd talk*, *jealousy in children when the newborn gets all the attention* and *desire to kill* stand out and will be among other findings that are peculiar, used to eradicate this callous behavior because the root will be eradicated. *This is a true natural chronic disease (**A78**), arising from a chronic miasm, which without the specific remedy will continue to increase indefinitely, tormenting the patient with even greater suffering till the end of his days,* ***despite the best mental and dietary habits*** *(emphasis added by author).* I also want to assert that Hahnemann was the first physician in his time to treat the "insane" with respect, psychopaths included, rather than flogging them and locking them up. In **A208** (and **A5**), Hahnemann again looks at the man in his totality, paying more attention to the person who has a dis-ease:

> The age, way of living, diet, activities, **domestic situation**, and **social circumstances** must be considered, to ascertain whether these things aggravate the trouble and to what degree they might help or interfere with the treatment. Similarly, one should not overlook his emotional and mental disposition, to ascertain whether it might be an impediment to the treatment and whether **psychological attention might be necessary** to guide, encourage, or change it *(emphasis added by author).*

This was written in the *Organon* in 1843, centuries ahead of the present Western approach. Remarkable also, is that this was worded already by Daldianus Artemidorus in his *Oneirocritica*, in the second century of our era, where he almost literally wrote the same to be known about a human, in order to make a correct interpretation of human dreams.

As mentioned before, Hahnemann used the Aphorism 153 symptoms of the patient with psychopathy, many of them which can be seen early in the child: fascination with knives, early violence, cruelty to animals (I had a patient, a 5-year-old sweet girl, who poked out the eyes of her favorite live rabbit with the justification, "This way it cannot run away from me anymore"), interest only in violent films, making drawings of killings and cruelty, *sardonic laughing* (a laugh that gives one chills), and *laughing at the misfortune of others.* I had another little patient who, when her sister was born, looked at every opportunity to hurt this baby (*jealousy in children, when the newborn gets all the attention*). Another child, when punished by her mother, quite deliberately destroyed her mom's most precious china vase (*destructiveness in children*), while another child would tear every paper, even a whole phone book, into little strips (*tearing things in general*). I also saw children in practice who would resort *to biting themselves and others*, or *use sharp objects to cut themselves*. And all these behaviors were without remorse (*malicious*). The homeopathic remedy is chosen especially on several of these syphilitic miasmatic symptoms, and remedies like *Tuberculinum*, *Stramonium*, *Hyoscyamus*, *Tarentula*, *Belladonna*, and *Lachesis* stand out. (For an in-depth picture of these remedies consult my book, *Discovering Life: Homeopathic Portraits*). Only the indicated homeopathic remedy, based on the syphilitic miasmatic symptoms (perversion, hysteria, destruction of self/others/things, fancies, cruelty, delusions) can "rewire" the brain of these children, otherwise they create exhaustion, havoc, and despair for themselves and everyone else in their orbit, while in spite of the best intentions, the darkness and tension of the shadow side builds up, leading to incomprehensibly violent, amoral actions.

To recapitulate about the shadow:

- You cannot get rid of your shadow: it is not only impossible but also not advisable to try (it only would mean projection or repression). You need to ask the question, "Where is my shadow now and in what circumstances can I see its activities?" It is too bad we don't ask each other this question on a first date with someone (*both* parties need to be asked that question)!
- The shadow appears in dreams as a person of the same sex, as an inferior being or someone we dislike, often as a criminal, a thief, or someone shocking or

perverted, as well as a man's brother or a woman's sister. The shadow in a series of dreams can take different forms: it might first appear as a brother, then as a villain or a peasant.

- The shadow may also contain undiscovered and archaic treasures which can be a precious source of guidance in our life.
- When we despise someone for a certain characteristic, we need to make sure to explore if this trait does not belong to us: it is the only way to recognize our projection!
- Not acknowledging our shadow will isolate us from mankind and makes us look arrogant and haughty —not humble. Acknowledging our shadow is needed, to know that we are a normal imperfect being.
- Acceptance of the shadow is the beginning of salvation. We must be able to say, "This is mine, this belongs to me," so we stop projecting our business on anyone else. Elimination of the shadow cannot be done, we can only try to achieve a homeostasis, a balance between the light and dark.

In this chapter, I have tried to show extensively the many characteristics of the shadow and the way mankind deals with it. The next topic will be a closer investigation of the other collective unconscious elements: anima and animus.

11

ANIMA

"The advantage of the emotions is that they lead us astray."
— Oscar Wilde

The Magical Feminine

It is interesting that many cultures—American culture surely one of them—teach young people from early on that "real men don't cry, ever!" as if a male is formed *only* of masculine genes, and that emotions, empathy, and love for Nature should not be the territory of men. Only leadership, competition, decisions, and fortitude in actions are expected. To avoid a dangerous crack in a carefully constructed edifice, the anima, being a personification of feminine psychological characteristics, is mostly unknown by modern man.

Derived from the Latin word for "soul" (the Greek term is *psyche*), *anima* expresses a man's soul and is the invisible woman in a man, the image of the unconscious in man. Every human is androgynous (from the Greek *andros*, or "man," and *gynos*, or "woman"), analogous to the word *hermaphrodite*, derived from the Greek god Hermaphroditus. (The son of Aphrodite and Hermes, Hermaphrodites merged with a water nymph who fell in love with him and prayed they would be united forever. Thus, he came to embody both sexual characteristics.) In our society, the anima is denied by most men with contempt and violent reactions, as if she is a spineless ghost possessing men in general, and needs to be ignored—even repressed at all cost—or at least, it is projected onto women in general so that men can tolerate their own archaic feminine side.

As this was always the case of the old guard, the idea is still roaming in modern man's unconscious, even when there are enough instances in his life where some other psychological tendencies are required—such as compassion, intimacy, sensitivity, warmth, artistic qualities, and deep feelings (the Latin word *anima* also means "breath of life," animating things in life; Vital Energy). Even now, it would be a mistake to think that young men have accepted the Boy Scout creed to be loyal, kind, and courteous, as young adolescents describe a narrow road to successful masculinity, one that is paved with aggression, dominance, sexual prowess, and stoicism (to "suck it up"). These attributes for the "ideal guy," recalibrating the style and scale of ambition, belong more to a stunted masculinity, relegating these teenagers to an impoverished emotional landscape, often encouraged by other males (starting mainly with the father), creating an ill-equipped feeling function, leaving them unable to identify and express their emotions. Their archaic anima reveals its presence even more when they are suddenly overcome with vague mood swings, impulses to anger, and irrational thoughts (animosity). Such emotional reactions are always immediately said to "not belong" to their real Self: "I was beside myself," is the cry. Indeed, it can be the shadow showing, which is an ego-adjunct (consisting mainly of all the repressed conscious contents), but mostly it reflects the untamed and undifferentiated anima—chaotic, moving with an autonomic character not belonging to the ego—that momentarily took over the reins of his ship, the Self. It is as if he has suddenly been taken up by a violent storm, becoming "animated" or expressing animosity. In these instances, the anima becomes a personal demon not obeying any specific rules.

Either sex is inhabited by the opposite sex as a smaller set of genes (their archetypal background), forming in every man a feminine character; there is no yang without yin and vice versa, and this femininity will undoubtedly be part of his personality. His femininity will be constellated in women to which he is attracted—"she is my type"—the result of projection (see Chap. 13). The strength of this anima-complex gains power as the amount of his repression of feelings increases, therefore leading to distortion of feeling. In other words, a weak unbalanced inferior feeling function will result in an exaggerated anima-complex, hindering and spoiling all genuine relationships, never achieving a truce.

Being just one of the different unconscious archetypes, anima always has a positive and negative aspect, the dual nature of good and bad, as good and evil function together (hopefully as a balanced cooperation of moral opposites), but should always be accepted as a partner. Above all, anima's negative traits reflect changing moods, spontaneous impulses, and childish reactions, overwhelming the possessor at inopportune moments, changing him suddenly into a stranger, even a hysterical woman—a being quite different from his ordinary character. Most men resist the appearance of the anima, which always acts with reflex-like speed as an emotional reaction. But eventually—especially around middle age—this archetype, the anima within, will have to be accepted and integrated, or the individuation journey will hit a wall and recurrent dreams about ugly, diseased, repulsive women, witches, or evil animals like a dragon will appear in higher frequency in which the dreamer attempts to kill them.

As Jung mentioned, "Younger people who have not reached the middle of life (around the age of 35) can bear even the total loss of the anima without injury. The important thing at this stage is for a man to be a man" (Jung, 1990, Vol. 9, Part I, p. 71).

TCM would have put this age for men at 5x8, or 40, and for women to accept the contra-sexual figure around 5x7, or 35 (7 being the sacred number for women, 8 for men).[1] Although it would not harm a man to allow his anima to be part of his life earlier (being sensitive, or the willingness to accept anima as an important partner)—as this would avoid the divorce catastrophes we have, with 60% of people divorced in Europe and the United States after being married more than 16 years—up until age 40 a man's anima participation in his life is mostly limited to projecting her onto external women while the internal anima remains hidden.

However, acceptance of this anima too early might distract a young man from his own future and plans. The following is such a case.

Male, age 28: He had this dream four times a year, with very little difference, indicating an urgent message.

Dream

I am floating in the air going to a house situated on the full moon; in front of the house is a perfectly grassy yard. I open the door of the house and see my sister in the living room. She says, "I want to show you a trick" and I see her with a dragon. I wonder, "How did he get in here?" The dragon is taking my sister in his mouth and tossing her around, rather gently and calmly, and my sister was roaring with laughter. She seemed to enjoy it. I was very confused, and that's how I felt waking up!

Conscious situation: He had a younger sister who in her teens got off track in life, abusing drugs and alcohol. She was now two years sober and doing well, but he told me how anxious and worried he was about her still.

Analysis

Floating in the air: His body feels lighter than air, a typical inflation of his persona. Was he trying to play the hero? Who is the trick played on? He is a sensitive guy, and as a man he took his role as protector very seriously. This is reflected in the fact that his **house** (the Self) was on the **moon**, the latter standing for a strict female or yin symbol, for love and nourishing, but also symbolic for *luna* ("lunatic"), the abode of the crazy. It was even a full moon—when lunatics reign. **A grassy yard:** This is where we can plant seeds to grow, reflecting new possibilities in life. Inside the house he meets his sister (his anima) who is with a **dragon**, symbol for evil, a destructive entity, reflecting (as for any animal appearing in dreams) a deep instinct.

His sister (his young anima) is telling him, "I will show you a trick," which is the dragon tossing her around while having great fun, puzzling the dreamer. What is this confusing situation? Jung told us that a man till age 35 can escape unharmed when not meeting his anima, saying, "A man needs to be a man." So apparently being only 28, this man focused too much on his sister's situation (although she was sober for two years), seen by situating his house or Self on the moon instead of concentrating on building his own house from the foundation up, and instead of planting new seeds to grow in his little yard (signifying new possibilities for him, which he holds off for now). Being in the air, he cannot build his foundation on Earth, or conscious, and is floating towards unconsciousness. So, the trick is played *on him*, saying in effect, "It is foolish to build your house on the full moon." This is telling him to worry less about his sister and concentrate more on his life, that his sister is OK, and integration of his anima is too early. This did create an "Aha," so we will see if further dreams will revolve in a series of dreams as the message is understood.

In the second part of life—in order for the male to cultivate his relationships and his spirituality, to let his life become less rigid and to soften his character to be kind and flexible—there is no choice other than to gather the courage to accept that siren, that serpent, the demon-woman, the Goddess, the unknown woman or spiritual adviser, psychopomp or messenger, the "One-That-Shows-The-Way," the "One-Who-Needs-To-Be-Obeyed," in whatever form the anima might appear at the stillest hour (midnight or maximum yin time). The anima compensates and complements the masculine consciousness, trying to force a change in his personality. If men want to pursue continuation of their individuation journey as a matter of psychological development in the second half of their life, they have to give up the fight with their magical feminine and welcome her with open arms, a *mandatory partial feminization* of the man, so that the chaotic tale of dreams and the disordered capriciousness of the anima reveal a deeper meaning. Here are two consecutive dreams on the same night from a middle-aged, intelligent man who questions the loss of his early love felt for his wife.

Dream

I leave my hotel room and go down to the breakfast buffet on the ground floor. In between I meet a male friend. He joins me for the breakfast as well. When we arrive there, we meet two more male friends. All four of us sit down at the same table.

Analysis

Hotel: The Self in a transitional stage.

Going down: Going towards the unconscious.

Breakfast buffet: He is seeking nourishment (there is food for thought; food for growth as an individual).

Male friend: This is his shadow.

Two more male friends: This brings us to the number **four**, the number of completeness, but unfortunately there is no female present. So in spite of being middle-aged, the anima remains in the dark and archaic, and the dreamer's whole personality and approach to life is based on Logos—the masculine principle of knowledge, literally meaning "word"—not Eros, the principle of relatedness and receptivity. **Two** males show that the animus is split in an active positive and a passive negative side.

Dream two

I have an emergency kit for a couple in crisis. This looks like a medical bag which doctors carry for patient visits. When I open the bag, I find memories from the early phase of my relationship with my wife during which we took care of each other very well, notes which described why we loved each other and photo albums. When I wake up, I only remember this bag and no stories along with it, unfortunately!

Analysis

Emergency kit: Indicates indeed an emergency in his relationship with his wife (couple in crisis). This emergency kit, contained in a **doctor's bag** (showing the need for repair and healing on the emotional plane), contains no meds but only **memories**, referring to instructions or memories of the times he was happy with his wife and the reasons why they loved each other very much—in other words, the key to return to Eros in his relationship with his wife. However, when he wakes up he cannot remember the message from the unconscious, the content of the emergency kit, so there is no Guiding Self to renew a fruitful union between the dream-ego and Inner Healer, no guiding light from the unconscious, only an indication of how times used to be. This dream connects to the previous one where no anima is found. In view of this, it shows he must reconnect to his feminine side or anima and integrate this side from his unconscious.

Next dream, after his simillimum

I see a hedgehog covering my cat's face and even biting his left ear, causing dark red blood to appear. I am wondering for a short time if I should take a picture or hit the hedgehog to rescue my cat. But after just a second of reflecting, I take the hedgehog away immediately. My cat's left ear is wounded but he keeps very calm and quiet as usual.

Personal association: "My cat seems to be a symbol of Mother Earth: quiet, calm, and peaceful. On the other hand, the hedgehog that bites his ear does not seem to represent an evil, but is more a symbol of a young boy making foolish jokes. I do not have any negative feeling towards him. A spontaneous desire to take a picture of the hedgehog biting my cat's ear is a symbol of my selfishness. From my childhood up to now, there are many occasions at which I laughed at unfortunate situations of somebody else (*laughing at the misfortune of others*). Sometimes I did not express it, but only thought about it. It is the same feeling I had when I was thinking about taking the photo. Therefore, somehow, I feel happy that I did not take the picture but helped my cat in the dream. The dark red blood on my cat's ear seems to be a sign of sacrifice of the mother whose love is not understood by a beloved son. It hurts my cat (the mother) but does not disappoint him as he knows it will be understood one day."

Analysis

The cat (see further) is bitten by a hedgehog. A **hedgehog:** Looking at its characteristics, this is an animal belonging to the feminine, or unconscious, an image of the dreamer's anima. The hedgehog was so named because of its peculiar foraging methods. These animals root through hedges and other undergrowth (=exploring the unconscious) in search of the small creatures that compose the bulk of their diet—insects, worms, centipedes, snails, mice, frogs, and snakes. Some people consider hedgehogs useful pets because they prey on many common garden pests. While on the hunt, they rely upon their senses of hearing and smell because their eyesight is weak. Here again the accent in this animal is on the unconscious: weak eyesight (=symbol of unconscious) and using other means of getting his prey (to fish for unconscious elements). They curl up in the day, sleeping, and awaken to search for food at night. So, the activity is mainly at night, representing the unconscious. Although the hedgehog bites the cat, which for the dreamer stands for Mother Earth—the positive protective and nourishing Mother archetype belonging also to the unconscious—the man does not consider the act evil but rather the action of a young fool. This hedgehog appears to tell the dreamer to investigate and clean up his unconscious (just as the hedgehog roams underground chasing his food, so must the dreamer investigate his unconscious to integrate some dark and destructive elements). At first, the man wants to take a picture of this scene (when one has a photo, one can remember) but then decides against it and takes the hedgehog away. Although the cat's left ear (the female, feeling side or yin side) was injured, the animal (now the anima figure of the dream) remained calm despite. There is a good lysis in this dream, as the dreamer wants to integrate his anima rather than continuing to follow his deepest instincts, which were injurious to him. Indeed, deciding not to take a picture tells the dreamer that he is serious in integrating his anima right away—he does not need a picture to remember, and understands that laughing about the misfortunes of others is not a nice trait. He is reflective as he says he used to "be selfish" that way. It is interesting, but not surprising, how his asthma has improved the past year with his indicated remedy but is not completely gone. Most likely, as this dream indicates, he must let go of the destructive instincts that "suffocate" him to be fully healed. It is not just the remedy that helps him, but by being liberated from the negative complexes he possessed before, he is now able to integrate elements from the unconscious.

A hedgehog can also symbolically refer to being sensitive to offense (*easily offended*), a state in which we sometimes react by "prickling," a response that causes us to hurt others. *The fourth undifferentiated conscious function appears in a dream as a child, or expresses itself in an animal form, and only rarely will we see animals and children as symbols of differentiated functions!* So, the hedgehog points to the man's archaic fourth function that needs to be further differentiated. And indeed, by repeating the same remedy (that, in turn, allowed him to further differentiate this function), that summer for the first time he had no asthma attack at all.

Another example is from a professor of literature, who at age 40 had seizures that robbed him for short periods of his memory. His first wife had abandoned and divorced him at that point. At age 67, his seizures (suppressed with allopathic meds of course) became worse, and he was put on a new medication that caused him to finally retire from the university where he taught, as he would have sudden episodes of being completely lost in his thoughts, losing big chunks of his long-term memory (a fugue state). These tonic-clonic seizures caused what allopathy called transient epileptic amnesia, or TEA. The present meds (taken for seven years) suppressed these seizures, but the side effects were not conducive for his life: not only did they cause incoordination, but also more permanent amnesia (not communicated beforehand by his physician!). This whole experience caused much anticipation anxiety in him, and he told me about a recurrent dream he had at least twice a week since age 67, when he started taking these new meds. Before, his seizures had an aura always occurring in the chest.

Dream

I am walking in an unknown city and I get lost. I want to return but I cannot find my way back. Initially I am accompanied by a female, but she disappeared, so I do not get help from her. At some point a lot of people walk with me but no one seems to have a clue! I wake up in an anxious state.

Analysis

This recurrent dream sends him an important message. So far, he had not understood its meaning, hence a recurrent dream, twice a week for many years. However, the message is clear. Here we have an intellectual person who conducted his whole life with his dominant conscious thinking function. His seizures started at age 40, an age when he should have integrated his anima and exercised his feeling function more. The lady in his dream was his anima, but instead of the psychopomp and psychic helper she usually is, she leaves him, so it is clear that integration—even at age 67, when the seizures became TEA—has not happened, as he had not exercised and grown his archaic feeling function. So, no important guidance is offered to him, hence the onset of recurrent dreams, trying to convey to him the important message to change his life by exercising and accepting his anima. (Being a thinking person, he thought this lady was his present wife—an example of objective dream analysis.) He is lost in the city (the Self)—resembling the fugue states he has on and off in real life. That this is a collective dream and not just a personal problem posed by this dream is evident when many people walk with him, who are also lost by not accepting their counterpart! This man was just an acquaintance of mine, not a patient, so no homeopathic therapy was given, but a gentle explanation of his dream was provided which created the useful "Aha!"

The world is full of men who have no idea about their inner woman, permanently losing their anima, and therefore at a later age become rigid, irresponsible, insensitive, and old crabby children, often resorting to alcohol and drugs. The positive side of the anima corresponds to what Jung called *Eros*, the function of relationship and the principle of unconditional love, a readiness for love in general towards humans, animals, and Nature. Eros is usually more developed in women and more a quality of a woman's true nature, whereas animus is an expression of the paternal *Logos*, a quality usually more developed in men, and formed more freely by the father's example.[2]

Other positive anima traits are compassion, generosity, altruistic feelings, and a desire to give the intuition and feeling conscious functions a voice rather than delegating them to the background, as well as a desire to investigate the unconscious, that "ghost land," using it as a psychopomp and spiritual guide and, equally, as a source of creative values. Worse than disregarding the anima, as we will see—men being unconscious of their own undeveloped femininity—non-acceptance will lead to a *projection* of their archaic anima onto the women they are attracted to and will marry. This kind of projection happens in every beginning relationship (see Chap. 13). But what else happens if the contra-sexual partner, a man's anima, is not accepted and integrated? We are alluding to midlife crisis, an event common amongst men. This will be extensively addressed in a further chapter (Chap. 14).

But first we need to address the making of the feminine. As the integration of anima and animus are essential in finding a meaning of life and developing the other-half of one's conscious being, it is important to find out who is responsible for the formation of these archetypes.

Formation of the Invisible Partner, Anima

Who is the maker of this magical woman in men? Who do we blame when the anima is malformed or absent? This has much to do with the lottery of life: what you were born into—illegitimate, or not, in a poor environment, or a stimulating one. For a good outcome, a human being's needs are ideally met by two parents who care and respond to all the child's psoric needs. Because of the intimate connection of the child to the mother, the mother is always the first and most important person to fulfill those needs, while forming the child's anima. The Divine Mother (the Great Mother, Mother-Of-All-Existence or the Mother of Compassion) is or rather should be the protective and nourishing power, most critical in the first years of the child's life. No doubt, the first picture of the anima is hidden in the dominant power of the mother, because the child at first lives in a state of unconscious identity with her, so the anima image is innate in every child and further develops from the mother's actions on her child. Nietzsche even expressed it with a negative connotation: "Usually a mother loves herself in her son more than she loves him" (Hayman, 1980, p. 202). The process of separation from the motherly love, as a child moves away from being dependent on the mother and towards adulthood, can be difficult for the mother, but a truly loving mother will love the child and at the same time will want to let her child move on to full independence.

The influence of motherly love was succinctly expressed by Oscar Wilde in one of his most celebrated epigrams: "All women become like their mothers. That is their tragedy. No man does. That's his!" (Redman, 1996). Wilde was very close to and much like his mother—a flamboyant and famous poet—and her death while he was imprisoned for two years was one of his most devastating events, wracking him with guilt about his past life filled with erotomania and his mother's futile efforts to bring him off his destructive path, as well as her desire for his reconciliation with his brother Willie. Fatherly love is usually different. According to Seneca, the father's first important task is to show manly love, the formation of a balanced animus, so that the child can acquire a skin thick enough to deal with upcoming misfortunes in life.

As we will further see, depending on what form the first encounter with the mother takes, the relationship between child and mother leads to either serious impairment or the contrary; the child is guided to the higher Self, determining the fate even of the adult male. To affirm the positive or negative influence of a mother on her child, Nietzsche claimed, "Everyone carries in himself an image of woman derived from the mother; by this he is determined to revere women generally, or to hold them in low esteem, or to be generally indifferent to them" (Hayman, 1980, p. 58, A380). In other words, the anima for a male has the power to be a spiritual guide and psychopomp, offering him a capacity for relatedness, or it can seriously impair his masculine development for the rest of his life in the case of a negative (as in the case of domination or over-protection), and can even lead to a pathological mother-complex, like incest. Indeed, the duality of an archetype is always present, and while most mothers are known to their family as the one who was nourishing, kind, wise, protective, and always ready to give good advice, some other mothers were demons, an indifferent presence from hell.

The interaction between mother and child, and father and child, is where the potential for growth or devastation can be.

Rightfully, medical science admits that it can neither predict human behavior nor match resources to those predictions. As "proof," scientists and psychologists say that there are less-than-perfect families with kids who are OK. Yet in another family, with the same kind of less-than-perfect parents, the kids seem unable to function. For allopathy, the risk assessment remains a murky science. It is here that the lack of allopathic knowledge is exposed: with the broader genetic aspect of the homeopathic miasmatic theory, coupled with the true or deviated constitution in utero, the homeopathic physician not only has powerful tools available but can assist the patient in fulfilling his road to self-realization.

In the case of a domineering, bossy dragon-mother (*Kali-c, Sepia, Lach*) and a weak father, the strong masculinity will come from the mother. It is not only the environment, however, but also the constitution and dominant miasmatic personal trait that will determine the outcome for the child. Characters with a weak ego (*yielding*: *Pulsatilla, Palladium, Lac-c, Thuja, Bar-c*), will grow up with no legs to stand on, being castrated, their individuality destroyed. If this person is an *Aurum* personality he might rebel from time to time, but eventually can be overcome by guilt and the *Delusion, he has neglected his duty*, which in his mind is, "He ought to obey his saintly mother, he ought to listen to her as she is the adult who knows best." These syphilitic reactions lead, over time, to a deep state of self-doubt and depression. Then there is the constitution who is inclined to have his or her own opinions, desires, and goals in life (*Sulph, Lyc, Phos* come to mind). They might react with a hypertrophy of ego as a rebellious gesture—depending on the degree of the miasmatic syphilitic dominance—not accepting in any way the clutches of an overpowering mother, to the point that they will show no reverence to any woman (*Phosphorus* is here the exception, with her true love and empathy, but as she is tubercular—

psora-syphilis—negative reactions like *indifference to family* can occur).

There is also the difficulty of having had an "ideal" mother, one who can be glorified because she truly fit all the characteristics of the Divine Mother. That child as an adult can have difficulties in relationships because of unrealistic expectations put on his wife, demanding from her to be the saint his mother was! And the opposite—when the mother failed to provide the nurturing of the anima—can lead to the same situation, as the adult, resenting this shortcoming of his mother, expects future females to fill the hole in his heart, an unreasonable demand. In both situations these children become adults who look for the perfect mother in every female they meet, being possessed by the past and wanting to hold on to the unconscious, the "Glorious-All-Forgiving-Serving-Mother."

But can the mother also be a negative source of anima, handicapping her child from a young age on for the rest of his or her life? One of the most moving examples in my practice was an encounter with an 80-year-old woman, who was overcome with tears when she told me that she realized that she was never loved by her mother who dominated the whole family with her one-sided animus, neglecting her Eros. What a tragedy! Approaching the evening of her life, the sun setting, and still a traveler in the desert looking for a sip of water! Even worse! She was still convinced that it must have been her fault that instilled such cold behavior in her mother, so her dreams were full of magical thinking, picturing a child being held lovingly, the result of the compensation law.

Another tragic incidence in which the mother has a hard time openly loving her young *Phosphorus* daughter, because of the absence of her own *Sepia* mom when she was young, is expressed in the following recurrent dream. The conscious situation is that, in her late 50s, this woman is trying to fulfill her dream of learning to be loving towards her daughter without neglecting her domestic duties. She finds it difficult to find a balance, while raising a sensitive adventure-seeking *Phosphorus* girl who perceives her mother's attempts as domination and control. This mother was raised by a *Nat-m/Sepia* mother, and therefore finds herself at a loss when trying to show/express love to her daughter and meet her emotional needs, because she has never seen it done in her own life and surroundings. Here is her quest to understand the dream's message.

Dream

I wonder what the subconscious is trying to communicate through a recurrent dream—things that need to be done and not being able to do them due to lack of time. Many times, I have to travel and realize that either I have not bought the plane ticket, have not packed, or there is so much to pack, or I have no time to arrive at the airport. Along with this comes the fact that I must take a shower but do not find one, go around the house looking for one, and when I finally find it, there are no curtains. Then I decide to take a shower anyway but then don't have shampoo, soap, or towel. I go to find those things, then get distracted by other responsibilities, and the feeling of never being ready continues.

Analysis

Although she herself is a feeling *Phosphorus* person, she never received the archetype or formation of the Mother archetype from her own mother as the latter was absent (*Del, mother is dead*). And for any person, the formation of the anima is first and foremost achieved by their own mother, who did not provide it in this case. And if there is not another female present in her further life who can replace this mother figure (grandmother—the grand or mother of all mothers—sisters, or female friends), then she is indeed unprepared to choose between duty —following her Logos or reason (principle of knowledge)—or following her heart, as she possesses an insufficiently confident anima and animus! It is also visible in this dream that she is in a *Sepia* situation herself: chaotic, unprepared, overwhelmed by responsibilities, struggling to start on a "clean sheet" with her daughter. She can't find a shower in her house (or Self), nor the accessories she needs to bathe, suggesting that she is not able to start afresh, as again her scattered busy mind takes over. This recurrent dream tells her to slow down, so that she does not fall into her mother's situation permanently, and to be able to deal with her young daughter lovingly, which in reality she desires foremost.

Is there not a saying, "The way to a man's heart is through his stomach," referring to the nourishing role of the female, as the first role of the mother was feeding and keeping alive the unborn baby in utero. No wonder the anima develops from the mother; anytime the child wants to function with his feeling, he will get into his mother's feeling. Man expects from his wife in the first place to be fed and loved, which is no different from the primordial role of any mother. The real mark of a good mother is to not always give in to her children and please them in all their little whimsies. Otherwise they would be handicapped for life, always looking for the partner that fits this "ideal, all-giving mother!" The true mother will always show a spirited interest in whatever ails her child, setting aside the trifling matters from those that are important for further development of his/her individuation. This means connecting to *any* kind of expression of feeling—be it anger, joy, foolishness, shouting, sadness, or frustration—encouraging the child to find a place to express his/her feeling, and gifting that child with a mother who is a wise counselor, the *Magna Mater* or Divine Mother. As seen further, depending on the relationships with these anima figures, man's anima is shaped in a positive or negative way, an inheritance that influences his life more than he realizes. The anima is the result of all the experiences of that man with women, good or bad. Additionally, the way one's father treats women and what he thinks of them will leave a strong impact on his son's anima formation. In fact, it is equally important that a father not be just a stern presence, never professing the love he feels for his children, even a son.

An anima form in which a tyrant is easily seen is in the *Arsenicum* mother. Her house is always spectacularly clean (*mania for cleanliness*). There are things on the mantelpieces, little porcelain figures collected over time that never can be touched. There are also drawers full of silverware and fancy plates that are not used except for Christmas. But each week they are cleaned and dusted off, as if there would be a sale that week (which would be welcomed by her children!). Such a mother is not prone to sweet nothings, but sometimes voices coldness or disgust with her children with a sharp, exalted tone that pierces the clean, dead silence in the museum-like house (*censorious, critical; aversion to those around her; contemptuous*). She thinks that it is a tradition never to kiss or hug her children except on New Year's (*reserved*). Her concerns are only important to her; they are mostly invented, something to keep her preoccupied (*anguish with restlessness, driving her from place to place*).

Another form of malnourishment of the anima by the mother is caused when she suffers from her own neuroses, being neglected by her husband and overwhelmed by loneliness, when she can turn her son, especially, into a love-object. Such a child becomes overwhelmed with spoiling love, which is not true love but rather a quest for satisfaction of the mother. A spoiled child is of course not sad but bored like a king or a dog. Although it does not look like it, the child is still a hapless shipwreck. As a result, because of a created inferiority complex, the son often rebels against the fatherly demands, not holding any job, flunking university, changing school continuously, and even resorting to alcohol and drugs—all signs of protest, always forgiven by the "loving" mother.

Other mothers who fail to have the all-enveloping, all-protective role of the Divine Mother, nourishing and protecting her child in the first years of life, are *Platina* and *Sepia*. *Platina*, with her delusion to be an empress, instantiates herself from the natural maternal role to focus on her sexual and spiritual needs (*aversion to children*). She is perpetually exhausted and overloaded, with every muscle and nerve pulled taut. Rubrics like *Del, does not belong to her own family; Del, being noble; adulterous* and *aversion to her own children* come to mind. *Sepia*, although a very conscientious mother (*too much sense of duty*), is overwhelmed by her daily work load (*Del, feels every fiber in her body on the right side*—right side being the yang or masculine side) and sexual demands from her husband (*aversion to husband and members of family; Ailments from sexual excesses*), so her feeling function suffers from these circumstances (*consolation, kind words aggravate*).

And then we have the *Pulsatilla* mother. Such a mother always demands attention and love (*craving for attention; kisses everyone*), rehearsing a dance of changing emotions (*moods changeable; weeping alternating with laughter*) her whole life, as these are the building stones of her existence, creating in her children an intense fear of losing her, but also keeping them in a psychological, compulsive battle that cannot be won, reflecting the mother's manipulation to ensure her demands. A *Pulsatilla* mother remains in a childish ego-state—is a pseudo mother—incapable of performing the necessary functions of a nourishing mother. Towards her children she acts as The Supreme Giver and Comforter, reflecting her own need to be the Perpetual Taker and Sufferer, although Support-Through-Non-Reassurance, impossible for her to offer, would be a better solution. With her yielding, soft character she will cultivate the same characteristics in her son: to be always peaceful and voiceless, using weeping as a weapon, to not express his opinions and to be non-aggressive, imbuing him with an identification of the anima and creating an effeminate person who will often be bullied and teased, while looking for protection and love in a male.

We must not forget the *Kali-c* mother, a perfect example of a mother who thinks she is a super-mom but fails to create harmony and self-confidence in her children. Without knowing it, "in the name of love" she is an ogress and condemns her children to exile as they are not allowed to have their own Self; she rigidly controls her children's actions, questions, and words. There is too much charm and sugar under the guise of authority in her feelings "for others, not for me," but we should be suspicious of this selflessness and invite caution, not admiration. This controlling mother "loves" her child with such intensity that this young child feels morally indebted to her love, feeling sorry that she is such a nuisance to her, not realizing that it is not love but her mother's insecurity coupled with extensive control, snuffing out her whole future life, reducing her to a soulless mass of flesh and bones. What a horror for a *Phosphorus* or *Sulphur* child to grow up in such a wasteland of boring, yielding, stifling, and oppressive passivity! The *Kali-c* mother shapes the destiny of her children who, once they escape the claws of control, exhibit mixed feelings of hatred, compassion, and suppressed rage, trying to glue the pieces of their shattered life together. Such an over-bearing mother creates the devouring aspect of the mother image. At whatever age the rebellion starts, that person needs not only courage to cut the cord and open new doors and choose freedom, but also knowledge and communication skills to flee the desert of his existence, to wet his lips with the water of life, drop by drop. He will have to become the hero who slays the dragon like St. George to free the maiden (his anima), to regain a sense of reformation and freedom. Otherwise there will be a continuous hindrance to his true capacity for relatedness to women. Once there is a liberation from the devouring aspect of the mother, the dragon in dreams will be substituted by a real woman, his new anima.

Eventually, anima is an archetypal image resulting from all the experiences of man with women. Further, by way of the stepmother, mother-in-law, sister, and any woman with whom a relationship exists (babysitter, au-pair, nurse, neighbor), the image of anima is transferred to the lovers, and finally the wife has to take over the magical role of the mother. But what about the total absence of the Divine Mother figure?

Absence of the Mother: The Injured Anima

A man whose mother was non-existent has not experienced the primary encounter with the first carrier of his anima, because his "mother is dead," in actuality or because she was absent due to illness, alcoholism, drug use, incest, or was simply too busy or pregnant to bother. In Western medicine human behavior is unpredictable, and matching resources to predictions for the protection of children is equally unpredictable. Allopathy is still far removed from the knowledge of true miasmatic influence to avoid broken families and their tragedies. In this case, if the mother's role was not taken over by another female figure like a grandmother, older sister, or another nourishing female figure, the anima will now appear in his dreams or in daydreams as a fascinating attraction, leaving him forever longing for that image of security—an image of what she would be if he could ever find her, an image that remains archaic and out of touch with reality. Even as an adult, he will keep looking for this fantasy person and never find her. Compensating dreams contain only intimate and sexual situations where the dreamer finds himself in a long embrace from which he does not want to let go, especially when such a man's world is ruled by Logos. Of course, the damage was done earlier.

When a child lacks maternal warmth and protection, he is often unable to turn away from the world of images of the collective unconscious and face life, expressed in homeopathy by *Delusions of fancy illusions*, an escape in a dream world. Also, by not having experienced the "primary" encounter with the mother, it's image can appear also in dreams in a non-human form such as a horse, frog, siren (winged creature), or any form representing the anima. What will be the result of absent motherly influence? The man, because of his wounded and immature anima, will be seized by touchiness and inexplicable moods, highly elated one moment and in the deepest depression the next, the expression of an assault by his anima. Looking at the statistics of the prevalence of diagnoses of manic-depression and bipolar disorder (BPD), this lack of positive mother-bonding is all too common in children and adults.

Another manifestation of an injured and infantile anima, and the incapacity to practice Eros (to find nurturing and rewarding relationships), is seen in the epidemic of erotic fantasy where men are preoccupied for hours on the internet with pornography, a crude aspect of the anima related to their infantile feeling attitude. To such people, the anima presents itself in the form of a femme fatale, or in the Greek mythological sirens, luring victims to their unexpected demise, symbols of destructive illusions. But the formation of an archaic anima due to absence of the mother (and any substituting female) in childhood can also lead to revenge when that child grows up.

As Eros, the capacity for relationship, is not a natural trait for the average man, it is no surprise that many succumb to the castrating power of their archaic infantile anima. Both animus and anima have peculiar irritating effects, and many fights in a marriage in which cheap twisting of the truth or effeminate remarks occur have their origin in an attack of the anima in men and animus in women when confronted with an emotionally charged situation. To present one such simple incident: who has not forgotten the birthday of his wife or, (in the woman's eyes) the all-important anniversary of your wedding day, the crowning of her love story? I do not know many men who keep a special calendar with what his wife considers, "Not-To-Be-Forgotten-All-Important-Moments," which of course are the first ones they always forget! Then the wife bursts into tears when her animus takes the lead, "How *could* you forget"—to which the husband gets into a state of disbelief, discomfort, and is truly dumbfounded by "What is this all about?!" However, this situation for the woman is translated as a "lack of relationship." The husband's initial reaction is always automatically and inevitably followed by a response coming from his archaic conscious function—that dwarf from his unconscious, the feeling function and the infantile anima—always an unsatisfactory and stumbling answer! Stung by his wife's remark, the man's anima may retaliate, and as a result his anima might drop a match into the gasoline with erupting affect, the result of many animus-anima battles.

Being possessed by a witch inside himself, the husband might hurl irrational insults in revenge—childish in nature of course, and often of a personal nature. Identifying with the anima creates neurotic, unreliable behavior and nothing but trouble! Then the wife's animus is awoken, coming back with a sharp sword and club to let him have it and yes, the result is an exhausting battle, poisoning the family atmosphere for days to come! Unfortunately, these projections are the negative images of the archetypal soulmates dominating this destructive scene, which often have the effect of driving man and woman apart (see Chap. 13, "The Human Love Story").

Indeed, it is not comfortable for a man to cultivate a healthy relationship with his soulmate, his anima. A better solution for a man in this case—before falling into the clutches of his inner woman—would be to apologize for his insensitivity/forgetfulness (yes, swallow his pride and mean it) and to make up by telling her what his true feelings are and what a happy day their marriage was. It is then not his anima in her destructive devious way that speaks, but *he* who is talking. He might also ask: "How can I make it up to you? Is there anything else that is bothering you? Where did I disappoint you?" Or simply apologize and follow it up with a good deed and thought, like dining out. Analogous to the *Ailments from*, or "Never Well Since" in homeopathy, if we get to the trigger of the hurt, the soulmate projection will disappear. How does the anima appear in dreams?

Appearance of Anima in Dreams

With exception of the mother figure, these soul images always appear in dreams as *contra-sexual figures*—contrary to the shadow, which carries the *same gender*. In a man, a woman or female symbol will be called anima, a representation of his ideas about women and his own feminine attitudes; in a woman a female appearing in her dream will be called shadow or alter ego! Anima's versatility to appear in dream images is spectacular! In a man's dream the anima can appear in many forms of the woman. The anima is not a single image representing only one aspect: she appears in innumerable images of enchanting, frightening, friendly, helpful, or dangerous feminine figures, and we must examine what sentiments she arouses in us and what role she plays in our dreams and ultimately in our life. Is she Marilyn Monroe? Or the Kali god in India—a god who is neither good nor bad but both good *and* bad, as she appears as the symbol of destruction but also as the "loving and terrible mother." Other anima images include the Eternal Mother, the Seductress or Temptress, the Divine Harlot (=the embodiment of a romantic idea of passionate love), the Witch-woman, the

Angel-woman (blue-eyed with golden hair), the Priestess, the Spiritual Guide, the devouring Vampire-woman, She-Who-Must-Be-Obeyed (I bet that is an archetypal figure welcomed by some animus-possessed women!), the Virgin, the Woman of Mystery, the peasant woman, the lady next door, a nymph, the elves, a dancing maid, a nurse, a martyr, a muse, a saint, sirens, femmes fatales, etc., or even as *animal figures* such as a snake, rat, horse, tiger, cow, hare, dove, owl, cat, toad, kangaroo, doe or fawn, as well as *objects*, such as a cave, a ship or vessel, hollow and womb-like objects like bottles, a cup, an oven or cooking vessels, and the uterus—all representing the Mother archetype or anima as they are feminine objects. Other forms are strange *mythological creatures* like a mermaid (a woman who is beautiful on top with a fish-tail bottom), or a half-serpent, or half-bird. In these latter pictures, we have a connection through the head with human consciousness, while below, this figure extends into the spinal cord or sympathetic nervous system, controlling our lower instinctive centers.

A common representation of the anima is the *damsel in distress*, frequently appearing in so called hero myths. A recurring theme is that of the hero rescuing a beautiful young woman and sometimes marrying her. So, the damsel in distress is the man's anima, which because of neglect or repression, is (metaphorically speaking) either dead or in danger of dying. The rescue or kiss of life means that the man has now lifted his femininity out of its dark prison and welcomed it and even submitted to it. A famous dream of Socrates referred to this representation, indicating, however, that his anima remained in neglect. In his normal life, he paid no attention to his feeling function as he had a bad relationship with his wife Xanthippe. Even when his son Sophroniscus died, he did not interrupt his philosophical discussions. Three days before his own death, a white lady appeared in his dream, telling him that in three days death will come (white for the Romans was the symbol for the realm of the dead and of mourning), and indeed she was "The-One-Who-Must-Be-Obeyed," prophesying the actual time of his death. In real life he did not pay attention to his anima, as he was "squandering" his time with philosophical ranting in the marketplace instead of working on his feeling side.

In my practice, I have often met "hero figures" who were trying to play the role of a valiant knight to rescue the damsel in distress. Upon examining such a patient's life, it became evident that identifying with this heroic figure was only to lift himself up from his own misery. Each time he was divorced after a short marriage, he did not hesitate to dive again and again into a new relationship, as he thought he had overcome his misery, a belief contradicted by the next action of his archaic anemic anima. It is common in these cases that the anima appears in dreams as a little girl or as a multiplicity of women, as such a man is utterly unconscious of his anima. This multiplicity of women becomes one if we become conscious of our anima. In general, when we dream of women, we usually refer to women we know. But sometimes, it is a woman totally unknown to us, and there is no direct and intimate connection or anything that feels personal to us. She is not our wife, a friend, or acquaintance. This "unknown woman" stands for a figure from a fairy tale, the language of the collective unconscious, and therefore also represents the archetype anima.

It is important to realize that anima and animus always have two aspects: a benevolent, or positive, and a negative aspect. Always determine what side they represent in dreams. Is the anima/animus appearing as positive (nurse, friend, helper, adviser) or negative (wicked woman, a witch, or ogress, chasing you, killing someone)? Evil anima figures are the witch, the dragon (also a symbol of the devil), the grave, and sarcophagus (from the Greek *phageo*, "to eat," and *sarka*, or "flesh"). We cannot predict the way in which the anima will appear, but in pre-adult years a maternal anima is common, while as an adult, our anima will take the form of an attractive woman. In our advanced years, the anima appears as a young girl or child.

Let's examine now the four configurations of the female archetype.

Anima and the Four Basic Types of Configuration of the Feminine Archetype

Besides the great variety of images in dreams, the anima or eternal feminine can also be represented by a combination of the *four types of femininity*. I mentioned "combination," or variation, as we have seen that no one is a pure image of a certain type when it comes to the four conscious functions, just as no one is a 100% *Sulphur* or any other basic constitution. Sometimes, at first sight it may appear that one is an outspoken introvert thinking type, or a flamboyant *Sulphur*, but upon closer examination there is always another aspect activated—somewhat tempering the single picture—creating an individual closer to the normal imperfect human being who indeed has to abandon his dominant conscious function, or has to appeal to the other side of his temperament, when caught in different changeable life situations. It is the same with the four types of femininity. Life circumstances push us to adapt and be more flexible if we do not want to be isolated in a community, and to act in life as human as possible. The role of one type, for instance the Mother type, is not the only form to express the feminine. Women often are a combination of some of these four types, one more predominant than the other depending on the feminine role and the circumstances in which more of a nourishment (yin in TCM) or action (yang) is required.

Jung's colleague and great psychotherapist in her own right, Toni Wolff (1888-1953), wrote a wonderful book about it, entitled *Four Eternal Women*. As we will see later, a similar structure will apply to men. A short description related to some of these four types is included in the following paragraph, using the homeopathic constitutional types.

These four types form pairs of opposites, referring either to the collective unconscious archetype, or pointing to aspects of femininity functioning within the realm of the personal. There is the Mother type, and its opposite the *Hetaira*, or Daughter. As well, there is the Medium and Amazon duo. The Mother and Hetaira are *personally* oriented, while the Amazon and Medium types are more *impersonally* oriented—the Amazon type related to the outer world, the Medium type to the inner world of the psyche. Just as with the four conscious functions, the opposite pairs reflect the dominant and least adapted or undifferentiated function, as this female typology is formed by fundamental instinctual or archetypal traits, by miasmatic traits and constitutional ones, and also by those traits formed by culture, race, and environment. When a woman is predominantly a Mother type in her approach to life, her least expression will be described by the opposite of that adaptational form —the Daughter type. As seen further, the Mother type is all about protection, security, and interest in family and close friends only, where the Daughter type is the opposite, with an interest in making as many friends (and lovers) as possible. The world is her stage, rather than the personal home her comfort. However, according to circumstances, this Mother type can turn into an Amazon (secondary adaptation) if required. For instance, this Mother type will fight for her kids as a lioness for her cubs when she perceives them to be in danger or mistreated. We can also find this Mother type (*Calc-c*) having another possible secondary adaptation—becoming the Medium type— as she is even interested in connecting to dead people or animals (*magnetized, desire to be; talking with dead people, Calc-sil*).

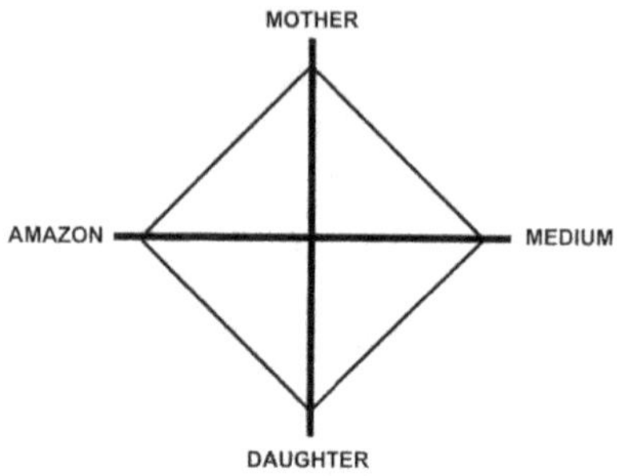

The Four Feminine Types

The Mother Type

The Mother type is easily recognized in the homeopathic world in the *Calcarea carbonicum* personality. For this type, life takes form through living for the people around her (men and women, mainly family and close friends). Mother represents the collective orientation towards protection—warding off all dangers by her presence, nourishment, and love. *Calc-carb's* worry is always personal and close to home (*talking of nothing but murder, fire and rats*)—not for the rest of the world (her "world" being nothing beyond her own neighborhood)—indicating *affectations from egotism.* She avoids bad news on TV and in newspapers (*sensitive to hearing bad news*), but when something happens to any of her family members or close friends, it hits her with hurricane force (*Ailments from grief; despair with fear of death*)! In these days of ubiquitous communication through social media, it is difficult to avoid seeing bad news, as the *Calc-c* person stays in close contact with friends and family. For example, she posts endless pictures on Facebook: of her baby with food smeared on his face, of reunions, of gatherings with family and friends, as if life were nothing but a never-ending party. Life for her is mainly about bearing and raising children—even when those children get married—with the risk that she might be overbearing, crippling the development of her "angels." It is easy to see that a depressive situation (very similar to an *Aurum* depression) can arise due to excessive worry and excessive responsibility (on a small, family-oriented scale versus that of the larger worldview of the *Aurum* and *Causticum* personalities). We find *Calc-c* simultaneously under the rubrics *duty, too much sense of duty*, related to her worry about domestic issues only, and *duty, no sense of duty* regarding world issues or even any matters beyond those affecting immediate family and close friends (so not so expansive as for the Daughter type).

Unity with other living beings is an imperative for any human being. Of course, different people achieve unions in different ways. For the constitutional *Calc-c*, an attempt to become one with her limited world is to submit to a person or a group (family) and most often to God (*religious affections, wants to read the bible all day long; religious affections, metaphysical concerns*). In this way she transcends the separateness of her individual existence by becoming part of something bigger than herself (the family unit and God), strengthening a perceived need for protection. *Calcarea* has great fondness for food and drink. She tends to overcome anxiety (which is everywhere!) and depression (always looming) by eating and drinking. The mouth is a prominent feature, often the most expressive one: lips tend to be thick and open, as if in a state of continuous expectation of being fed. To her, this is a symbol of being loved. She is always nibbling on something; even more, she is driven to eat. She has to eat to quiet her anxieties about being unloved or about the calamities that are so visible in this world (avoided at all costs by the *Calc-c* person as they belong to that "foreign" world, too calamitous to consider). Food is like a drug for her, acting as a tranquilizer: a refrigerator full of food and drink is her medicine cabinet in case of worry and/or depression (to which she is quite prone)! The collective orientation is also extended to God. God is the almighty protector (*religious affec-*

tions, in children; religious affections, alternating with metaphysical concerns [black type, only remedy]; religious affections in puberty) from whom she expects everything; it does not occur to her to put forth an effort. Faith allays *Calc-carb's* deepest fears and mitigates unbearable losses. She is always searching for the magic helper, as in the fables and dream worlds that she likes so much, looking for the paradisiacal existence she had to leave coming out of the womb. That *Calc-c* is not a pure Mother type is seen further when discussing the Medium type to whom many *Calc-carb*s belong. As mentioned before under the archetypal symbol of mother (see Chap. 2, under "Relative Fixed Symbols"), the duality can be at work when the nourishing mother turns into the Devouring Mother when she is overprotective, robbing her child of his individuality and smothering him at her breast, minimizing the relationship with animus in her child (*Kali-c* is an example).

The Daughter or Hetaira Type

This type resembles most often *Phosphorus*, the individual form of personal functioning. This contrast with the Mother type is outspoken and opposite, as connecting to people in the world is desired (*love for travel; Delusion, is on a distant island*), rather than strictly with close family and friends. She represents a woman of a fairy-tale character, possessing and radiating anima as a quality of herself, exemplifying the Aphrodite aspect of the feminine archetype, the Goddess of love, desire, and beauty, who finds her main fulfillment in seeking union with the masculine, an irresistible attraction for most men saddled with an archaic anima. Just like Aphrodite, the mythological goddess, she not only has many natural gifts and all the mythical attributes of desirability, but seems to have a "magical girdle" that compels anyone she wishes to desire her (*Sulphur* and *Lycopodium* types mainly), as *lasciviousness*, *lustfulness*, and *nymphomania* can be part of her fabric. She truly is a representation of Eros or function of relationships, having the sexual appeal, the affection, and the attraction that binds people together and draws out the Eros in men. A *Phosphorus* person is born for company and loving relationships. She is a woman who is fond of travel, and has love for the strange, the mysterious, and the unknown, so there is nothing that will keep her at home. As is the case for any archetype, she exhibits duality: she can be the nymph and the seductress, moving from one relationship to another. Needless to say, this kind of woman does not win any popularity contests among other types of women! It is not just her smile or shapely body that is beautiful; her whole appearance—soul included—silences praises of her parts. A closer look at *Phosphorus* will demonstrate the characteristics of the Daughter type.

As D. H. Lawrence once said, "The great home of the soul is the open road." This can be said of any *Phosphorus* person! She travels through the universe as if she is walking in the garden of an estate which belongs to her! Even when at home, resting between her treasures, she can summon whole countries and vistas of beauty. She relaxes and strolls through the world with a mixture of exhilaration and relaxation, bringing with this attitude a childish delight, seeing everything afresh. Above all she enjoys being lost, a nightmare for her *Sulphur* husband who usually walks with a map in his hand. She loves to dive uninhibited into a souk like the Medina of Fez, which is like a human beehive with each bee sitting cross-legged in its own little cell while thousands of others pass to-and-fro gathering their honey, the "necessities" of everyday life. She does not hesitate to be "stung," as the merchant offering a cup of mint tea is enough for her to sit down for a genuine conversation about his family history and where they gathered the honey—aka, family treasures. *Phosphorus* is characterized by a tubercular *dissatisfaction*, a fidgety character, and quickness in shifting interests (*capriciousness*); therefore, a need to change physically (restless traveling from one city to another) as well as mentally (changing study topics or interest all the time) and emotionally (easy connection to others but very often tires of and dispatches them) is not uncommon. Being averse to subordination, and driven by her dissatisfaction, she will find it difficult to commit herself to a permanent relationship (*capriciousness*). The whole psychic force or libido of the *Phosphorus* person is aimed at connecting to others—to as many people as possible—including not only those in her neighborhood but to anyone in the world in general (*desire for company, aversion to solitude; Del, is on a deserted island*). Love and personal interaction are her ultimate goals, rather than being contained in social or family settings like the Mother type (*estranged from her family*). She lives only in the present and does not care for the future or the past. Her chief urge is to scatter as much sunshine and brightness into the lives of her friends as she can.

Phosphorus is a mixture of delight: refreshing nonchalance, possessing a natural class and culture, going from frivolity to gravity with ease, always adjusting to the atmosphere around her. How envious to many people is *Phosphorus's* easy way of enjoying life, her independent persona, her radiant outlook! For a *Phosphorus* person, the cultivation of strong social connections in general are not only important to living a fulfilling life: they are vital to *Phosphorus's* healthy life. *Phosphorus* is a *compassionate* person, which means that she does not make a distinction between her own ego and that of others. For *Phosphorus*, the suffering she sees in others touches her almost as closely as does her own. Her acts of compassion are not oriented to each situation individually but to the world in its entirety, as she has boundless compassion for all living beings, humans, animals, and all of Nature's beauty. She is mindful, which makes her more connected to other people—an empathetic feeling of being at one with the universe. Conveying the contents of the

Phosphorus soul is not only done through talking (*loquacity*), but is commonly expressed through a love for drawing, sculpting, theater, dancing, clay model making, crafts, painting, and writing in verse. *Phosphorus* is not only intelligent (*active concentration* and *easy comprehension*) but also interested in all kinds of extracurricular activities (*desire for numerous various things*). It is a pleasure merely to be in her presence and hear the sound and excitement of her voice with which, like an instrument of many strings, she can pass from one language to another. These are all forms of communication, which is the major compensation of the *Phosphorus* child and adult, and when such communication is lost because of moving, the loss of a friend, or the death of a family member, the ensuing grief easily sends this child into her own dream world, reflecting autistic characteristics.

Some lucky souls are born with a brighter outlook than others; they simply see beauty and opportunity where others see flaws and dangers. *Phosphorus* belongs to the first category. *Phosphorus* is derived from the Greek words *pher* or *phoreo*, meaning "to carry, bear" and *phos*, or "light," which defines this person perfectly. In her pure state, *Phosphorus* possesses genuine personal advantages that mold her personality in the broadest sense. She *is* the way of lightness, playfulness, charm, attraction, and sensuality. She is wholly awake and fully alive. She is attuned to beauty, pleasure, and enjoyment, the play of love and life. She is the radiant vision, appearing as an angel of beauty and love. Life looks worthy and bright to her. She gives lightness and poetic inspiration, enjoys and grieves easily, loves and rejects often, connects and repels even more. She dances and plays with a life that for her is simply a game and an illusion. Happiness, for *Phosphorus*, comes from within as well as from without: she avails herself of the manifold blessings which surround her and has a personality that allows her to appreciate them. She feels that life is indeed a glorious inheritance to be enjoyed!

She is a person who, when in balance, loves life to the fullest; she is capable of wandering, always ready for an adventure, and to see something new rather than being tied to the security of finding confirmation in the old. She is satisfied with minor goods or position in the world as she is always capable of satisfying her needs, meaning traveling and meeting new people, regardless of fortune and economic circumstances. With readiness to see beauty, she looks at the world with refined observation, immersed and intoxicated by moments of splendor and beauty. For *Phosphorus,* life seems full of fortuitous circumstances, as she is fearless (despite the many fears she has) when it comes to trying something new. If an opportunity appears, *Phosphorus* will usually take it, as it allows her to live in a sort of never-ending fantasy world. Instead of giving in to worry about what could go wrong, she says to herself, "Isn't that interesting? I'd like to give it a try." Variety in life increases her day-to-day happiness. She maximizes her chances of good luck by maintaining a large network of friends and acquaintances. Serendipity smiles on *Phosphorus* and her relaxed approach to life. If our world is shaped by our perceptions, then the world of *Phosphorus* is interesting and full of beauty and meaning, an exciting adventure; *Calc-c* might see the same lifestyle as shallow and superficial, because *Calc-c* wants a steady home and security, not an adventure!

A love of life can be contagious—and *Phosphorus* is its permanent messenger! She has constant readiness to love, the kind of love that can be experienced towards many others, but loves her own Self equally, out of a necessity to love others and not an expression of selfishness! There is a theme of *diffusion* in *Phosphorus.* She wants to spread outward into the environment. She finds joy in being friendly, being warm, in considering and respecting another person and making him or her happy. She organizes her life around goals such as fostering community, connecting to family, and engaging creatively. *Phosphorus* is a person who experiences falling in love as exhilarating and intense. As it quickly loses the desired intensity, this love ends in the wish for never-ending conquests, always with the illusion that the new love will be better than the previous one and will result in finding *Phosphorus's* soulmate. In this conquest, this tubercular person is greatly helped by her beautiful physique: *fine eyelashes, tall figure,* beautiful eyebrows and angelic face. Lucky women like *Phosphorus* have big, beautiful eyes—the flames in her eyes outshine the twinkling of the stars—while other constitutions just seem to have big eyes thanks to the clever application of eye shadow. Trying to explain *Phosphorus's* appeal is very much like attempting to justify one's fascination with a beautiful song. The melody haunts and the lyrics tantalize. There is not just one portion of the tune that stands out, not just one single, compelling line among the lyrics that will go down in history. Each note and word are part of the whole, and the whole mesmerizes and is unforgettable. And it is this way with *Phosphorus*!

Her chest is usually unremarkable and even boyish (although she is the first one to correct this minor mishap of Nature by getting breast implants). Her arms and legs are slender, and neck photogenically firm. The chin is determined. The mouth is enchanting, small and drawn, turning up at the corners only slightly, almost royally, when she smiles. Her eyes are captivating and seductive, and her voice can be soft or enthusiastic, with a tone always comforting. Nothing can exceed the grace of her movements and the charm of her manner, both of which give her the delightful distinction of being different from others. Her heartfelt laughter brings sunrays on a dreary day. When she reads, she continually comments to herself, as she feels present in the story and cannot fail to participate in the topic. Any "labor" in the house becomes a product of an accomplishment of beauty: she gazes with joy and pride at a well-placed vase with beautiful organized flowers. It is not boasting, as her creation will be complimented on by others as something that pleases the eye. And when she does an ordinary job of dusting her precious objects of travel (although a *Sulphur* husband would not see any dust), for her it is reconnecting to her treasures, which means of course reliving adventures and meetings with her many friends abroad.

A *Phosphorus* person communicates more than anyone else through her well-developed conscious functions, including all her sensory senses for sure! Her speech is both "with it" and educated. *Phosphorus* is little impressed by fame and only slightly more by fortune. Her abundant beauty and inviting charm easily capture the imaginations of *Sulphur* and *Lycopodium* men; they are carried away and wish to support her honorably in some form or other for the rest of her life. Beauty is indeed like an open letter of recommendation, predisposing the hearts of others to favor the person who presents. Her secondary adaptational structure is especially the Medium type as she is very interested through her intuitive nature to delve into the ESP world. We find these characteristics in the rubrics: *magnetized, desires to be; mesmerism ameliorates; introspection; meditation*, and in the rubric *sensitive to external impressions*, reflective of her susceptibility to environmental vibrations. Less frequently present for *Phosphorus* is the Amazon type, although her desire to be regarded as an individual and not subordinated to people and their strict rules points to a fighting spirit when a need arises to preserve her individuality and her emotional wandering spirit.

The Amazon Type

Amazons, mythological figures, were women who were artful and brave in single combat. This feminine archetype represents force, strength, and power. Were they a figment of Greek imagination or was there proof of their existence in the past? The 8th

century BC poet Homer, in the *Iliad*, mentioned the existence of women who were "the equal of men," worthy opponents to compete with men, as is the case today. In the 1990s, 2000-year-old burial mounds were found in a remote Russian outpost near the Kazakhstan border—graves of warrior women who had been buried with their weapons, daggers and bronze-tipped arrows. When we analyze the etymology of *Amazons*, we see the Greek words *a*, or "without" and *mazos*, or "breast"—reflecting the idea that they removed the right breast in order to have better bow control. In the 1960s, with women's emancipation, these heroic warriors were found in the tomboy next-door, becoming the prototype for the independent wonder woman, a woman who can achieve fulfillment in the outer world in some type of career in which she is the equal of men.

Such a figure dominated by a strong animus makes us think of *Sepia*, a person who will not back off from any battle between the sexes when it comes to success in life, pursuing a career, and being regarded as an equal partner in marriage and career. Even her physical appearance shows the dominance of maleness with flat breasts, narrow hips, and hirsutism. To many, she appears as a person with poverty of emotions and lack of Eros. Poverty on the emotional plane does not mean a lack of emotions in general, but a lack of positive or anima emotions (warmth, love, etc.). Her emotions go from violent anger (*Ailments from emotional excitement*) to absolute *indifference, even to loved ones*, and sometimes inability to bond with children and husband (*aversion to family members* and *aversion to husband*). These last emotions are linked to her drive for individuality and self-expression, which also explains her *aversion to sympathy, consolation, and company*. These emotions are outgrowths of repressed sexuality, and of the eruption of the unconscious personality, a mixture of the animus and the shadow.

Sepia can come across as bossy, because she says what she

thinks and what is necessary and does not pad it with extra fluff. She can be sarcastic if people talk down to her (*mocking, sarcasm, with great intuition concerning other people's weaknesses*). She can become an overwhelmed mother who is prone to flipping out, running out of the house screaming that she is not coming back and that she will kill herself, leaving the rest of the family shattered and helpless. Many miles have been added on the family car by the exhausted *Sepia* mother on her escapes! Several rubrics reflect this exhaustive state: *nothing suits her, she finds fault with everything; she has the greatest irritability from the slightest cause; she is very indifferent towards everything and has no proper sense of life*. She may say things like, "I have no more ambition. I simply don't want to do anything, either work or play. It is even an exercise to think. I feel like quarreling with everyone and became very excited about a mere trifle and said some sharp things (feeling ashamed of it at the same time)." This *melancholic depression* and *adynamia* stem from hypo-adrenalism. *Sepia* has a high affinity for the thyroid and adrenal cortex. This dutiful person is dependable, precise, and punctual. At the same time, she sets high standards for everyone and follows societal rules. The other side of the coin is that determination may give way to obstinacy, censorial behavior, and precision to the point of preoccupation with trifles and even OCD behavior. An overactive sense of duty can lead to lack of adaptability in new situations, rigidity in views, and inflexibility in approaching problems. It may lead, in that situation, to a life filled with burdens rather than joyful accomplishments—a life filled with guilt because of a perceived neglect of duty and being insensitive to relationship needs. Such an individual becomes sensitive to criticism because anticipated praise is not forthcoming; this leads to the creation of the delusion *she is not appreciated* (*Aur*, *Pall*, *Thuj*; to these, add *Calc-s* and *Lachesis*). This can result in smoldering, unexpressed feelings of rage, resentment, and depression in otherwise seemingly well-adjusted people.

Her secondary adaptation is the Mother type but in a very different form than the traditional mother. Even as a child, *Sepia* demonstrates the extreme opposite of the passive immobility of the *Calcarea* child/Mother type. *Sepia* is a *serious child* that is called to duty far too early in her individuation path because of a noble misfortune (*Ailments from early responsibility*), like the absence of the mother (due to death, alcoholism, sickness, drug addiction, etc.). Early on, the put-upon *Sepia* child becomes the sterner mother who rules the household with a practical, no-nonsense approach, void of warmth and emotional values. As the oldest child, she takes over motherly duties (*maternal instinct exaggerated* and *too much sense of duty*). Initially, this type is an extravert. In other words, everything is aimed at the object, not the subject, aimed at the goal to be reached—this is not done with much introversion, but with a plan of action, a plan of attack that secures the best result for everyone involved. The least occurring adaptation therefore is the Medium type, the Amazon type's opposite. Small wonder that someone whose anima (her female side) had to be suppressed from a young age in order to respond to her animus (her active male side and sense of responsibility), should have difficulty expressing her affection for others. Rather than kissing and hugging her younger siblings, she will be overprotective of them, a kind of displacement, as this overprotection takes the place of expressing deeper feelings, which she is unable to do. Her emotional side has been stunted: if someone in the family dies, *Sepia* will not say or ask anything, but will remain emotionless.

The *Sepia* person becomes the stern mother who rules the household with a practical approach, not a warm one. She has this fixed idea that rest is not possible, that she can't let her guard down; she fights inattention with every fiber of her being (*Delusion, feels every fiber on **right** side* and *duty, too much sense of*)! The right side stands for the active side, the yang side, the sword, the consciousness: it is here that *Sepia* wields her animus, her maleness, to get things done! But because of this relentless feeling of being needed, this delusion will change in the syphilitic phase to *duty, aversion to* and *aversion to domestic duty* as well as *escape from family*.

Sepia can be a great companion: she is active, and practical; she is a go-getter, a mover and shaker, a person whose business is also outside of the family—and no male is safe from her competitive mind. *Sepia* is ready to fight for her own needs and rights, for cultural achievement, human dignity, and noble causes. For the sake of her convictions and needs, she is willing to neglect relationships and disregard old patterns that have outlived their usefulness (like those patterns expressed in the old German adage, "kinder, küche, und kirche"—"children, kitchen, and church"). She is the quintessential career and pioneer woman. She also has the capacity to structure and order her environment. She can be a wife and mother, but also a competent administrator and the creator of home and soul. She responds to practical and concrete rather than abstract situations, and to the requirements of the moment. She listens, receives, carries, nests and nourishes, protects and promotes growth. Rest and standing still are things *Sepia* hates in any situation, personal or otherwise. When this type is unadapted, she can become the feared steam-rolling bitch, charged with dogmatic convictions that leave many amputees in her path.

The Medium Type

This type, opposite of the Amazon type, is deeply interested in the deepest layer of the yin, in the world of visions and recalling the dead. *Calc-c* and *Phosphorus* come to mind, although both personalities are quite different even in the formation of their ego. Where *Calc-c* has an absence of ego firmness, *Phosphorus's* quest, as seen before, is to be an individual, showing a strong ego that cannot be subdued (she would become sick if she was dominated and hindered from branching out into the world). The *Phosphorus* Medium type will be an inspiration to others (*femme inspiratrice*) with her upbeat and extravert intuitive character welcoming ESP, while the *Calc-c* Medium type can create confusion within herself, as *Calc-c* in general can be overwhelmed by these extra sensory perceptions, imbued as she is with an inability to avoid psychic infection. While the *Phosphorus* Medium types are the seers and prophetesses, the *Calc-c* type seeks refuge in this unconscious world to connect with dead family members and pets. The Medium's secondary adaptation is most likely the Mother type for the *Calc-c* and the Daughter type for the *Phosphorus. Calc-c* is extending herself to family, dead or alive, and staying in contact with them, reminiscing about the "good times" they spent with dear family and friends. For *Phosphorus,* it is an extension of the world to which she communicates feverishly, to make sure that no one is entirely forgotten in her support system, and to not succumb to her cyber delusion, *is on a distant island.* It speaks by itself that the *Phosphorus* Medium type is not likely to succeed in business —except when tailored to her talents of art, jewelry, and writing, and supported by a business partner when dealing with the daily entanglements expressed by the rubric, *Delusion, is doing business.* The *Calc-c* Medium is not any better, although being a mother, and bringing comfort to people by connecting them to their dead relatives and pets, play an enormous role in the lives of Earth types. *Calc-c* also has the *Delusion, of being sick and for this reason will not work,* expressing her desire to be nourished and protected in the safe home environment, to ward off the numerous fears she suffers from (*fear of death; fear of impending disease; fear of infection; fear of her confused condition being observed; fear of hearing bad news,* among many others).

Men would do well to understand these different types and aspects of women. As noted before, even a Mother type can become at some time an Amazon, when she feels she needs to evolve to fulfill another part of herself, and woe is the man who wants to suppress this aspect of his wife: vicious wars will result! Let's investigate now the connection of men to the activity of their anima.

Unbalanced Connections to the Anima in Men

With most men, the anima has a strong autonomous personality (unconscious to them) and is not always a smooth relationship function between the conscious and unconscious. There are three unbalanced connections in man to his anima: identification, inflation, and projection—all of them leading to their own kind of misfortune in life.

Identification with the Anima

In identification with the anima, the anima is abnormally abundant in the male—in other words, strongly constellated in the man, when the Self is contained in the anima—causing the anima identification, often pointing to a mother-complex. Such anima will distort him into a kind of "hysterical woman," exposing the weak spots in his character with fits of *changing and alternating moods*, unfounded fears and anxieties, feelings of distrust (*suspicion*) and resentment, *being easily offended, brooding, jealousy as foolish as it is irresistible, vanity or narcissism*, and sudden bursts of *passion and rage alternating with affectionate disposition*—all well-known rubrics for remedies like *Crocus, Nat-m*, *Pulsatilla*, *Lachesis*, *Kali-c*, *Mercury* and *Lycopodium*. "Passion" in this sense often drags its victim down with the weight of his/her folly. Identification with the anima can occur when there was a father with a weak animus or an overly one-sided, overpowering imbalanced animus. It also can occur if a mother becomes overprotective, often in reaction to the latter situation, even when we could call this a positive encounter with the mother anima where "children always come first."

An ideal and idyllic paradise family upbringing can stimulate a man's anima but ill-prepare him for challenges in life, for letting go of the mother relationship, to face hardships in life, or even to find his own goal. Such a man in the first half of his life (or forever, when the anima does not find the balanced relationship), through partial identity with the mother and failure to form a sufficiently masculine ego, can become *effeminate*, submissive (*yielding*), sentimental with a moody and uncontrolled disposition (*moods alternating; reproaching others*), or too *easily offended*. This man at such moments, while losing control over his thinking function, acts no better than the animus-possessed woman with her dogmatic, prejudicial opinions.

It is not uncommon that such a man, under the spell of his unconscious feminine side, has rather boyish looks not revealing his real age, and that a high degree of aestheticism—even wanting to dress beautiful and neat—is the result of his close mother bond. This he exhibits amply in his good taste, tender feelings, sensitivity, charming manners, great capacity for friendship, fine appreciation of all the fine arts, possibly artistic achievements, and gift for poetry and design, while demonstrating interest and great capacity in connecting to the unconscious. He is usually distinguished by a certain artistic sympathy, and often by many attractive intellectual qualities. These epicures have soft voices and ingratiating manners and are bold enough to make a direct appeal to the heart and emotions. Such a man can be classified under the *passive-feminine* character: besides softness and excessive politeness and devotion, and a friendly, submissive, shy, awkwardly accommodating and humble demeanor, he may also display a feminine facial expression and bearing. He can be bashful and ceremonious, ready to please his physician with ostentatious gestures and long-winded excuses and explanations. He may have an exaggerated readiness to help, a seeming inability to assume an aggressive or even decisive attitude, and a great need to *cling* to people and constantly maintain and establish contact with other people. This attitude of devotion has nothing to do with love or helpfulness, but more to do with warding off strong hidden envy, and inhibited aggressive and destructive tendencies, like the sycotic and syphilitic characteristics of *Pulsatilla* for instance (*abrupt; anger when obliged to answer; being besides herself; chaotic behavior; fastidious; hatred of women; Delusion, women are evil and will injure his soul; impulsive; hysteria; kleptomania; misanthropy; morphinism; rage in paroxysms* and *indisposed to talk*).

That such a male with plentiful anima—leading to an effeminate personality—is not always well-received by society is expressed by the following example, as noted in a "Dear Annie" column in the *New Mexican* of December 8, 2017, with the headline, "Father hates his introvert stepson." Although the stepfather is well aware of and even ashamed of his bias and judgment, he wants his stepson to be "normal" like his two other sons, which for him means being interested in sports, hunting, girls, and cars—something he calls being typical rough-and-tumble boys, and something he wants to impose on and discover in his stepson, an extremely effeminate and sensitive being, respectful and open-hearted, who is more interested in baking cookies with his mom and reading books than doing outdoor things and exercise, which he claims he hates. His stepson's sensitivity was discounted as weakness, but obviously the stepfather denied his own feminine side, archaic as it was. He feels embarrassed by his stepson when he meets friends and the boy is present, and admits to feeling hate and not love for him. The answer of Dear Annie was: "Hating something in others is actually something that one possesses oneself." While this can be the case (disliking something in others indeed can reflect the same characteristic that one hides in one's shadow side), in this case I rather suspect that the stepfather is also a typical male dominant thinking person with a poorly developed feeling function. What we lack the most, we hate to see in others. In this case, one with an undeveloped and unbalanced anima hates to see an exaggerated anima in others (his stepson). Rather than despising the teenager, which no doubt will be acutely felt by this young man, the stepfather would do well to incorporate newly discovered entities into his own life, like love for the arts, cooking, and reading (book reading, but not just novels). Doing so would enrich his own life, and lead to greater respect and love for human beings that do not follow the "norm," especially not that of his warped, male-dominant viewpoint.

The Native American Indian tribe of the Lakota summoned the aid of the spirit world to tell them what to do in battle by giving the task to exactly such a man, whom they called *winkte* or "two-souled person." By this was meant a man with a great deal of anima, or womanly qualities—an effeminate man, an ego structure identifying with a hermaphroditic nature—which is not surprising, in view of the anima's luminosity that can exert profound influence on certain men's psychology. The tribe called upon this *winkte* also for certain kinds of magic or sacred power, to read the future, and even to name their children, as well as to serve as matchmakers. These men were perfectly accepted and not ridiculed among the Native American Indians.

The effeminate man, or man with feminized masculinity, might look for his masculinity in another man of rather crude nature, someone inferior and rather aggressive, trying to balance his own lack of vigor and assertiveness. Homosexuality is usually characterized by anima possession or identification with the anima: the patient has the desire to change himself into a woman through extensive operations or worse, self-castration.

There is however a positive side (as there is never yin without yang) to identification with the anima. The anima can become a spiritual guide in life, and the world is full of artists, sculptors, writers, painters, dancers, and teachers who put their soul, or anima, in their work, living a fulfilling life.

Inflation by the Anima

Inflation is a body that becomes too light, rises too high, as expressed by the delusions: *Del, body is lighter than air; Del, is floating in air* and *Del, is flying*, in which we find *Lachesis, Opium, Spigelia, Verat-a*, and *Tarentula* among other personalities. Here, a man's anima voice puts him in a state of exhilaration and an unquestioning feeling of assurance, with exaggerated expectations and a feeling of power that nothing is beyond his grip and capacity. When it pertains to inflation by his anima, such a man denies having feminine characteristics, which he shows all the time when he has delusions of grandeur and a hefty dose of autoeroticism. He is the chosen one, the anointed one, the savior of all women! We see it most often in men where ambitions, hopes, dreams, and desires are confused with real accomplishments and realities, the eternal daydreamers who remain living in that dream: fame has not arrived yet but it is just around the corner and it is only a question of time before people recognize their genius (*erroneous and haughty notions*). His anima constantly praises him (as if it was a real woman!) about his potentialities and glorious achievements, all just preparations in his mind and not yet actualized, but it is his archaic anima that keeps on whipping him, creating clouds around his consciousness. Of course, such men feel cocksure and righteous and behave as if they are rich (*Delusion, of wealth*), and *boasting* is more to convince themselves that they can spend now what they don't have (*thinks himself distinguished, squanders his money*). Or, they go wild after receiving an inheritance (*insanity after gaining fortune*), dressing with flair (*extravagance*), *gossiping, finding fault in others,* and *attempting a great many things but accomplishing nothing*, as well as *lying and never speaking the truth*—the grand master, Pinocchio—and may have the *Delusion, he is hard at work.* All these expressions are produced by the inflation of the anima, as well as religious delusions: *imagines himself in heaven talking to God,* and *Delusion, he considers himself to be Christ.* The homeopath recognizes the portrait of *Veratrum-a,* the prototype of identification with the archetype of a deity, therefore bringing him far removed from the unconscious, his shadow, as seen before (Chap. 7, under "Identification with the Persona"). In this case, when a man goes up in a balloon, his anima, his Achilles tendon, can even cause him to marry a person identical with his shadow.

This inflation of the anima can easily lead to being possessed by the anima at inopportune moments, where the feeling function is archaic and Logos rules. Here is a dream representing such a situation.

Conscious situation: This was a 50-year-old man, engrossed in a life of reason as CEO of a big company. He was married to a tall, beautiful wife, and since they were both my patients the contrast between the two was easily observed. The wife clearly had climbed up the ladder of self-realization much higher than her husband. Two days after an insanely jealous attack on his wife (*jealousy as foolish as it is irresistible*), in which he accused her unjustly of having an affair, he had the following dream.

Dream

I am on my wedding day, and a lot of people are present. It is time to have a picture taken with my future wife, and everyone is looking at me. I am aware of the repulsiveness I feel towards her, as she is obese and hideous looking. I put up a fake smile but can hardly hide the real disgust I have for her as I cannot understand I am going to marry someone like that. I woke up in horror!

Analysis

Of course, this Logos-oriented person did not come on a visit because of this dream—which he dismissed as pure nonsense—but rather for hypertension and heart problems. He had no idea that the dream was about his "inner woman" (subjective dream analysis) rather than his real wife who was well-rooted in her four conscious functions (objective dream analysis); the woman within who possessed him in his irrational jealous rages. This person is unable to distinguish between his actual wife and his personal and mythological projection. It is here, under this circumstance, where we can help him understand the differentiation between his wife and his projection—where homeopathic treatment, with judicial doses of the simillimum (which will cover every aspect of this person), will be readily accepted by this patient and faster working than if I made him feel small by explaining first the urgent message of his dream to exercise and integrate an improved anima.

The third unbalanced connection of men with their anima is called *projection,* often the start of any romantic relationship with women. This will be extensively discussed in Chapter 13, "The Human Love Story: Projection of the Sygizi." We have brought our discussion up to the appearance and influence of the anima, and will now proceed to discuss the other sygizi, the animus.

12

ANIMUS

Going over a bridge and going down and under,
is the road to completeness.

The Man Within: The Fight for Emancipation

When we look at characteristics of the animus, we see that it is more likely a naturally active and even an *overactive* archetype of males, but "the man within" refers above all to the male personification in the woman's unconscious—a voice that should be heard and practiced in order for a woman to have a fulfilled life, and to be able to play an equal role in the matrimonial relationship. In past times, the role of the woman was at home, and certain professions (physicians and lawyers among them) and positions of leadership (CEO's in business and high-ranking officers) generally were not open to females. Even in the field of science, women participated in advanced science and technology for centuries but their achievements were not recognized, as men controlled everything—the press, the church, and every political office. Several papers by female scientists were presented in conferences but wrongly credited to men. Marie Curie, two-time winner of the Nobel Prize, was dismissed by many as merely a helper to her husband, considering him the real genius. Till the beginning of the 20th century, schools to educate women had one goal: to confirm that God intended the female to be "Adam's helpmate," to develop "neat handwriting," and "skillful needlework." The pursuit of intellectual ideas by women was considered dangerous, as overtaxing their brain would lead to "a deficiency of their reproductive power." All females had to do was make room for the desires of men.

Gertrude Bell, called "Queen of the Desert" (1868-1926, British explorer, diplomat, and archeologist), scion of one of England's most prominent families in the Victorian Age, ended up with the cold reality of spinsterhood in spite of initially walking the marriage market, from one ball to another, as was the custom of ladies from influential families. Armed with a very strong animus obtained from her father, who encouraged her to follow her own choices, anyone she met (with few exceptions) was turned off by her sharp tongue, impatience, keen intellect, willfulness, and her high-spirited, commanding personality and competitiveness as well as her strong, often snide opinions. Few men (or women) could match the high standards set by her father and herself. A similar figure was Florence Nightingale (1820-1910), called the "Avenging Angel," who was tutored by her father in mathematics and the classics, defying Victorian conventions that suppressed intellectually powerful women. She broke out of her gilded family cage to care for prostitutes during the cholera epidemic of 1853, and to care for the British soldiers in the Russian-held Crimean Peninsula in 1854, facing the resentment of officers and bureaucrats who regarded her as an interloper when she single-mindedly broke down barriers. She remained unmarried also, ambivalent about the compromises she would have to make as a married woman, and died at age 90, suffering from spondylitis that kept her in pain and bedridden much of her life.

Before women's emancipation (Queen Victoria called it "the mad, wicked folly of 'Women's Rights'"), the female role was limited to the nourishing aspect of the family: taking care of the kids and husband (which often meant being continually subordinate to the spouse and lacking a point of view), feeding them, tending to the garden, and bringing the family to church on Sundays to keep up saintly appearances for the outside world. Indeed, as the German slogan described the woman's role in the Nazi State: "Kinder, Küche, Kirche," or "Children, Kitchen, Church."

This adage was reflected long before by the Stoic philosopher Seneca (4 BC-AD 65) when he stated, "Women are born to be passive," and that their role was to obey, consent, and accept. Women's expressions and wishes were kept like the top shelf of library books—hidden and neglected—as women were hustled off to the knitting room after dinner so that men could smoke cigars and talk business (and gossip), before female persuasions and awakening took place in the world as a whole. Too long—in matters sexual and social—women were mostly unfairly judged by men who made all the rules! Wives had one master, while husbands could enjoy many mistresses. It was the French existentialist Simone de Beauvoir who created a sensation in 1949 with her book, *The Second Sex*, a very influential work about the role of women. She exposed the myth of a woman in a position of a slave/master relationship, merely an object of attraction and sexuality, with her famous statement, "One is not born, but rather becomes a woman." She created an uproar and received nasty comments and resentment from the male society, as her treatise broached so many subjects taboo to women: sexuality, lesbianism, abortion—all topics hidden in the closet till then.

Why did it take us centuries to let women vote, and to

accept them in certain professions and positions (medicine, science, military, CEO, etc.)? Even now some men prefer to be like the rooster, and when it suits them, they've never heard of women's emancipation. They turn up their nose when asked to bring out the garbage, preferring to go fishing with male friends on the weekend, leaving the care of the children to their exhausted wife. The struggle for emancipation still goes on behind closed doors in many households. Now, as in the past, a woman has the sacred role as a mother, and is expected to maintain consistent fidelity during marriage and to be an innocent virgin upon marriage. Of course, at the same time, great liberties are allowed men. This can continue today because personal relationships for many women are more important than making their stamp in life, although economic necessity and true personal desire to step out of the background into the world activity have made great changes in the old status quo. Today, there is no earthly reason, biological or otherwise, that men should have more power than women. Unfortunately, if married to an excessive persona partner (*Lycopodium* for instance), some women still must repress their masculine aspects, leading to a *Staphysagria* situation where the animus becomes a little voiceless dwarf, disallowing the person to reach equality in her relationship.

It is not uncommon that a couple has many fights early in their relationship, but if the husband has all the power and his animus is over-controlling, either the marriage bursts or the woman does. If the latter, caving in is to agree with everything the controller desires, relegating the victim to a helpless child dependent on the husband for everything—money, friends she should or shouldn't have, who she talks to or doesn't, how to dress, and the very life "she should live." This typical *Staphysagria* situation will doom the soul of the victim and halt any spiritual growth of *both* partners involved. Often when women free themselves from such an abusive or deceitful relationship, they do it with vengeance and determination; nothing wakes up the woman's animus more than confronting control, deceit, and betrayal. But is there a useful, balanced amount of animus necessary for a woman, and is excessiveness a hindrance rather than a tool for going through life?

Animus in Women: Balanced or Unbalanced? A Crook or a Saint? A Bitch or a Warrior?

As for any archetype, the duality of the animus has to be taken into account and the "man within" has to find a healthy balance in a woman to achieve peace, harmony, and a feeling of equality, before it becomes the master of opinions in a woman. In order to be able to feel part of life, any woman needs to have an urge and freedom for action, and a capacity for judgment, making choices with deliberation and discrimination, without being immediately suppressed or ignored by her male counterpart. A woman with a good relationship to her animus speaks her opinion and demands the right to be heard and to be taken seriously. In what circumstances is animus required? Animus (meaning "breath or spirit") should have the freedom to enter automatically into any situation that requires action or initiative, determination and authority, rationality and understanding, critical thinking (greatly absent in our society), creativity and judgment, and makes its appearance in philosophical and religious discussions—conducting, in other words, a "spirited" conversation.

At this time in history, a taboo has been lifted. In almost any arena—the movie industry, the media, the political environment (Senate and House), colleges and the military—where men used to be in a dominant superior position, women have suddenly found their voice or animus, and a flood of women are "coming out." Hopefully, this trend continues; women should be able to stand up and speak up and make their oppressors accountable. Women's speech has been undervalued for a long time, and hopefully individual takedowns and the #MeToo movement will positively affect working environments that until now only paid lip service to the cause of gender equality. Obviously, the entire present work environment must change, and women will have to use a *balanced* animus to be empowered now and in the future.

Animus is like an assembly of judges who, when adequately represented, always brings a fair, competent, and balanced judgment, but turns into an inner accuser and prosecutor when the woman has an unbalanced relationship towards her animus. Through integration the animus becomes the Logos of consciousness, where anima is the Eros of consciousness. Logos means literally "word"—that which gives order to chaotic elements in life. In dreams, for women the animus always appears as a *contra-sexual figure*, speaking always in a deep male voice, one speaking with authority within the woman, a voice whose advice needs to be followed. This does not refer to the homeopathic remedies in the rubric *dictatorial, speaking with a voice of command*, which is an aberration of the idea "speaking with authority." Dictatorial people shout because they can't speak and need to convince themselves. Their words sink in an immense ocean, having no visible effect or result. Their voice is harsh, hollow and bossy, coming from feelings of inferiority coupled with a power attitude, a vicious cycle.

So it becomes obvious, that just like the anima in men, the animus in women has to strike a fine balance in order to be effective and to avoid evoking a man's wrath, his archaic anima (although we would hope he is aware of needed improvement in that aspect). After all, males and females both have an individual responsibility to guide their soulmate in the right direction through such psychopomp, and to use it with the right amount of intensity and integrity. At home and outside of the home, in modern life a thoroughly feminine woman learns all too fast that she must integrate at least a minimum of her animus, rather than only project it onto another man and others. When successful at integrating her animus, a woman feels counted as a human being, can assert herself, has independent reasoning and judgment, and does not let herself be pushed around as happens in some cultures around the world where the woman, once married, discovers that the old German adage ("Children, Kitchen, Church") is still at work. She must have the freedom to explore, "What is *my* opinion? What am *I* thinking? What is *my* judgment and does anyone respect it? What would *I* prefer in this situation?" Life indeed must include a certain fulfillment of personal desired goals and aspirations. If someone is caught in a marriage situation where the husband is continuously belittling his wife (*Ailments from mortification* and *Ailments from indignation*), undermining her self-worth and self-confidence, as in the following patient's history, her animus is nothing but a silent dwarf, which is the goal of the controlling abuser. This patient's dream tries to give her a wake-up call, showing where she is after many years of abuse.

Dream

I am in a car but not in the driver's seat. I think I am in the back seat and the car is rolling slowly forwards. I try to move to get to the brakes but can't seem to move, no matter how hard I try. I am frantic as the car gets closer to a car in front of me. No matter how hard I try to wiggle my way into position, I can't! My car does hit the car in front … not hard, but I bumped it.

Analysis

It is obvious that she is not in control of her destination, as someone else is at the wheel of the car and she is in the backseat allowing someone else to drive her car or take care of her destination in life. She cannot get to the brakes, although the car goes slow, but obviously needs to stop to avoid a car in front, expressing how her individuation journey is on the wrong course, waiting for a catastrophe to happen. No matter how hard she tries, her animus (willpower, drive, decision making, a voice that needs to be heard) is too weak to act and her car bumps against another car in front of her. "In front" denotes the "process of becoming conscious," not a smooth process for her but a frantic attempt to move forward in life (hitting an obstacle). The dream does not end completely in a catastrophe as she is not killed or hurt, so it is still a lysis, one telling her where she stands in life—a dream warning that something must change; that she needs to gain control over her life.

As with any archetype, we have the other side of the coin. Women in a *Sepia* state especially personify the exaggerated animus in women, where it is often clear that the animus becomes an inferior Logos with ruthless intellect. In that case, opinions are hurled towards the opponent that often have nothing to do with the essential nature of the topic but are, instead, outbursts of futile and childish emotionalism. Not only does this dominance of animus show in *Sepia's* physical characteristics with hirsutism, narrow pelvis, and addiction to exercise, but also and above all, in the emotional sphere of the psyche: a mother who acts fair but rather cold towards her children, in a business-like way, where there is no place for negotiating. To her, "Mom is always right." As a spouse, any attempts at sexual advances—except for the sole purpose of procreation—are met with an ice-cold attitude. The unbalanced animus shows intolerance to others' opinions, *obstinacy, intolerance to contradiction* and *contrary behavior*. Such a woman is most pleased with herself when she is most in the wrong. Every argument is considered a battle where an exaggerated, unbalanced Logos or the conscious thinking function will rise to the occasion and at all cost victory must be achieved, leading to dogmatic dictatorialness, generalizations, and apodictic assertions.

It is not that her arguments are necessarily wrong, but they are without feeling, without empathy, just factual! "Facts are facts, how can you argue with this," is her motto! She exclaims, "Is it not obvious? Why even further discuss this issue! Get on with it. Don't argue with me. Pay attention. I could not *have acted otherwise*." She hisses with the ferocity of an angry cat, and we realize that no one *can* argue with her! Of course, these are only sterile intellectual discussions, satisfying only the woman who misuses her animus. In fact, any decent discussion ceases instantly when an exaggerated anima or animus enters in. There will be no chance that a conversation will take place, as conversation means "in a discussion, we say something to each other, taking turns," from the Latin *cum*, or "with," and *versare*, or "turning": "turning over with." "Now I talk, then you talk." I make this clearer by citing below the experience of a woman in whom the image of excessive authority and judgment was completely hidden from her consciousness, an appalling disproportion between her feminine side and her unconscious masculinity, leading to many misunderstandings and even hostile responses.

Suppression of the animus from childhood on leads often to hostility and resentment for the offender. I remember a female patient, born into a traditional family with four boys. She was supposed to be submissive and feminine, encouraged by her mother, but all she wanted was to be one of the boys. As a protest towards her mother she used feminine diseases to evoke sympathy and get all her wishes fulfilled. But in the following dream the message became clear that she needed not only to accept her animus but to use it in an appropriate way.

Dream

I am in a room with a man. I am afraid that my mother will see him, so I hide him under the blankets. But then I said to the man: "I don't care if my mother sees you, I am not hiding you any longer."

This dream encouraged her to get her balanced voice (opinion) back, which ended the stream of female illnesses and was the start of a more confident and worthy life for her.

Another patient reacted quite differently to her possession of animus. Here is her story. On my yearly vacation to a resort, I always met a female, a super athlete, forceful and energetic, who sized up the tennis attendants the first day of her vacation. From the moment I saw her, her conversation was seized by her animus who spoke through her teeth as she announced, even within earshot of the victim, "Don't ask that one to play with us, ask that other one, he/she is better!" Now this was not a request, it was an order to be obeyed (*She-Who-Must-Be-Obeyed*). In the pure sense of reason, it was logical to her (and maybe others too), as she wanted to have a competitor at least as good as she was. Alas! She did not consciously and adequately relate to her animus but had fallen under the spell of her animus's absolutism! She identified with the archetype animus; she was imbued with its contents, as her mouth blurted things out like the flow of an untamed river. Such a formidable animus goes very much against a woman's instincts and interfered with the feminine side of her character.

To deal with such an animus-possessed woman is very confusing for a man. Anatomically she looks like a woman, but when she is talking, he finds that it is a man who is talking with an inferior feeling function. The air of authority has become one with her personality and her pronouncements are therefore indisputable. She does not adequately investigate her feeling function and sacrifices her human side, as she does not spare the feelings of the person who looks forward to playing an insignificant tennis match with a better player. Fat chance: if such a person dares to ask, she will say directly to his/her face, "You are not good enough for me, you are not in my league!" Not a statement from a female with a warm natural anima, as she always talks through the medium of the archetype animus! Of course, this does not make her many friends; she is generally referred to as "the General," "the Great Exterminator," or less flattering, "the Bitch." A general only issues orders, not requests!

It is no surprise that she remained unmarried. She asked me to find her a suitable husband, not understanding that being possessed by such animus leads to a loss of femininity, forming a destructive element to any future relationship. What should have remained inside (animus) had been turned outside, obliterating her natural anima, ruining her personal relationships. Her negative animus—which she should have whipped, with its sweeping statements and banal opinions—had robbed her of a life with warm and meaningful relationships. The heart has reasoning the mind will never understand. It is the secret source of a will that speaks through the head. Unfortunately, because of such an animus she will remain bewildered by men and eventually die not knowing herself, forever linked to the female stinging bees and black widow spiders. A positive animus should direct—not order—and encourage people to go forward without pushing them. This is a woman who is *dictatorial, speaks with a voice of command* and is *censorious.* She will overgeneralize with unshakable opinions, and at all cost wants to win the battle with certain statements of which she is very fond of: "You should do this!" "You would be better off if you would listen to me!" "You are a failure and cannot do anything right!" "You are not worth much!" "All you do is trivia!"

Dominated by and identified with her animus, her rationalization is only reasonable to her and no one else. She fails to realize that her only rebirth could come from her neglected conscious function, her feeling. Any possible relationship coming her way—which she so craves—is immediately violated by the poison of power, chasing most men away as they do not want to be entangled in an animus battle.

I asked her in an innocent way if she had any recurrent dreams! The unconscious seems to never rest, and here too was a letter in her mailbox on a regular basis. This is her dream.

Dream

About three times a month, I have the following dream. I dream I forgot to take my medication or forgot to do something and as a result I will die. I am very scared and then wake up.

Analysis

Knowing something about her conscious behavior, this dream is self-explanatory and not unexpected! Naturally, she is shocked and scared by this dream, as most people would be. I refer to Chapter 4, "Common Themes in Dreams," where death in dreams usually means that a certain attitude or characteristic is in strong need of change. First there needs to be a "death" before "rebirth" can take place; a certain previous position or attitude must be destroyed in order to produce a new possibility, a new human. This urgent message, to take her medication because she has an illness, means that she needs to tame her animus and cultivate and display more feeling function and anima. Since this is not heeded despite repetition, the mail carrier keeps bringing additional letters with the same message. She is unconscious of her conscious behavior, so only understanding this dream will bring respite. But she had no curiosity about any possible explanation, as she thought her attitude served her well in life. As a result, her conscious dream of finding a life partner will go up in smoke!

Women usurped by the animus are no easy patients for the homeopath, as every truthful fact is met with a flood of resistance (*contrary*) and a desire to draw the homeopath into endless sterile, semi-intellectual discussions (*intolerant of contradiction*). Discovering the truth for an animus-possessed woman is not her goal; winning is, and feelings are not spared to achieve it. Good arguments are met with counterarguments because the animus-ridden woman is a fierce warrior and invincible lawyer, a typical *Nitric acid* person who encounters and sees lawsuits everywhere (*Delusion, engaged in a lawsuit*). As animus also means spirit and breath, such a woman can also be called "spirited." With men, a strong animus is usually a question of vanity, to be the "king" of the household, as his animus is an expression of his true nature. No matter how natural and obliging a woman's Eros might be, if she is possessed by her animus, hers will be a fury that cannot be tamed, not subject to any reasoning power!

Sometimes possession by the animus is subtle, as the person can use many sophisticated rational arguments to support her behavior. But such "reasonable" arguments become sterile if they are not balanced by the opposite conscious function, feeling. Only the unconscious through dreams can rectify this attitude, as shown in this example of a 55-year-old woman.

Dream one

I am at a gathering with many women. Suddenly a man appears and asks if anyone wants to accompany him to have breakfast with him. I am the one accepting his offer and we proceed to go to an unknown part of the city to find an eatery. The weather is very cloudy, almost dark as we proceed. Once we find the café, I order a coffee and suddenly this man disappears. I am waiting for some time, and he comes back and orders a coffee himself. Then before we can order our breakfast he disappears again. This time, I say to myself, "This man is flaky, so I am going home."

Analysis

The dreamer did not recognize that this man represents her own immature flaky animus as the dream offers her its message. She accepts the offer to meet with her animus only to receive the message that he is flaky; she should consider trying to balance her animus in an appropriate way. He even comes back and disappears a second time, confirming the defective animus, but she instead goes "home," to the motherly womb, preferring to remain inactive and unaccepting of this message to integrate a balanced animus. The foreign part of the city refers to the unexplored part of her Self, and the dark environment refers to the invitation to visit her unconscious. She rejects this dream with the usual disbelief, thinking it utter nonsense, and will maintain her sweeping arguments no matter what. Her conscious situation tells us that the dream was a reaction to a one-sided attitude of seeking power, like an Adlerian-complex *Lycopodium* person who is a coward on the inside (*lack of character*). But in this case, it is a reflection of a woman—although naturally a very sensitive, empathetic *Phosphorus*—who had suffered abuse from controlling people early in her life and thus developed a strong (albeit unbalanced) animus as a defense mechanism: "No one will mess with me again!"

The latter is easily seen in the common event when a man expresses to his animus-possessed wife that he feels discouraged about something in life or at work. The ill-equipped feeling function of a woman with a strong negative animus may respond with a generalized remark like, "Everyone feels like that at some moment," stopping any further genuine expression of the husband dead in its tracks. And sometimes, if a man has courage enough to occasionally let his feeling function operate in the right manner, confessing to his wife that he was not always sensitive to her needs, the animus-possessed spouse comes back swinging, immediately responding by reciting a list of "sins" he committed! Logos, without tempering its masculine sweeping judgment, can indeed be a force to reckon with, throwing a man into turmoil and incomprehensible messes! One of my *Sepia* patients with an excessive animus said it this way: "Unfortunately I am always right! I always have done it this way and it worked well for me!" For her yes, but how for the others? It takes a strong man to spar with such a woman! In the same way that a real mother defends her own children even when their conduct is not always perfect, a woman at the mercy of her animus will fight to the death for her talking points! Eventually though, the negative animus will have a paralyzing effect on the woman's energy.

It was a subsequent dream that brought a change to this patient's character. One year later, she had the following dream. (She did not remember dreams for quite some time, so this archetypal dream was obviously bringing her an important message.)

Dream two

I find myself in a large paper product and hardware store with many aisles. I am wrapped up in a white sheet all around my body with no clothing underneath. Coming down the aisle from different directions towards me are two men. I avert them by fleeing out of the store. They do not follow me out of the store. While walking down the sidewalk, I decide to go shopping with money in my hand. I briefly encounter an old bearded man on the street who tells me that it was perfectly acceptable to be walking down the street wrapped up in a sheet.

As I continue walking, I realize that I have no pockets for any of the change I was to receive from shopping so I return back to that same store in order to take the elevator up to my apartment to retrieve a purse. I enter the store and start to walk to the elevator when I spot the same two men coming towards me, again from different directions. They are both young, in their early 20s, clean cut, short hair, wearing white, long-sleeved shirts and dark trousers. You never see people dressed like that working in that kind of store. As I stand in front of the elevator, waiting for the doors to open, I decide to confront these men to find out why they are chasing me, so I decide to come to them. I go to an aisle where I can see them both as they approach me. When they finally come near to me, the dream ends.

Analysis

Large paper and hardware store: The Self of the dreamer, with many aisles, containing tools to make changes in her life.

Wrapped up in a sheet: A sheet is part of the bed, the birthplace, also belonging to the unconscious (where one sleeps). It is white though, reflecting more the innocence, the truth, not black, and there is nothing underneath it. She is apparently ready to be almost naked, to let her hair down, so to speak; to be vulnerable, to make a change in her life, to appear as she is.

Two men coming towards her: Her newly forming, non-fused animus (two men) coming to her. They are wearing white shirts and black pants; again, a combination of the conscious (white), and the instinctual life of the unconscious (black pants, signifying the lower part of the body). This also symbolizes unification of the opposites, the undifferentiated dark with the light, as they appear when the dreamer is in the grip of the unconscious. *When something unconscious tries to become conscious, it is automatically split in two, the pair of opposites.* It is an attempt at reconciliation of the pair of opposites, part of the integration process. They are both young, so are in the process of growing up towards adulthood. But she averts them by fleeing out of the store. Her first reaction is to feel threatened and flee from her Self onto the street; in other words, to initially not accept her burgeoning animus. They do not follow her: they do not pursue her because the acceptance must come from the dreamer.

Money in her hands: The money signifies psychic strength, or psychic libido/energy to move forward. When we put or have "money in the bank," we have psychic energy in the storehouse of the Self, the unconscious. Money means power to change things, to do things. The dream further tells her, in symbolic language, what she needs to do: accept her animus.

Old bearded man: Personification of the wise old man, one of the animus configurations, who is mostly the advisor as in this dream, a psychopomp or guide, who tells her it is perfectly fine to be dressed like this (to let your hair down and be open to change).

Pocket: A sense of ownership. "It is in my pocket and I want to make sure I don't lose it (her psychic strength or money), nor that anybody can steal it."

She returns to the store and takes an **elevator to her apartment:** Her apartment is in the upper part of the store (the most conscious part of the Self) and she takes an elevator to get there. In other words, she needs to ascend, to go to the light in order to reach her "home," the place she calls home, a secure place.

Then the same young men approach her again before she can even take the elevator. This time, instead of fleeing them (we flee something that we usually should incorporate in our Self—see Chap. 4, "Common Themes in Dreams"), she confronts them and asks the question, "What do you want from me, why are you chasing me?" This is an excellent lysis of the dream as the dream tells her that she needs an urgent change. In order to go "home" (to become a more complete person), she needs to integrate her burgeoning, forming animus that is not yet fused. Rather than exercising the unruly animus creating havoc in her life, she is finally willing to accept a new animus and to ask the inevitable question: "What do you want of me?" The answer: to integrate her newly forming animus, which now is in the process of fusing to a sensible proportion, so the tyranny of the animus will stop, bringing more peace to herself and others. By confronting these dark figures, they usually turn out to be helpful for the dreamer.

The same woman had the next dream, two days later.

Dream three

I find myself in the early morning hours of the night in a hallway of an apartment building. I am in a semi-reclined position, propped up on my elbow. In front of me, I can see the steps through the front glass door that lead down into the street. The boulevard is wide, dimly lit with few cars passing and few people walking. To my left is a door that is closed. It is then opened by a man with dark hair, pale skin, and grey clothing. I can see that inside is only one messy, disheveled room and in it, a bed with a nude woman sleeping under the sheets. She, too, has dark hair and pale skin. The man is at the door looking down at me, and while doing so, he throws a silver pistol in front of me. It bounces and startles me. I feel great fear. Instinctively, I get up and leave the building as quickly as I can. He does not follow me. I hurry down the street to get as far away as possible, thinking of getting a cab in the dead of night when I see a woman walking in my direction. I immediately grab her arm, locking us together, arm and arm, and I make her change her direction to my direction of walking. Through my fear, I tell her what just happened and that I need to find a cab. She too, like the others, is dressed in dark clothing, with dark hair and pale skin. She says to me that I must go back and confront that man and sort it out. I tell her that the man was a stranger to me and that he has a gun and I have no intention of ever going back. Upon saying that, I let go of her arm and begin to hail a taxi and to my good luck one comes along just then. I get into it and tell the elderly taxi driver, "Charles de Gaulle Airport!" Without a word, he drives on. At that point I knew I was in Paris. In the next second, I find myself waking up on a narrow metal bed in a tiny, well-lit room, crammed with shelving and an orderly clutter of items everywhere. Everything is white. From where I lay, I could see to my left a large picture window, with the street below with the dimly lit wide boulevard that I had just come from, the same as the first time in the beginning of my dream. It seems to me that I must have fainted, and I think that the cab driver must have taken me to a hospital. I know that I must leave and then the dream ends.

Analysis

Is this dream another chapter of her Book of Life, or is the same question posed by the unconscious? This second dream, quickly coming after the first one, indicates even more the urgency of listening to the unconscious. Here is the analysis, well-understood this time by the patient, bringing an "Aha" of recognition and approval.

The dream starts at **night** (time of unconscious) while she is somewhat reclined on the floor outside of an apartment **looking down at the boulevard** (she is on the threshold of conscious and unconscious, the bottleneck or isthmus between conscious and unconscious), which is dimly lit, with few cars and people on it. To her **left** (the yin or feeling side), **a door is closed** (the door to her expressive natural anima from before is still closed), and is then opened by **a man** who is pale, with dark hair and grey clothing (her animus coming from the unconscious, nothing about him is "light" or "white"). She sees **a woman**, naked in bed (pale and dark haired also, her apparently real—nude—shadow). But this animus is even more threatening than in the previous dream, throwing a **silver gun** (silver: between black and white, as grey, white, and black are non-colors) on the floor in front of her (not putting it against her head, but throwing it on the floor—a warning). This makes her **flee** immediately (non-acceptance, and non-integration of this dangerous animus, which seems to be a normal reaction). However, when she comes down to the boulevard (in the unconscious), she meets **another unknown woman** (the positive side of her shadow), who tells her that she must go back to the apartment to confront her animus again. She thinks this is foolish, and she wants to leave town (Paris—**a foreign place** to her in the world—reflecting again the unconscious unexplored part of her Self), as quickly as she can. Miraculously she finds a cab, and tells the **elderly driver** (the wise old man, being at the wheel of the car, determining her destination) to bring her to the airport to fly **home** again (which would be like being entombed in the unconscious again, having not progressed in her journey as nothing is achieved). But this wise old man, her spiritual animus guide, advisor and figure, does not drive her to the airport to go home, but instead brings her to a well-lit room, with orderly clutter (bringing her back to that bottleneck), which she recognizes as a **hospital room** (to be evaluated and healed, so she can continue her trip to wholeness). And the dream ends as it began: looking through a window on the left, down onto the boulevard dimly lit with few people. It is obvious that this dream repeats the message of the previous one, with even more details and more menacing, telling her, "You need to tame your animus and take it with you on your journey, in order to be successful in life; (in other words) integrate a more balanced animus." There is no lysis, no new chapter has started, so this is a repetitive dream. Only when in the next dream(s) she will be able to integrate this unbridled animus, and the next chapter of her Book of Life will be written. But all in all, there is movement towards healing, so the indicated remedy from before might be repeated.

Dream four, the following day

I dream that I am near the elevator on my way up and in a measured hurry. My husband is there and so is a younger man. I need to take one bottle of shampoo that my husband gave to me and one bottle of hair conditioner that the young man gave me. I then leave and go into the elevator to go upward and upon my journey upward, I look at the bottles and realize that neither had their bottle caps on and so I needed to go back down and get the caps to the bottles before continuing my journey. It seems that my mission was aborted, if only temporarily.

Analysis

This is only the next day, so now we see more movement as she takes the **elevator upward** in a measured hurry (desire to go to consciousness) with a bottle of shampoo and conditioner, given by **her husband** (old animus or wise old man) and new animus respectively. As she goes up, she sees that these bottles have no caps on, which the dreamer translates as having been giving something incomplete, hindering her desired new journey to enlightenment. Without caps she could spill the content, so she feels she must go back to get the caps. It also means she is not ready to make this trip, that she needs perfect tools (bottles with caps), so she aborts her trip for the moment with the intention to continue it when she gets the new bottles with caps. In other words, she needs to spend some more time in the unconscious before ascending. Why washing the hair?

Washing the hair: Changing one's attitude, altering the way we think about something or changing our viewpoint. Head hair symbolizes spiritual higher forces, and a full head of hair represents joie de vivre, linked with the will to succeed. Washing the body may symbolize getting rid of old habits and emotional reactions.

In a future dream, she might take the new animus (the young person) with her in the elevator up, completing her journey.

A strong animus can even be seen early in childhood. No words offend such a child more than phrases beginning with "You must" or "You must not," enough to raise the anger that is always at the surface and produce screams of rage thought to win the argument! Such a strong animus expresses itself also in temper tantrums (*Tuberculinum*), when the child with flailing arms and legs throws himself on the ground, resisting with all the weight of his body to be moved, as if he was glued to the floor—all to win the argument. And when parents give in, another battle is won, and animus never leaves the house again. Such a distorted animus, with convulsions and tears, howls and screams, cannot stand losing a battle, and will shatter any resistance of the finally yielding parent. It is as if a spell has been put on the child changing him into an animal, although it might just be an expression that this young child already feels as a complete individual, knowing what he wants and what he is like inside. There is of course the danger, seizing upon the successful battle, that now all excesses are justified, and no laws bind him anymore.

As times have changed in comparison to Jung's century, there are plenty more women who, out of necessity or ambition, helped by women's emancipation, have replaced the animus's little mouse voice with a roaring lion's battle cry. Competitive tendencies, and business and material success, have made inroads in the outmoded "comfortable" family environment, and women now rightfully demand to be involved, even in politics, which for the longest time was only male territory. Of course, such an animus-possessed woman can sometimes evoke a paternal benevolent reaction—especially if she is pretty—but more often she will unleash great irritation in the man who feels threatened in his traditional role and state of manhood. This is most visible in the office, in the workforce of this world. Women with a strong (and perhaps unbalanced) animus invariably get cataloged in the "aggressive, passive-aggressive, and indifferent bitches" group. Surprisingly, female bosses seem to be the worst and the toughest, not accepting even the most justified excuses, with words like, "How can I work with someone as incompetent as you?!" or "Your questions reflect the lack of confidence you have in yourself." Not infrequently, this mirrors their own past struggle to get to the top, which means, sadly enough for women, that being a "Dragon Lady" or a "Softie Who Nices Her Way Up," and not competence, were the only choices.

Sometimes, in order to survive, the woman must train her animus at the expense of her anima. Here are some dreams of a 44-year-old woman who moved to France from a Slavic country. Although very intelligent, as a stranger she was not appreciated nor acknowledged at work, causing her great stress. After the indicated remedy she had a sequence of dreams, starting with an all-important archetypal dream, often appearing at moments of change and distress.

Dream one

I see myself in a house, it must be my family house just before our departure. I can see the scene from above and inside at the same time. The main part of the house is at the right side. On the left and in the center of the picture there is a patio; on its left there is a small shed with a snake. This snake is my snake. I remember during the dream that first she was in the main part (right side), had fascinated me, and at the same time I had been sort of careful with her. Now she is on the left side, has liberated (freed) herself and is about to go on (continue her way). A deep voice in me is saying something very clear. I am about to wake up and try hard to memorize it, after I have asked, being half asleep, what I shall remember from this dream.

These words came: "You have held the snake tight. This is good for you, but you have not relaxed, you have wanted to keep her. Now she is free, and you let her go, and this is better for you." The snake is white.

Analysis

House: Symbol of the Self of the dreamer; can represent the self-image too; how you see yourself or want to be seen. If it is the parental home, it says a lot about your childhood feelings. The main house is on the right side: meaning the person's main conscious function is the thinking function and reflects a dominance of the animus- driven person. But on the **left side** (anima, female side, unconscious, emotions) there is a **small shed** (small structure, again representing part of her Self that has broken off from what was once a solid structure; a new evolution; creation of more feeling and anima).

Snake: Great archetypal figure as discussed before in Chapter 2. This is an important archetypal dream. It is a symbol of healing-spiritual awakening and healing-transformation and resurrection; shedding of old persona; kundalini rising: in Kundalini yoga, the snake climbing up the spine and touching the various chakras; also symbol for female; darkness; night; yin; death; fear; cold blooded animal. **Black snake:** represents evil, a demon; creates a sense of danger, the integrity of man is threatened. In this case it is a **white snake:** white is purity, healing, innocence. It is the patient's snake, part of her Self. It has a protective and transforming meaning that refers to the female sex. White also signifies absolute truth. Originally the snake was in the main house, but now is on the left: a split has taken place as the snake is on the left, the emotional female side. Finally, the female side has liberated herself from the overpowering male or animus in the dreamer.

The voice from within: A voice from the unconscious. In dreams, the animus always speaks with a voice of authority, a male sounding voice, and the voice tells her that it is for her benefit that she has to let the snake go in spite of her tight control over it (tight control over the female side, and her emotions).

Furthermore, this next dream came to her the night after the snake dream.

Dream two

I am a child and play outside with my siblings. We are all around 7-10 years old. The landscape: meadows, fields, grass, shrubs, some mud. Suddenly I realize it's war and we have to hide. We were playing hide and seek but things get serious and we have to escape and find a safe place, as planes are coming, menacing us with bombs. Suddenly a narrow hole opens in the earth and without hesitating I jump into it. It's like a mouth swallowing me, getting narrow (like a throat) and then widening up again further down. I have the reflex to jump heartily down, feet first, arms joined above my head to make myself as thin as possible. I'm able to pass the narrow passage and I land safely in the bosom of the earth. Safe! I look for my family and find them all there again; I'm reassured. Then there comes a threat: enemies are down there, too, so we quickly imagine a fence, and it appears between them and us. We have to be very careful that it holds against them, that they cannot trespass the fence, and all is fine.

Analysis

Child: 1. Can be a childhood experience. **2.** A symbol of the true Self of the dreamer, which she can unfold. The fact that the real Self is represented by a child suggests that the true Self is a beautiful unspoiled product of Nature, that it needs the nourishment of true love if it is to grow (child representing innocence). **3.** It might also represent a new beginning, a new development in her psyche, a new attitude in life, a new balance of her psychic forces. **4.** In all of us there is a child, our emotional Self, that often needs reassurance, to be told that all is well and that there is no cause for fear or anger.

Meadows, fields, grass: The dreamer's contact with what is natural in her—freedom from social pressure, sense of herself when away from other people with her natural inclinations. **Mud:** deepest part of the unconscious.

War: Internal conflicts: could be a battle between one's moral code and sexual needs; or a battle between intellect and bodily needs or emotions (in her case!). Conflict can also occur between her personal drives and the social, political, or economic regime she lives under, again the case in this dreamer!

Narrow hole: The entrance to the unconscious. She lands right into the vast world of the unconscious and feels safe except there are some dark elements in there for which she erects a fence to protect herself, so she does not get overwhelmed or swallowed by the elements of the unconscious.

Dream three, the following day

I'm walking around in nature, it's quite dark. On my right side I see a concrete construction with water in it. Coming closer I see it is divided in squares. In two of these squares I see a cat, so two cats in all, still alive but drowning. One has a necklace, the other one does not. They are greyish-brown and a bit white, of an indefinite color. My feeling is, I cannot touch them, it would not be good; for some reason I cannot say. My first reaction is to go my way and think well, they will just die, that's part of it. Then after some steps I start feeling bad about this thought and feel pity for them. Nobody has seen them, only me, and dying slowly like this is too cruel. I ponder on the idea to go back and give them a push so that they die immediately. Interestingly I don't think of pulling them out of the water. It seems to be OK they are about to die. Thinking about all this I reach a house at the edge of the woods and come in. The door is open; the ground floor is a big room, sparsely furnished. At an end there is a desk; two men are sitting there, waiting. I go to them and tell them about the cats. I ask them to take care of the problem; they agree, nodding. One of them stands up and goes in the direction I have indicated. So, I'm reassured, I know I didn't just let these cats alone with their sure death, but I also didn't have to take care of the problem myself. I'm relieved and somehow glad I didn't have to pull them out of the water. My last thought is: maybe they were injured, or some other problem would have arisen, maybe they were sick of a very contagious disease, and what would have I done? Then I wake up.

Analysis

Nature, in the dark: Refers to preparing to investigate her unconscious.

To the right a structure with water: Her animus is taking command and now she sees the unconscious in compartments. Two of them have cats: the representation of her natural emotional state and of her anima, though two means not fused yet and therefore not part of her natural unconscious state. As the dream goes further, she walks further, reasoning that it is not right to save them; they are dying or sick, what is the use.

She realizes it is a non-union, not a balanced female side yet, and she does not have any desire to save them. But as mentioned before, everything that wants to become conscious is split in two, the pair of opposites. **Water:** Symbol of rebirth.

House at edge of the woods: A border between conscious and unconscious. There are two men, again showing the non-fusion of her new forming animus. One of them resolves the problem, going to check out what is going on. She feels relieved, or should we say, is silencing her guilt for leaving them as her split animus will check it out. You can see that she is not sure of her conduct, as her last thoughts try to convince her she did the right thing. But there is a partial lysis.

Another prototype of the animus-possessed woman is the dogmatic *Kali-c* mother, who, because of her personal excessive anxiety (*cyber delusion, there is an abyss behind her*), becomes the great moralizer, aimed at stilling her *excessive anxieties about the future and her health.* She is an imposter, and the rigid warden of the home that can be called a "prison," depriving her children of her affection as they encounter her blocking animus repeatedly, with hard discipline and dogmatic unchangeable opinions, which effectively cuts them off from motherly emotional nourishment and tenderness. And then of course, she complains that her children don't love her while she is always there for them, "guiding" them in every aspect of life. She thinks she is a martyr, but really, she is the animus-ridden mother! *Kali-c* is never at peace and neither are her children! *Kali-c* is a person who is confined in an emotional straitjacket and does not hesitate to do the same to her children.

With *Kali-c, conscientious about trifles* is not an option (*Ailments from mental work)*—she voices dogmatic ideas about what *ought* to be and opinions about people whose attitude she feels to be entirely wrong. Hers is a ruthless, power-driven dogmatism and domineeringness, a devil of an opinion, quite unconscious as far as its owner is concerned, and all in the name of righteousness, truth, "motherly love," and angelic goodness as *Kali-c* proclaims. It is an attitude consumed by opinions, moral-ethical discipline, routines and conformism, rights and wrongs and nothing in between, in which the *Kali*-parent pushes her virtues on her children for the sake of "their welfare." *Kali-c* rejects the live-and-let-live attitude, revealing her own rigidity instead. As she censors the morals of those living under her roof —being so highly conscientious—she takes life very seriously. Combined with high anxiety and low agreeableness, you have a person who is always critical of others (*censorious*). She wants to be valued by the family, a social power grab within the family, and to gain respect with those she holds to impossible standards —even when she wears a smug mask of moral superiority mixed with high anxiety. Bubble-wrapping her kids to shield them from failing does them no favors. Without the trial-and-error learning from gradual exposure to risk, children become vulnerable to anxiety disorders. What's more, harsh discipline and repression of desire only lead to her family's frustration, resentment, and a sense of emptiness. It does not cause them to look up to the *Kali-c* person as the one taking on the role of moral authority and discipline. Yes, children cannot be raised without learning discipline and responsibility. Yet if stigmatizing rigidity is to be avoided, value judgments will have to be offered as models—not inflexible prescriptions—to be observed in their spirit, not followed to the letter and by rote. Children need to find their own standards and emotional values with minimal physical and emotional punishment, otherwise emotional security, self-confidence, curiosity, and autonomy will be the first casualties. *Kali-c* does not harm her children consciously in any obvious way, yet she slowly strangles the family's joy of life, as her negative attitude towards living is contagious and infects her family like an insidious, slow growing illness.

A *Kali-c* mother creates a field or atmosphere of dogmatic, oppressive restraint, a disabling barrier, that keeps her children from establishing a conscious individuality of their own. Age-inappropriate over-parenting leads to aimless children (and ultimately adults) who are prone to depression, with diminished self-efficacy, lacking the ability to put a plan in place to achieve goals. By not letting children stumble over little things, a *Kali-c* parent prevents them from developing coping skills. To not acquire a sense of mastery and self-confidence fosters long-term dependence on parents, and that is what the *Kali-c* mother wants. She ends up trapping the child in what she views as a pampered life, but her actions are more like those of a prison warden.

Much smarter are characters like *Phosphorus*, *Pulsatilla*, and *Silicea* women who are a different stereotype of animus possession, called the *Strong-Weak-Women*—great seducers and actresses who use their abundant anima to evoke the protective animus qualities in men, who feel they can't refuse these angelic figures anything. These women often identify with the man's expectation, and make sure to incorporate the man's ideal prospects and needs. These women know that men consider them goddesses, princesses, or baby dolls, and make sure that full advantage is taken of this projection. As much as they look weak and in need of support, they are the winners in life. They know just what buttons to push in their husbands or friends to get what they want! The real balance a woman should seek is to come to terms with a fine-tuned, working relationship between her anima and animus, a bridge to the unconscious, just as the balanced anima in man is the function of a correct relationship to his unconscious, not a force that disrupts his life! No doubt, *Phosphorus* with her naturally ample anima and intellectual capacity is often successful at this, as not only is she a very feminine woman, but can also speak with power of inspired wisdom (*dictatorial, speaks with a voice of command*). Only by understanding our unconscious do we set ourselves free from its frightening domination!

Here is a repeated dream of a 36-year-old woman, who by integrating a new animus starts forming a better Self, an attempt to join the anima with the animus.

Dream one

I am working with my sister (I do not know about what) and a young man comes to help us. Then I ask him about the "monastery of light." How to get there. I knew it was in Spain and it was a beautiful place (she cried when saying this). When I come to the monastery, I see a crater with water in it, and in the middle of the lake is an island. I try to get in, but the door is locked, and I cannot climb through the windows as they are too high.

This dream repeated itself for quite some time, until I consulted a male hypnotherapist in a dream, who I asked for help to get in. Interestingly, while in his presence, before he did anything, I got in.

Dream two

I get in and it is a beautiful round room (circle) with mirrors on the wall all around. I am changed into Aladdin's lamp where my head is a little flame and the rest of my body is the body of the vase. The small flame reflects on the mirrors; it gets through the windows and spreads through the world.

I feel fantastic about this dream and this dream still repeats itself (less frequent than in the beginning) till this day.

Analysis

Locale: Persons—**Sister:** her shadow side. **Young man:** a newly accepted animus; there is a meeting of animus/anima as he wants to work with her. This is favorable as there is acceptance of the animus.

Monastery: A place of rest, harmony, and peace, where one goes to restore; to get away from all the noise of the real world. Personifies the unconscious (withdrawal from the rest of the world).

Light: Consciousness, life, insight, giving answers: "Bring light to me!" She wants to go to the monastery of light: she wants to go to the unconscious that has the answers to her problems, to be able to integrate dark elements into the conscious, to be enlightened. She can't get through the door at first: she is not able to withdraw into the unconscious. Until she meets a male **hypnotherapist**, a man who helps people connect with the unconscious (a personification of the wise old man), and his mere presence is enough to get her in.

She saw a **crater:** The moon is full of craters, and craters reflect vessels. Further, there is water in the crater; all these things represent the unconscious. In the middle of the water-filled crater is an island (the consciousness). She is changed into Aladdin's **lamp** and her head was the light, signifying the conscious thinking function (which was still small). The rest of her body was the body of the lamp (unconscious). The room was round, like a **circle:** a place of protection—the womb, representing a return to the warmth and protection of the mother figure, the unconscious, or rather the love/protection of the mother figure of the collective unconscious. A circle or mandala is also a place of perfection and wholeness but mainly of safety.

Mirrors: Looking in the mirror to see the real you, without a mask. Mirrors stand for consciousness too, and the "mirror" in this dream amplifies the woman's light, making that light go through the window so she can get it to the world. In a further dream this light becomes a golden child which she nourishes (she cries again when telling this). **Golden child:** New archetype, ideal and precious (gold) which she wants to nourish and bring to life (her path of individuation).

As men and women grow older, the animus seems to take on a different attitude. Through integration of the anima and a softening of their animus—which should normally happen around age 45—men tend to become more home-oriented, and show newfound kindness and sentimentality, especially to their grandchildren. In turn, it is not uncommon that women's animus shows a positive stronger side. Older women often become interested in the family's business and financial responsibilities—preparing them for widowhood, as statistically most women outlive their husband. This brings forth the question: who is responsible for the animus's creation?

The Formation of Animus

How do some women get endowed with a strong animus, while others (as if by a stroke of lightning) renounce any voice of self-confidence, initiative, and judgment, often for the rest of their life? Just as the man's relationship to his mother or sister serves as the first model for his anima, so the relationship to the father shapes the woman's animus. It is further shaped by her grandfather and brothers, as well as by lovers, teachers, and friends. Or, her animus is formed by the ideas she receives from other people, especially the mother. I knew of a young girl who received the conviction from her mother that "all men are bad," since her mother divorced her father before this girl could have known him (she was only 1 year old). For a long time, distrust and hatred of men was injected into her, like a contagious disease, before she could see the reality of where it came from and free herself from the possession of this unconscious animus voice telling her to "distrust all men." Only then could her animus become an invaluable guide for her life, providing her with a sense of individuality, a grown-up with her own voice, responsible for her own actions—freed from the anxieties and fears of her mother who "only wanted to protect" her daughter from the evil in this world.

A weak father presence can create havoc in the future relationships of his daughter. We would think that as a reaction to having had a weak father, a woman would look for a strong man to be married to—a hero figure, the knight on a white horse—so that she can finally relax and provide the lucky man with her abundance of natural femininity, a horn full of tenderness and nourishment, supplying the hero with the well-deserved praise and admiration. Paradoxically the opposite is often true, as there remains an infantile remnant of desire to see the father as a semi-god, he who was always present to protect her, even if he was nothing but a voiceless being in real life. Her incorrect estimation of him is just the result of her projection, and so she remains unaware of the fatal mistake of marrying someone more akin to her weak father, not the hero type who roams in the underground of the infantile tale of her unconscious.

Even more destructive for the woman is a negative experience with her father. *Ailments from domination*, *betrayal*, and *discord* often lead to long-lasting hatred for men as a result of the possession by her animus, to the point that the opposite of her natural temperament is created, inhibiting the natural Eros from developing. Therefore, any relationship with any man is not only doomed for her, but also leads to pathology that can be predicted. I remember such a case from my practice.

The patient was successful in business but impoverished in terms of feeling and interpersonal relationships. She married for the first time at age 40 but soon divorced, and then married a younger person whom she dominated in the same way her own mother was dominated and cheated on by her father. As a young girl she could never understand why her mother could not stand up for herself, so unconsciously she took on her mother's silent indignation. Here is the dream she had.

Dream

I am driving my car uphill as I have a date with my lover but suddenly a deep voice warns me that all men, my lover included, are the same as my father. Then I woke up, confused and thinking, "This is utter nonsense!"

Analysis

Her lover: Her new animus, to complement her; the meeting of the contra-sexual figures.

Going uphill: Becoming conscious; an attempt at making unconscious things conscious; there is an obstacle, something needing energy to deal with and overcome it. Going uphill can also mean difficulties, hard work or effort; a task of long-term undertaking ("I have a mountain to climb!"). We can feel that life is an uphill struggle. A hill also symbolizes the climb to higher attainment, with a wider view of life or opportunities. It also reflects the first half of our life, while going downhill reflects the second part or old age.

Her car: Not surprisingly, with her kind of animus, she is in control of her destination; she would not have it any other way!

Solemn voice: Animus speaking.

What is the message of this dream? The patient told me, "I knew this voice told me that all men were cheaters and that I could trust no man. If I married, I would only repeat the tragic experience of my mother." Her hatred of her father (a negative father-complex) became the idea of identification with all men in life. In a way, as seen in her relationships with men, possessed by her exaggerated animus she became her father without knowing it, letting her animus dominate every relationship (which was of course doomed from the beginning!). She was highly sensitive and would overreact to anyone who behaved like her father (*easily offended*). While business was booming, the business of relationship or Eros—because she refused to listen to the woman voice within herself—was doomed at the first strong opinion she uttered! The woman in her had long been repressed out of fear of becoming a helpless abused creature like her mother. Her anima, built from without—influenced by her mother's example—has warned her to show resolution and opinions, not empathy and unconditional love. Not unexpectedly, while disgust for men might have been lurking in her unconscious, her chief complaint, severe pain and bladder infection after each sexual encounter, revealed the hidden disdain and repulsion she felt towards men, experienced as a physical violation or rape. Hostility towards her father was now projected on every man she met.

If not derailed by such a negative experience, however, the animus represents for the woman the capacity for reflection, deliberation, decision making, confidence, and self-knowledge (the thinking function). In the case of a negative father-complex, leading to a distorted animus, there are often various disturbances of the sexual function. Examples of this are menstrual disorders, *vaginismus*, and *honeymoon cystitis* because the anima has been injured. Unfortunately, such a woman is really possessed by this negative animus figure of the unconscious. A negative animus expresses itself through brutality, dictatorial behavior, empty talk, overzealous criticism, needless defensiveness, recklessness, and salient, obstinate evil ideas. Just as a negative anima robs a man of possible creativity, a negative animus will have the same negative influence on a woman, pronouncing to her that it makes no sense to follow this or that future ambition. "You can never achieve this," a deep sounding voice says. "Many people already tried this. There is no sense in pursuing it. You are not intelligent enough to do this, don't even think about it," or any other discouraging message plays on her psyche. As we can imagine, this happens mostly in women whose animus was never stimulated—if not totally suppressed—creating a voiceless dwarf for the rest of their life.

It would be a mistake to think that the animus of the son is not influenced by his father. All things mentioned before (for the daughter), equally influence the son's animus.

How does the animus present itself in dreams?

Images of Animus in Dreams

Archetypal images come from the deeper layers of the unconscious, the collective unconscious. Any archetype can appear as a positive or negative figure. The father archetype can appear positively as the father, lover, hero, scholar, a council passing judgment, the Spiritual Guide (appearing as a priest, a sage, a bird, a messenger, or a loud voice bringing information), and the Man-Of-Wise-And-Benign-Authority—a representation of experiencing the archetypal father in the role of support, objective wisdom, and benign guiding authority, who will reveal the role in which a man's life is cast. In myths, a *negative animus* plays the role of robber, mafia, and murderer, while depicting fearsome destructive scenes. Other forms are strange *mythological creatures* such as beast-gods, like the satyrs (goat men) and centaurs, which were half human, half horse. Other examples of dangerous negative animus appearances are figures such as Bluebeard of the 19th century, rapists, dictators, mafia bosses, or evil magicians, who often provoke *Ailments from indignation, domination* and *mortification*, reducing the person in conscious life to a silent dwarf, undermining his self-confidence. Such upbringing often creates in the victim an inner voice of this overbearing negative father archetype, visible and audible in dreams as a male figure who constantly reminds the dreamer that there is no point in trying to achieve something, that he/she is nothing but a failure, robbing the person in her conscious life from any libido (from the Latin meaning of the word, "desire or urge"), unable to transform unconscious creative energy into a conscious content and preventing her from active participation in life, reducing her to a meek idle spectator. If the animus in a dream appears as a group of men, rather than appearing as a single individual, it demonstrates the animus as a *collective* rather than a personal element, which is often the case when appearing as a negative animus.

Animus also has *images from the Nature world*: an elephant, eagle, lion, dog, frog, bull, goat, or other male animals and also phallic representations such as a spear, or arrow—all powerful creatures and powerful forces in the unconscious which, when they are stimulated, may overrun the conscious position. A *folk tale animus* is the dwarf. Dwarfs and other little people work underground in mines out of which they bring gold and other precious things. This illustrates the way of animus. If cared for and nurtured by a woman (as Snow White looked after the Seven Dwarfs), this will bring up from her unconscious many valuable things that will serve her well in her daily life.

There are also four archetypal forms of masculinity portraying the animus.

The Four Faces of the Archetypal Masculine

Like the anima elaborated on before, the animus appears in dreams in a great variety of images. It often appears in dreams as a person known to the dreamer. It can also take the shape or archetypal form of four types of masculinity: *Father*, *Son*, *Hero*, and *Wise Old Man*. To be remembered is that these masculine types, as seen in the four feminine types, are not pure representations found in men, as most people are a combination and variation of these four types.

The *Father* (*pater familias*) prototype is the archetypal

authority figure of all sorts, protecting and ruling his subjects, ranging from the actual father or grandfather, to king, president of the country, president of a local bank or country club, ministers, bishops, and all the way up to God the Father and Zeus with his lightning bolt, as well as the great political orator (for instance Winston Churchill). Then there is Tsar Nicholas II, called "Little Father" by the Russian people; Ataturk, meaning "Father of the Turks," a name given to him by the people; and The Shah of Iran, or King of Kings. The father is he who leads his children in the family and his country, the ruler of his house and country.

The *Son* or *puer aeternus* (the child of the wise old man), is the opposite orientation of the Father (*senex*), having all the qualities of hopeful one-sided masculine adolescent psychology, and appears as a brother, son, friend, ideal lover and partner, the unknown lover, neighbor or fellow next door, the gentleman, Prince Charming or Adonis, the Seducer or Don Juan who lives passionately, though secretly in despair, the latter personified by the *Medorrhinum* type, "the one who loves you and leaves you."

It is *Medorrhinum* who will write the *Casanova Field Guide* or "How to Sweep Women Off Their Feet and Drop Them Fast." *Medorrhinum* is a person who welcomes the rapture of losing himself in irrationality, in pure emotion, in the drunkenness of passion and the abandonment of the ego sense. Thinking he is God's gift to women he wants to "be made mad with love (so-called)" and has no apparent need for knowledge or reason. Drinking alcohol with abandon, experiencing fleeting infatuations with as many women as possible, abstaining from sleep, and, above all, staying on the move (*unusually active, going as if on wings*), *Medorrhinum* resembles a person in a permanent state of *mania*. It takes gregariousness, a lack of inhibition, a desire for unrestrained liberty, impulsiveness and absence of deliberation, a highly developed sensibility to beauty and refinement and an appreciation for fine things to produce such a lively personality (*strange exhilaration of spirits*). As if taken up by a tornado, "carpe diem!" is his motto. He escalates and de-escalates in all his performances. In his turbulent, undisciplined life, he goes from one person to another, from one event to another, and always seeks the thrill in everybody and everything. He really thinks that life is 90% fun and 10% responsibility (*aversion to responsibility; libertinism*), the opposite of what life really is. He never does anything to find meaning in his life or to direct his life towards a worthwhile goal. There is no more mistaken path to real happiness than this kind of high living, for *Medorrhinum's* whole object is to transform his secretly miserable existence into a succession of temporary delights, pleasures, and amusements of every kind, a process which can only result in excess and debauchery, disappointment and further delusions. He can be the eternal seeker but also, on the other hand, he can be the dark side of the roaming knight unable to become a true human individual connecting to the soul of another human. Authority and permanence are not words found in his dictionary. Oblivious to collective concerns, he is the hunter who is hooked on the hunt and, armed with irresistible charm and charisma, only thinks about conquests; he leaves each conquest days later after breaking hearts and wrecking marriages. He proclaims to each new conquest, "You are the love of my life." What the innocent, swept-away woman does not know is that *Medorrhinum* has more lives than a cat. His love life is compartmental and short-lived, so there is plenty of space for many new "loves of his life." What longing-lust must he have, to see three hundred women in his Topkapi palace, disposable at the blink of his ever-changing passion.

The *Hero* type is the soldier, knight, boxer, wrestler, Sir Lancelot, Achilles, King Arthur, President Kennedy, or any exciting man appearing in the dream. It represents the aspirations we hold for ourselves and for establishing our place in society—in other words to go and get what we want. Hero represents the quest for personal power, competence, efficacy, and identity, even venturing into the world with some degree of naivety, simply being open to discovering life. And the grandfather is the first model of what a hero stands for. In mythology the hero stems from divine birth and must kill a series of monsters and perform Herculean tasks, often helped by friendly companions in different forms. A real prototype in life was Ernest Hemingway, a man of action, war hero, hunter, and writer.

The *Wise Old Man* or mana figure appears in dreams as the great and superior teacher, representing the timeless wisdom of the psyche and bringing guidance, new revelations, and healing in our inner struggles. He is a psychopomp and initiator, has the power of the word or Logos, and is the spiritual guide, other than the biological father, to assist us in the rite of passage from boyhood to manhood. He is the archetype of the *meaning of life*. As every archetype has a duality, he is worshipped *and* feared as he is gifted with witchcraft and magical powers. He is called upon in dreams when the person is full of doubt, confused and in a risky situation, when he is lost at what to do, because the wise old man knows how to deal with difficult situations. He is the person with mana, which is magical knowledge and power. He is also represented by the helpful old man, a sage, the god Hermes with wings, a priest, guru, pope (wise man by excellence), preacher, professor, magician, sorcerer, Merlin the Wizard (can also be the wicked magician), a judge, prophet, a philosopher, the initiator, a council of wise men, an archetype of the spirit, or anyone who claims to know, or one who has, all the answers and enlightenment (your physician, analyst). This archetype in fairy tales and dreams can also be seen in the motif of helpful animals, or he may come as a bird or a messenger. The wise old man represents wisdom and insight, he is the shepherd and leader of the soul, always following his moral insights as well as testing the moral insights of others (e.g., Gandhi) and ready to help in any way he can (positive side of this archetype). In dreams he can present as an authoritative voice speaking with the conviction of truth, the prophetic deep voice in the unconscious, or take the form in both sexes of the ghost of one dead, or a youthful person, even a dwarf (as Goethe said, "little in length, mighty in strength"). The negative aspect of this archetype (signifying then an infantile shadow), is the wicked magician, the concocter of poison, an inner voice that tells you "You are never going to be amount to anything, don't even try!"

Here is a dream of a female patient experiencing the positive side of the wise old man.

Conscious situation: This is a report from the patient after the intake of *Nat-mur.* She was one always searching for love which was not provided by her mother or her present husband. Once a week for many years she had a dance class (freestyle), during which she had the following feelings: "During my weekly dance I felt a strong connection with the Divine Mother. For a long time, I had this feeling, but now this reminded me of how much I had missed mother love. The next day I dreamt of a good female friend who is dead now and she told me about a wise man that I should follow. After the dream my back pain for a long time totally disappeared, and I felt a strong itching on my right foot." (*Author's note: Itching is psora and a sign of healing.*)

Following are dreams from the same patient after taking *Lachesis* (which helped greatly). "It has helped me to deal with a lot of anger," she said, but there is still confusion in the patient. "My relationship with my husband remains important and energy robbing! On a regular basis I am confronted with a certain theme that I can't neutralize satisfactorily, especially the sentiment of emotional neglect. In the last week I had two remarkable dreams."

Dream one

I am in my home, but it is a very luxurious version of it with extra rooms and windows and a big garden with a pond and beautiful tall trees—a manor sphere. A male friend comes on a visit and he acts in a physical way and gives me plenty of attention, which I like very much. I enjoy it but I am surprised about it as well.

Dream two

I am again in a big house, but not mine and I hear upstairs in a room a female baby crying. It gets my attention as if the baby is mistreated and I run to this room and knock on the door. A man opens and tells me to not worry about anything, that all is fine. I go away but the baby keeps crying so I return to the room and enter it and the baby sits in a highchair and looks at me. It is my own face as a baby!

Patient's remark: "I had these dreams about babies that I need to feed and for whom I could not find food, over the last years. Most of the times these babies were not crying like this, they were quiet, so this behavior is new!"

Analysis

House: As in both dreams, the house is her Self. The first one is her own house, but a better version—the one she wishes for with plenty of space, and with serene Nature surrounding her (**Nature** reflects the relaxed feeling, being in contact with one's own nature). We can derive a feeling of rest, happiness, and beauty in the background of this dream, compensating for what is missing in her real life. The **male friend** is a desired new animus, one that is nourishing her. This is a dream full of fulfilled wishes following the rule of compensation.

The second dream is more revealing, as it is "not her house." In other words, it is still the Self, but the Self that is not satisfied! She hears the **baby** cry (the new her, or the newly wanted one, a new burgeoning anima side) and a **man** (her animus) telling her, "There is nothing wrong." In other words, she tells herself, "Don't listen to these emotions, only let your head work!" (Logos and negative animus, which she had to overdevelop to survive). In other words, no matter how well her Logos works, she can't suppress her Eros (the principle of union and attraction) and feeling side, even now. It does warn her for the future that this (*Ailment from*) *disappointed love* must be resolved in a more positive way, not as it is now, before pathology strikes!

Another dream in a man shows the help of the wise old man to guide him in life and help him in moral choices when dark instinctual drives try to overtake his path to individuation.

Dream

I am driving my car with two other men sitting next to me. Although I am at the wheel of the car, I feel that it is not me who controls my destination. One of the men says that we are going to go to a woman to rape and kill her. I protest loudly to this plan and I let this man out of the car as I feel I cannot communicate with him. The other man stays with me as I trust him and feel I can reason with him.

Analysis

It is very clear that these strong forces of the unconscious (personal and collective) rule the dreamer's destination. We see the battle in this patient between good and bad, as his shadow hides deep instinctual and primitive desires, but the patient's morality protests against these crude encounters with a female (and his anima) as he does not submit to the impulses of the unconscious and deliberately leaves this man (shadow) behind and keeps the trusted advisor, a rescuing figure (the wise old man, representing the factor of intelligence, morality, and knowledge) as he feels he is the most reasonable of the two and he can talk to him. As we see, no one is free of devilish and cruel acts which are the embodiment of the primitive shadow (here in the form of a murderer and rapist), but the collective and personal unconscious can be the guiding light to remaining human and staying away from misdeeds.

The Balance Between Anima and Animus in Order to Succeed on the Road to Individuation

As I mentioned before, women need to reach a fine balance with their sygizi (animus and anima) in order to have a fulfilling life. This will be portrayed in the dreams of the next patient.

These dreams reveal the struggle of a woman to reestablish the balance between her anima and animus. She was a 53-year-old intelligent woman, without any doubt *Phosphorus* is her constitution, with great interest in dream interpretation and connection to the unconscious (originally a feeling-extravert intuitive type), who had entered menopause for some years and after brief episodes, hot flashes ceased, but her main problem became chronic sleeplessness. She could not fall asleep till 2 a.m., which of course caused fatigue (not always) in the morning upon awaking. Some rubrics of this insomnia in her case are to be found under sleeplessness: *Falling asleep difficult; Sleeplessness till 2 a.m.; Sleeplessness before midnight; from activity of thoughts; from anxiety; after domestic calamity; chronic sleeplessness; from suppressed discharges; excitement aggravates; from fear; from grief; from irritability; from mental exertion; alternate nights, periodical; thoughts, from activity of; after waking aggravates.* Other characteristics: she had a *dictatorial, speaking with a voice of command* attitude caused by self-protection issues (*Delusion, is about to receive an injury; Delusion, is being injured by her surroundings*). Few other symptoms presented themselves except that her mother, who divorced when the patient was only 2 years old, instilled in her the fear of men, betrayal (*Ailments from disappointed love*), and domination (*Ailments from domination*), which undoubtedly had stifled her abundant anima as a retreat in self-defense. Otherwise she was a well-adjusted, world-minded woman with a capacity for languages, art and culture, and love for people. *Phosphorus* seems to be the indicated remedy. After *Phosphorus* 30C, 2 drops from the first cup, she had the following dream.

Dream

I am in a well-lit room with a girlfriend. There is a second room connected to the first and equally well lit. I meet a man in the second room, a *Sulphur* type and we converse a bit. I don't know what about, but we agree to meet in the second room to watch a TV program. Instead I choose to watch the TV program with my girlfriend in the first room, being totally oblivious to my commitment in the second room. When I finally became aware of my commitment, I leave my girlfriend to look for the man and find him under a small low table in a fetal position! When I approach him, he hands an envelope to me. I take it, and he comes out from under the table. He is understandably upset with me. My eyes tell him I am sorry, but he leaves anyway. Before he leaves, another woman comes in the room and looks at me as if she knows me. When the man leaves, she follows the man, not because she knows him or is with him but only to see where he is going. He is unaware of her following him. I open the envelope he gave to me and it is full of money. I don't feel right keeping it and it is too late to return the money to him, but I know there is a good chance I will meet him again in that other room. On the other hand, if he really wants to avoid me, he can choose not to come there or at least not to be there for a long time. Meanwhile I fret on how to return the money to him as it does not feel right to keep it. I do not count the money nor do I remove it from the envelope. I proceed to tape up the tattered envelope and put it together as well as I can. The dream ends here.

Additionally, this patient writes how these figures in her dream appear, and what each meant to her:

> Including myself, these women were all *Phosphorus* constitutions and we were all the same height. My girlfriend in the first room is tall, lean, fair and blond with straight hair. She is wearing loose, soft feminine clothes of the palest pastel colors. The woman in the second room was tall, lean and fair with straight medium brown hair. She has on a distinguishing pair of leggings/tights that had wide bands of horizontal stripes on them. They had alternate colors of black and beige. Her top was an average nondescript T-shirt. When she moves, one notices most the bold stripes on her legs and the pointed tips of her long hair swinging back and forth freely. Of the two women, the first is the most feminine, most attractive and the fairest. In the dream I had the same build but with long black hair, and olive skin. The three of us are all similar in age, in our 30s. The man was a few inches taller and had short brown and slightly curly hair, with a fair complexion and a muscular build and was wearing a fitted T-shirt that revealed his upper body shape and well-developed arms. Colors of his clothes were of a universal and nondescript tone, such as white T-shirt and black pants. He was in his 40s with average features.

Personal associations, described by the patient

Girlfriend: Feminine, slender, attractive, draws everybody to her. This person is like me and I am drawn to her and want to be with her.

***Sulphur* man:** I am also drawn to certain (but not all) *Sulphur* men and he draws my interest but only to a certain point where I become conscious of my actions of meeting him in that second room where I feel I am betraying the trust I have with my girlfriend. Furthermore, I do not know him, so why I am so spontaneous? Once I meet him, I no longer feel comfortable in his presence.

TV program: It equals a date at the movies for me, not about anything special. It is just an object to lure me into this other room. I question myself why I accepted this, going to meet with a man I don't even know. Who is he? Will I regret this? Am I in danger? Why did I not think this more through in view of my experiences with men in the past? I feel apprehensive and some fear.

Table: It signifies that my suspicions are correct; he may not be benevolent, as he hides from me. He seems to know I am apprehensive of him, so he decides to hide under the table rather than to face me.

Fetal position: Rather than thinking he is suffering I see him as a coward hiding from me and plotting.

Money: I really do not know a reason why he gave me money; it cannot be for a positive reason! I am suspicious of his motive to give me money. Nobody gives me money just like that. I fear this implies that I will have to do something that I don't want to do. It can be evil.

Tattered envelope: The envelope is only tattered because I ripped it open and the edges of it became tattered. Originally it was whole but to open it, it had to be broken apart. I neatly try to tape it together and make it whole again. I saw it first as a present, but it became an unwanted present.

Analysis

The **well-lit rooms** are the different levels of the Self (or house) of the patient, and as they are well-lit, part of the conscious or upper level of her Self or the light (attention), is on the people that are in this room. She is there with a **girlfriend**, her shadow, while **a man**, her animus, is in a second room which is connected to the first room. This connection tells us there is no obstruction between these two levels and there is a good connection possible with the archetypes, anima and animus. She meets her animus and after conversing with him, she promises to watch a TV program (might be symbolic for aspects of oneself–of her past or character) that she does not wish to acknowledge (certain moods or realizations). For the dreamer it is more like "having a date" for a movie, a meeting, to see what is going to happen. But she forgets her animus's promise and instead watches the program with her shadow till she remembers and goes to find her animus **hidden under a table** in a fetal position: her animus is dying off. "Table" can indicate social connections with others, and hiding under the table is a self-image of the status of this animus: disappearing in the background and in danger of death. Her personal associations (more important) evoke more aversion to him, considering him a coward (*lack of character*) with sinister plans, who wants to obtain something from her that is not right, revealing aspects of her own animus from which she wants to liberate herself.

The figure of a man in the dream of a woman represents not only her animus but also the principle of Logos, and apparently this dream tells her to leave this dominant function and concentrate on her natural neglected Eros principle. He hands her an envelope (a hidden message, a present maybe) and then her animus leaves her in spite of her apologizing (disconnection with her animus, on purpose or unconsciously, as she is trying to get more contact with her anima with whom she watches the TV program due to her fear and mistrust of her animus, feeling that he has something else in mind). Then **another woman** comes in the same room and from appearance and dress described further, it is the other side of the shadow, the dark side in contrast with the nice looking and fair girlfriend (duality of archetypes) as she has a hard look, with long hair and pointed, swinging brown tips and a normal T-shirt (not soft like the other woman); she is more the one who is *suspicious*, not trusting, acting and following the man. This female follows the animus to see where he is going, trying to protect the dreamer or wanting to make sure he is gone (most likely the latter one). The envelope is full of **money**, which is psychic strength or symbol of psychic libido and psychic energy to move forward. When we put or have money in the bank, we have psychic energy in the storehouse of the Self, the unconscious. Money means power to change things, to do things. It might also be used to bribe people, to be able to obtain favors from a person. Money might also mean excrement or feces, something you need to get rid of, something from your past that has been poisoning your psyche ("stinking rich"). This might well refer to her fear and distrust of men in general.

As the money comes from her animus, which already was too strong in her present life and imbalanced, she does not even count the money (the amount of male psychic energy) or take it out, to make sure it is not added to her make-up of animus. She wants to return it and tapes the tattered envelope to make sure it is known that this "money" is refused. It tells us that the dreamer is mainly concentrated with watching the TV program (social connections) with her anima, and with making sure that her animus, with whom she is not in good relationship, is subdued to create a better balance between anima and animus. There is a good lysis so a further dream will bring the next step in this series of dreams. The women are all the same type, same age, indicating that they are indeed part of the dreamer. The description of the man represents the animus, a collective archetype as she describes him perfectly (she mentions "universal clothes, black and white": denoting the duality of the archetype). Also, muscular with short hair, symbolizing the power, action, and commitment we can link to the animus in general. Interesting is that the women are around age 35 and the man around 40, the age when these archetypes need to be incorporated into the Self of the dreamer in order to have a good balance in the second part of life.

The total of persons in this dream is **four**, **three** females and **one** male, so definitely a balance going to the feminine and feeling side, which was present in abundance early in her life but was restrained by early experiences with men which changed her as she felt the need to stand up for herself for protection, so as to not appear weak.

Next dream (dream two) after *Phosphorus* LM1, 2 drops from RSB, 2 drops from 1st cup

I am in a room with two other females, both lesbian-looking, with rather butch-like haircuts. They are looking at a map book to figure out how to get to the point of their destination. They go to different pages in the book to figure it out. Then I tell them I can draw this on one page and I do it, nicely colored and very precise: the whole itinerary on one page, which should make it much easier than having to go to these different sections of the map book. When I present my sheet to the oldest strongest butch, to my surprise she refuses to acknowledge the value of it. I turn around and see in the same room a small cafeteria and I feel hungry. I decide to eat something, and

I pick out the smallest bite-size muffin to satisfy me. Then I wake up.

Analysis

As mentioned, she was born a free-spirited *Phosphorus* woman, who first was somewhat controlled by her mother and afterwards betrayed by a husband and controlled by another. So contrary to her nature, she had to develop a strong animus (she never knew her father nor had any other siblings and grew up with her mother and a mean grandmother) in order to survive in this world and somewhat protect herself, as a *Phosphorus* person is very trusting and compassionate towards most people. But after the remedy intake it shows that she can relax, as here again there are three women (a dominance of the female yin), two with a strong animus, and herself with her intelligent artistic nature, compiling something complicated on one page. Not surprisingly, her animus—which before the *Phosphorus* intake had to be in charge in order to protect herself—can be let go somewhat, and now she can follow what comes naturally to her. Just like in the previous dream where she lets go of the man (animus). The man has become a butch in this dream, more towards the feminine. Then she eats just a little bit. Of course, the trip they try to figure out is her road to individuation, to become more the Self, more complete in correspondence to her *Phosphorus* nature. And the "little food" she needs gives enough energy to go on her further trip and to allow further growth as an individual as she feels more independence and freedom. There is an excellent lysis to this dream, so we expect the next chapter in the dream book.

Next dream (dream three) after LM1 *Phosphorus*

My husband and I are on a trip overseas together and we are supposed to have a room together. When we check in, I am told that my husband has a separate room in a different hotel. Meanwhile, I check in and he leaves to go to the other hotel. I know the name of his hotel and after I put my luggage into my room, I leave the hotel to look for him. On the way over to his hotel, along the way, I find coin money on the ground, one at a time. The first one I pick up is a USA penny. The next one I find is another USA penny. I sort of smile about this. Then I find another coin with the number 10 on it. It says on it "Old Town" and is from a country we have already been to. The last and final coin I find is from a country we haven't been to. A total of four coins were found. After finding the fourth coin on the sidewalk, I cross the street and there is the hotel towering tall in front of me. I go inside and find a lot of activity from tourists there. I go to reception and there is only one desk clerk reading something in front of her. I ask her for my husband's room number as I give her his name. She said it will take half an hour. I don't want to wait half an hour, but there seems nothing I can do about it. Meanwhile, many people are coming down the steps from the upper floor. I go to the stairs to see if I can see a glimpse of him. Maybe he will be coming down the stairs too? I go back to the receptionist and it is a different person and again, only one receptionist. I tell her the story of us being separated and that I need to find him now! She was also indifferent and said I had to wait. I feel frustrated by this indifference and that I cannot find him, so I resume my place by the stairs to see if he will walk down with others. I then wake up from the dream.

Analysis

Trip overseas: A journey away from home or an investigation of the unconscious.

Hotel: Checking into the state of the Self but hotel means a transitional stage.

Husband: Her animus.

Money: See before; money is psychic strength or symbol of psychic libido and psychic energy to move forward.

Four coins: The number of **individuation**; **four** is an ancient symbol of completeness or wholeness, the emergence of human consciousness or bringing order to the chaos—four corners of the earth, the four cardinal points of the horizon, the four winds, the four directions of the compass, the four seasons, the four humors, the four arms of the cross (the empirical basis that conquers the powers of darkness), the four phases of the moon, the four-petalled flower, and four-lobed leaf representing wholeness, as well as the mystery of birth, life, death, and rebirth, and the four main colors of the rainbow: red, yellow, blue, and green. The number **four** stands also for the four conscious functions.

USA: Birth country and present living country.

Old Town: The unconscious, what has been left behind; she is now in a different country and cannot use this money anymore, as with the USA pennies.

Coin of future country: What is ahead, the conscious world.

Crossing a street to reach next hotel: Approach to next transition stage in life (hotel=temporary Self). She is crossing a street used by many people, indicating the journey belongs not only to the dreamer but to many others (collective archetypal dream).

Many people coming down from the stairs: Again,

showing the collective nature of the dream as many people come down (meaning to investigate the unconscious).

Receptionists of the hotel: Those who give out information regarding other persons and rooms, but both are indifferent or rather saying to the dreamer, "Be patient, it will take a while."

Further clarification: There is a lysis to this dream, as she is waiting. It is a somewhat enigmatic lysis, but one offering possibilities. Comparing this dream to the previous dreams we can see many different positive evolutions: **four** coins, always a sign of completeness and individuation and the coins point to the past (Old Town, present [USA], and future [unknown future place to visit]). We can see the movement forward in this dream where the dreamer is traveling and has "psychic energy or libido" to continue her journey. Apparently, her animus does not check into the same hotel (indicating a new animus during this transition phase) and she knows he is in another hotel, another part of her Self, not united yet but she is desirous to find him. In fact, she is impatient to find him and the receptionists (the guides in the transitional phase) tell her to be patient, quite indifferent to her drive to find her animus or husband.

In the meantime, many people come down from the elevator or stairs where she waits (=border of conscious and unconscious) to join her to explore the unconscious. This shows the problem in life posed to many people, not just the dreamer—a collective dream of mankind, in search of exploring the unconscious and uniting with the contra-sexual figure, or animus in this case. Apparently, she needs patience to meet this newly formed animus, one who she wants to be with and not a threatening figure as in the past. All in all, a good direction of cure, and part of a dream series in which the next chapter needs to be written. As it is not a recurrent dream with no lysis, as a vital problem of the dream has been resolved through the intake of the remedy, no new remedy is needed but *Phosphorus* needs to be repeated when her Chief Complaint of "insomnia" occurs. It is remarkable too that this insomnia, when one needs to sleep and investigate the unconscious, meant the latter was in turmoil, causing sleeplessness, but on *Phosphorus*, her sleep has been deeper and longer lasting. Intake of the remedy, for the moment, is needed infrequently, not like other remedies (no doubt similes) that had to be repeated more often. What is the significance of the sygizi in modern times? Any changes?

Adjustment to the Sygizi (Animus and Anima) in Modern Times

Jung limited anima and animus to the unconscious dynamics of either sex. On the strength of clinical experience since his early formulation, this no longer appears valid. The evidence does not justify that anima exclusively embodies the non-personal unconscious of men, and animus of women. Feminine standards were devalued and rejected in the early 20th century. In our time, we have witnessed a reemergence of femininity (yin or anima qualities). So, man can be as animus-ridden, dogmatic and power-hungry as women: we have seen enough women fall victim to such male animus possession, when sitting at the feet of some guru who "really understands them and can guide them through life." Women on the other hand can be as anima possessed—moody, seductive, and depressed as men. While anima remains natural to women and animus to men, the quantity or intensity can still be abnormal in a person, either increased or decreased—if not destroyed. As one man stated to me when I pointed out that he was quite dictatorial towards others, "It is not a problem of being dictatorial, and it is not that I refuse to accept being dictatorial, it is just that I always want to get the issue right, because I *am* right." But upon further questioning, he had to admit that at a young age people told him he was authoritarian in his behavior. Obviously what we usually do with such "knowledge" or remarks is to put them in the unconscious as something that is "not nice" about our personality that needs to be put in a tomb, so that we can have the illusion of being "a nice person." However, he admitted to being a coward in some circumstances, and we can see that this dictatorial behavior and *speaking with a voice of command* is nothing but an Adlerian power complex at work to establish a foundation of a stronger ego to survive challenges and confrontations in life. "I always want to be right" is exactly a distorted animus at work, unbeknownst to its possessor, but visible to anyone around him. Alas, most of his family will sustain his illusion by telling him that he was, is, and always will be a nice person. And when he says something offensive, it was only because "he was clumsy, and his opinion was not well-expressed." Observations to the contrary from well-meaning friends will fall on deaf ears and be met with strong incredulous protest. "How can you think this of me when everyone else says the opposite?" Well, since when is a distorted animus deliberate, rational, and clear? Not when you express yourself with "always, everyone, ought, (or) should." That is the sole language of a distorted animus, seemingly logical but not fitting the actual situation!

The father's character and conduct will not only influence his daughter but also his son. Take my father for instance. He never had a job you could put a name on—or as they say, "twelve jobs and thirteen accidents." He was a figure straight out of Scott Peck's book, *People of the Lie: The Hope for Healing Human Evil.* Not only was it his habit to mesmerize and exploit people's weaknesses when he could, I was also at his mercy to be his "favorite" child and at the same time to feel his belt, without much reason, mostly just for him to vent his own insecurities and frustrations. This created some revenge in me towards authority (especially the army) so that, one day, I did not hesitate to incite my naïve younger brother, whose main strength and quality was a forceful stream of urine that he could whip up yards into the sky. I bribed him with a sweet surprise to urinate through the window while my father, unknowingly to him, was sitting on the toilet. I knew that this would create prodigious trouble and it did. But it was not in me to resist the temptation. I had to succumb to the law of my make. I forgot what the punishment was, but I was not the person at that moment to care about that. I had already collected my dividend. I am older now, but I confess I still see my brother swinging up his behind to produce a perfect arc falling straight on my father's head. What a glorious moment! My father's swearing was music to my ears and was worth all the forthcoming punishment I had to endure. Although my brother for a few minutes thought he was the star, I knew I was the brilliant inventor of my "justified" revenge, while my brother was just an accessory. No doubt, I retained a rather glorious memory of that day for quite some time. This exploit—at least in my eyes—surrounded me with a halo of pride and victory. And even thinking of it now, always brings a smile to my face.

This act of subordination became part of my animus when dealing with authoritarian and dictatorial figures, dulling for a long time my sense of diplomacy and strengthening my anarchistic sense of justice. Of course, my father made sure he had the last word as he sent me to a military prep school at age 13 to become at the same time the best academic student and worst military student they ever had. And when my father was trying to show his "good side," he sent me away to a summer camp, which was only two miles away from home. I know that now, of course, but being very shy at that point in my life, it might as well have been Timbuktu!

For my father, I found out that his motto was, "To beget children, nothing better; to have them, what iniquity!" As a true *Lycopodium* he was consumed by the canker of power, always waiting for the next opportunity to show off, as the alcoholic is always waiting for the next drink. He could produce a full act with a hundred varied sketches: forgetting the beating, he would praise me to his friends in my presence as his exceptional child because it reflected the superiority and intelligence inherited from *him*. I was the most obedient child, but of course the obedience was tailor-made by him. Any contradiction or the slightest protest was followed by serious punishment once out of sight of others. But among his friends, his eloquent praise of his "best son" would be so excessive that, after being so often terrorized and abused, I thought he was talking about someone else. I found my role so becoming that I did not dare to step out of it. Of course, my father's whims became my law.

Let's see an example about the sygizi in two dreams experienced by the same person in one night. We will not do a complete analysis but just confirm what I said before regarding the sygizi!

Conscious situation: This unmarried man, age 45, was raised by a typical animus possessed *Kali-carb* mom. Everything was decided for him "to make his life easier," as mom knew best. She was always right, and this made an indelible impression on this man till he had these dreams.

Dream one

I have to take a flight overseas and hurry to the airport with my wife at my side. Once in the airport, my wife takes charge of where to go, and to find the way to the airplane in this seeming labyrinth of entrances. She always stays ahead of me and knows where to turn and what next corridor to take in order to arrive at the plane. I feel secure but before reaching the airplane I wake up in a terror.

Analysis

We can easily see that this man is indeed still possessed by his mother: here we have a situation where the Logos or animus has to decide, yet it is his anima who takes over, indicating to what extent his animus was weakened if not destroyed by his mother. *This does not mean his anima is strengthened! This person does not have an anima excess but rather an animus deficiency.* What this created in him shows in the next dream he had, the same night:

Dream two

I have to take an airplane overseas and have to fly to Amsterdam. I am with my wife and another guy who lays eyes on my wife and tries to seduce her. I am so mad at him that at some point I take him by the arms and swing his head against the wall. It was shocking but he came to life again, to my surprise. Then we go to the airport and I see that I am the only one arriving at the counter to check in my luggage. I only have one hour left before the airplane leaves. My ticket was OK but my wife's is torn in two. The guy at the counter says to me, "I will keep your luggage here but you have to return from the city from where you came by bus to get a new ticket for your wife, and I am only here for another hour." I am taken by despair and cry as I realize that it would take me more than an hour to return by bus. Then I gave up and ask for my luggage back. I wake up in great anxiety.

Analysis

The other **guy**, his shadow, is the shadowy character of himself, containing secret wishes but also deficiency of character created by his dominant mother. As a compensation in real life, this created an Adlerian power complex in him, creating an excessive persona. As successful as he was in business, this dream shows how he falters and "does not reach his destination," or in other words, when faced with a challenge in life, his animus, weakened by his mother, is not able to overcome this obstacle and halts him on his way to individuation. There is no lysis in this dream, so it will come back until he is able to liberate himself from his mother, even when she was dead already a long time. He remains stuck and asks for his **luggage** back (whatever is in his unconscious) instead of integrating it in consciousness, as in "getting rid of your baggage". Of course, he could not kill his shadow as much as he tried: this shadow always remains his ever-present sibling, it is part of him. The *Kali-c* mother created a *Lycopodium* son!

While inflation and identification with the persona and anima/animus is not rare, the most common form of disastrous relationship to the anima/animus is the projection of the sygizi —in this case, anima for men, animus for women. This holds the secret to any relationship, which needs an in-depth investigation, worthy of a new chapter on projection of the sygizi in men and women.

13

THE HUMAN LOVE STORY: PROJECTION OF THE SYGIZI

"The joys and sorrows of life . . . " — Rousseau

Love, Marriage, and Other Heresies: "The Heart is Deceitful Above All Things"

If you are looking for a chapter about romantic-fantasy juvenile-dream-like love, a land of permanent ever-lasting fancies, then skip this chapter. As one innocent naïve *Pulsatilla*, who read some of it before I published it, exclaimed, "But there is nothing about love in this," not realizing that it was all about *true* love and how many pitfalls of love and marriage are due to projections of the sygizi. I say "other heresies" here in reference to the Greek word meaning, "opinion profoundly at odds with what is generally accepted," or maybe I should say, "hoped for." At the end of this chapter, the reader will see from his own unfortunate and fortunate relationship experiences that this definition will remain intact.

Anima and animus, also called the sygizi, or sygyzia, from the Greek *syz*, or "with, together," are true personalities and archetypes from the collective unconscious; instinctive, emotional, and connective urges, which make their influences felt in projections for both men and women. Unknowingly to men, when it comes to "falling in love," it is here that men's archaic anima plays a dominant elusive role. Women should ask, "*Who* is falling in love with me? Is it someone who wants to exert control over me? Or perhaps dominate me or consider me only as a sex object? Someone who needs inflation and undeserved praise? Or is it someone who never considers a wife to be part of an equal relationship? Does he want a wife that can be all at once—his mother, his best friend, his willing sex slave, his nanny, his cook, and a tenderhearted woman, who can listen to his ravings without rolling her eyes, without sighing?" If we really want to know our partner or people in general, we want to invite the animal part of them, which is not only the most interesting part, but also the truer human side.

The woman who is not a slave but an equal—who gives herself according to her own feeling—is infinitely more desirable to a real man than any submissive serf who is always waiting on his will. Is the partner expected to say, "I am as you desire me"? For some women, exclusiveness is the other side of their "devotion," even to the extreme for a *Lachesis* woman, who changes these tender emotions into green-eyed jealousy if she does not feel reciprocated (*jealousy, as foolish as it is irresistible*). Most men, knowing little or nothing about psychology, tend to project their undeveloped anima onto a real woman—his wife or another woman—experiencing her entirely outside as opposed to the woman inside of him, showing the anima as the personification of men's unconscious, that ghost land, that vast unknown and often terrifying cold winter land, the Antarctica of the soul.

At first this seems to be an ideal solution, as men, by marrying the opposite type, can now let go of confronting the nagging and tyrannical inferior function! So, this unknowing woman is forced to play the role made up in man's mind. At least temporarily, till an occasion comes up where the need of personal intervention of man's inferior function is required, which leads to nothing but trouble and fights in this "peaceful" household. What men don't know is that this projection of their anima is quite dangerous, as anima transforms everything it touches—almost reducing men to hopeless weak beings—not an exact replica of the strong sex to which they claim to belong. This is the source of moods in men, showing that they are possessed by their anima and emotions, leading to instant transformation into a hysterical woman. Of course, no man admits he has moods; he has reasonable explanations for his change in behavior: "Look at what happened," he says, "Look at what *you* did (or said)!" And as proof that he is possessed by the anima, he becomes a skillful lawyer, always talking for the sake of talking till the opposition finally surrenders. Really, such a man is a boy who wants to get what he desires, not wanting this projection to become conscious although that would be his only salvation.

Projection is used as an eternal excuse for mishaps and shortcomings of the individual. Projection is the apparent needed helper to get out of a situation that confronts the owner with the content of his dark side, but in reality—if continued—becomes the destroyer of happiness, progression, and life itself. It frees the owner for just a short amount of time—a Pyrrhus victory—but is really the beginning of losing the war on living. Of course the possessor is not conscious of having such projections (these events are quite autonomous!), as their presence comes in handy in too many daily life situations where imperfections, misdeeds, and shameful actions and thoughts can be transferred to the other person, the one with the mistakes and defects, as we can see only good in ourselves. And so, the projection goes on forever, often for life, causing incomprehensible moods frequently leading to depression, remaining unrecognized even on our death bed, after having created havoc in other people's lives. More importantly, it is sad to see how such persons wrecked their own life, going to their death with the conviction of the purity of their life, not seeing that they themselves had been the author of their greatest misfortunes (ignoble misfortunes). Only courageous and honest people recognize these projections after having used them, when they make these high feeling-toned complexes conscious.

Oftentimes parents are the object of projection. While the miasmatic family traits are indeed to be "blamed" and are transgenerationally transferred, it is exactly the goal of any human with the help of psychotherapy and homeopathy to smooth out the dark side of his family inheritance. But how many ever resort to such helpful action? It is much easier to use others as scapegoats for personal shortcomings. Projection, done by the unconscious, is also the constant source of the *initial* formation of any relationship, especially the "falling in love at first sight," and is something almost no one, man or woman, is initially conscious of when he or she finds a suitable candidate for capturing this projection. All they know is that the projected positive aspect of anima and animus is highly desirable to them. Eyes lock, hearts stop, and soon—a few months later—they are down on one knee, offering a ring and the prospect of a life together. "I don't need to think about it" they say, with a briskness befitting the confidence of the "One-Who-Is-Totally-Sure," so that is that! Except that it isn't! "Falling in love" delights a human so powerfully as to render him totally incapable of feeling anything else, or I might add, thinking about anything else, proof that this person has temporarily lost his thinking function or Logos. "I am so preoccupied with thoughts of her; I see her at every turn of the road, always creating a jolt in my brain, and yes, I am so tormented by unrest when I think someone else is in her presence." Well that must be love! But, no! It is non-love, an unhealthy bondage, a kind of love that lures the moth to the flame, unable to survive for long. Sadly enough, the majority of these moments of ecstasy are short-lived; such extreme delight cannot last a whole life! A second sight might lead to a brutal liquidation of Prince Charming or Princess Full-of-Grace, and to taking up arms against "love," a disaster that might and should shake this one-sided fixation that we initially thought would never disappear. What we failed to follow is the insight of the old Romans and Greeks who considered falling in love a divine act. As they described it, "the arrow of Eros hit him." But we can avoid the tale of "I was married once, briefly—long story!"

Falling in Love: Illusions and Delusions

Projections therefore—and the more we use them—are the source of numerous illusions, the fundamental cause of many man-made great ignoble misfortunes. As projections are responsible for many emotional states, they are also in constant use when we fall in love—having someone in our lives who carries the projected animus or anima image—the first earthshaking experience of adolescence. There are plenty of clichés out there: "I fell hard for her," and, "The moment I saw him I knew he was the one!" Maybe we did not fall hard enough to wake up. "Falling in love" is indeed the right expression as it reflects the suddenness and violence with which we were overcome, as if possessed by primitive passions and powerful life-giving emotions, resulting from the autonomous power of the anima (in man's case, animus in woman's case). We can only hope to be able to get up again when the blinding lightning of the sudden encounter with the soulmate (the soul representing the idea of unity) takes a more stable form—when blind emotions transform into genuine feelings. "I was struck with his or her presence," "It was like I knew this person all my life," or "I started falling for him," should be followed by another look when the eyes are wide open. Such passion can create suffering as it is easy to be burned by its flame. Love might sometimes be called the world's greatest illusion as most people are in love with the concept of love—which is far from true love. Pathological attachment is not love and love cannot live where there is no trust.

What we do not know is that we were knocked over by our inferior function and such a relationship, founded on projection, was mainly a relationship with our unconscious. How can we assume that we are totally in love with someone in those sudden whirlwind romances when we do not know the other person yet? A human, supposed to be a rational being, should not follow the dictates of passion in one of the most important acts of his life. Yet many enter willingly into a contract at first sight—almost without thought, and against the advice of well-meaning friends—at a time when they know they are not in their right mind. Love is not blind; it is *non-love* that makes us blind. And non-love monopolizes each other's affection to the exclusion of friends and relations, while passing the days in trivial existences, and the inferior of the two actors inevitably will drag the other down to his or her level. As Sandor Ferensczi, the great Hungarian psychoanalyst stated, "People want to love one another, but they don't know how!"

Alas, all too often the intense domination of the love emotion gives birth to feelings that are distorted by love's inflation. Opposites attract irresistibly—the charm of the unknown. *True* love will look more than once, looking for details with immense curiosity. Even when our friends take a more honest look at our new relationship, and caution us to go slower, *we know without any doubt*, she or he is *the one*, so no point in waiting, we just know! "I am madly in love," "She/he is my soulmate I have been waiting for," we say. Nothing could be further from the truth for this has more to do with madness than real love! Good advice would be to "sleep on it," when the frenzied unwise consciousness is extinct, and we can become acquainted with the voice of an archetype like the wise old man through a pertinent dream. Even in medicine we are taught to ask for a second opinion in the case of a serious disorder. Marriage can be considered "serious" and often can be called a "disorder" considering the pain and unhappiness it causes when followed by divorce—a common incident as seen by examining the divorce rates in Europe and the US, both at 60% for marriages above 16 years' duration.

Falling in love is mostly nothing more than the exchange of a person's package—his looks, charm, education, and seductive convincing smile—hopefully for a profitable trade, possibly a higher social position and lifestyle. The actual reality of the other person is likely to be quite different than what the *projected* expectation is, as well as than the continued projection (she is Greta Garbo, Elizabeth Taylor, May West, Marlene Dietrich, etc., and he is George Clooney, Brad Pitt, or Prince William). Once the magnetism of falling in love evaporates, we feel disappointed and disillusioned and let down by the partner when she or he fails to conform to this image and expectation. We must realize that an actual spouse is a combination of attractive and unattractive qualities, not the glamorous star we have in mind only. In the days of the honeymoon we should learn the art of living and loving as we all are apprentices! We need to prepare not just for intense love, but also for disagreements so that we are not taken unaware, and cultivate friendship with common interest, so that foolish fondness will not soon change into mutual dislike. Live with the person for a while and you will know that this person is all too human, no different than you. Pass through a time of trial and conflict first and see how unfortunate but common situations are dealt with. One of the gifts and mysteries of true love is that no feelings of envy and hate are entertained towards the loved one.

Nietzsche exclaimed when he spoke of committing to

marriage, "Careful have I found all buyers, and all of them have astute eyes. But even the most astute of them bought his wife in a sack" (Nietzsche, 1954, p.773). I guess he never took that chance as he never had a long-lasting relationship with a woman. With his Logos well in control (he was an intuitive thinking person), he had an explanation for this: as he had wonderful idealistic ideas about marriage and children, he said that such ideals were not accomplishable so he "preferred to die," foregoing marriage and an heir in real life. But this was only due to his inflation, to his identification with Zarathustra, the archetype of the wise old man or Super Human, who claims that he knows when to marry and when and how to die, rather than accept the series of life events not voluntarily chosen. There is at least one aspect I agree with Nietzsche on: that a degree of intellectual compatibility is necessary for a good marriage, otherwise the physical aspect will become a source of boredom, even disgust, as duration is not possible! How lucky we are if we find both aspects in a partner; in such a union the two people will strengthen each other!

What people don't understand is that the inner woman or man they loved, projected onto another, never really existed at all and was over-evaluated, but failing to have a conscious connection to their archaic inner archetypal images, their only solution was to find wholeness in an outer being. The false conception they clung to of the loved one—even in the face of all real evidence and common sense—was purely imaginary. Love, for men generally, is not equal to Eros, the capacity to relate, so women complain, "He is so insensitive to my needs," a battle cry I often heard in practice. The woman, the carrier of man's projected anima, initially flattered and valued by this powerful image projection, eventually becomes suffocated. Being the carrier of the man's soul, she finds out that things are not going so well when she is not available to his wishes or whatever one-sided character trait he wanted in her—taking care of him as a mother and lover starts hindering her own individual personality and freedom. Such a situation is not uncommon in mail-order brides, where a lonely elder man brings over a much younger and often poorer woman from a foreign country with the underlying message, "I wanted to marry you because I wanted to take care of you and of course (even more), have you take care of me—and that did not entail you going to college to get a degree!"

Now suddenly she is no longer the woman *he wanted* her to be! From then on, from the princess image, this woman receives the projection of the negative anima, the Witch! The result is a continuous conflict between a confused male and female who don't understand what each other's role is. Marriage has become a sick mixture of resentments over trifles as he has neglected to adjust his feeling function and is now caught in strange moods descending from that archaic feminine side and the shadow side, in the form of jealousy and possessiveness—the hidden real image of his "love." Momentary oneness only occurs for such a man while having sex, and that will eventually be resented and dreaded by his partner because of its compulsive expected nature. This results in terrible loneliness for both, the fate of too many married people. To expect that a human can surrender himself at any moment to the endearments of love, is like expecting that such love would impel a whole nation of atheists to worship God!

We have to understand that personal feelings can also be expressed in small personal ways: the soul of the body—the eyes, the facial changes, and above all hand gestures, can express either aggression or ridicule or soothing love, compassion and empathy. An extraverted intuitive type like *Phosphorus* always makes the other person feel special, guided by the effect she has on others when observing their face and voice change. Men fall straight away in love with such a female—at least they imagine they are in love with her, whereas I think she did the imagining for them. Couples would do well to understand that a well-operating feeling function is concerned about the quality of time, rather than the amount we give another. And to antidote the falsifying and exaggerated actions of this archaic anima, to produce clarity instead of fuzziness, men (usually saddled with an ill-operating feeling function, as seen before in Chap. 8, "The Four Conscious Functions") should be "man" enough to set the imagined fairy tale aside and express real feelings, even the negative ones, in a calm deliberate manner. To their great surprise this will be far more easily accepted by their partners, rather than lack of communication leading to silent or not so silent battles where men become chronically moody, sullen and anima-ridden, expressing opinions without regard to facts, relationships, or logic!

This possession by his anima was nicely expressed in the dream of one of my patients. After having a fit (*anger, besides himself*) over a small word by his wife, driven by his sense of *easily offended*, he remained sullen and taciturn the whole day, apparently not able to overcome this dark feeling. The same night, he had the following dream.

Dream

I am with my wife at a gathering. Another woman, to whom I show some desire, keeps throwing herself around my neck, kissing me on the mouth. When my wife happens to see this, I have that feeble excuse to her that I could not help myself, that I couldn't get away from this woman. My wife leaves in a fury, I try to follow her, and she arrives in a hotel. I am looking for her and see her leaving the hotel, far ahead of me. I follow her on a path along a river, where many people walk but I have a hard time catching up to her. Then I wake up frustrated.

Analysis

Obviously "he could not help himself"—referring here to the fit he had the day before and to the fact that this lady was throwing herself around his neck, indicating he was possessed by the anima. His wife (his archaic anima) was leaving the hotel (a temporary Self) and he tries to catch up with her along the river (the border between conscious and unconscious) but he has a hard time reuniting with his anima, a collective problem, indicated by the fact that many people walk with him on the same path. Apparently, he will have to unite with his anima, probably after investigating and making a plunge into his unconscious.

Of course, women are equally under the spell of their projection onto men. A woman's husband might have come into her life as the hero saving her from a desperate situation, such as poverty, lack of family love, abuse or even incest, or from the isolation of being the ugly duck at school and many other factors, but this can turn him quickly into a dictator telling her what to do, how to dress, and who to mingle with! Every man at some point feels (or wants to feel) that he is the rescuer of his damsel in distress, a troubadour traveling from castle to castle, singing love songs and telling romantic stories, convinced that the targeted lady will be grateful for this joy brought to her, as well as for new passion, before unknown to her, releasing her from boredom and simplicity of life. While words and ideas were initially an attraction, drawing her like a moth to the flame, they can suddenly turn into vicious weapons —swords that go for the jugular, extinguishing the creative flame within her, the flame of life itself! And now the husband represents the negative archetypal animus type—the figure of death—allowing no equal relationship and no blossoming of her personal life! For both men and women, such projections can only cease to exist when familiarity exposes the relationship to a dose of reality, not an easy task. I think living together for six months before tying the knot should be a must before any marriage! It certainly would be bad business for lawyers but a great start for a more solid marriage! Or is there no hope on the way to the altar?

On the Way to the Altar, Dead or Alive

While Nietzsche, in view of his life experiences, cannot be regarded as an expert in marriage counseling, he tried to give astute advice—which of course was dominated by his intellect and a conscious thinking function: "Before going into marriage, one should ask himself: Do I think I could have a good conversation with this woman, continuing into old age?" (Hayman, 1980, p. 202). This was of course the same man, while suffering terribly from the consequences of tertiary syphilis that occurred at age 23 (causing eye troubles, nightly headaches, and digestive disorders, eventually leading to dementia), who exclaimed that "His way of thinking, his reflections, were his main nourishment" (Ibid., p. 220). But any relationship with a female in his life was a disaster and clumsy—with his sister Elizabeth, with Lou Salomé and Cosima Wagner, the wife of Richard Wagner, the famous German composer. And Nietzsche's "love" for Salomé and Cosima were more a construction of fantasies and tidal waves in his unconscious, caused by his archaic anima in a mainly intuitive-thinking person. Unfortunately, his soul died even before his body, as he was overcome with insanity 12 years before he passed away in 1900. What a shame he did not receive homeopathic treatment for his syphilis at age 23, as it was readily available at that time in France and Germany (Hahnemann died in 1843). Homeopathy could have cured him at every stage of the illness, from the primary effect (Hahnemann cured primary syphilis chancre with *Mercurius* 30C in 14 days) to the very unfortunate retina involvement that reduced his eyesight to a minimum, and the severe headaches and stomach pains he endured from this "incurable" disease (by allopathy), to the sinking into an infantile state, hardly recognizing anyone. But how does someone become adrift, losing his way in love and finding the path of a wound in the heart?

There are those who marry out of sheer impetuosity. Unconditional love is universally desired—a noble concept, yet rarely accomplished as it does not come natural to human beings. Why does this concept remain mostly elusive? This pure love mainly exists between mother and child—even to the detriment of both—but between two adults there are mainly conditions to secure "love." We are always occupied with what love brings to us: a tonic for self-esteem, an increased sense of power and fake sense of being admired, an inflation of the ego when obeyed and rarely criticized and viewed as belonging to the toast of mankind. A man overwhelmed by his anima, upon falling in love thinks about the other person all the time, and hearing from her becomes like a drug he is miserable without. The desired object of love—the female—becomes alive, feeling wanted and exhilarated. Should we be forewarned about the pitfalls of Cupido, or should we think that imprudence and spontaneity is what makes us human, and what is life without illusions? Such "love" is, after all, a delicious feeling of being singled out for adulation and specialness, satisfying our romantic intensity and cravings. No doubt, all this is part of the initial falling in love at first sight. And who doesn't want to be wooed, to be insistently persuaded, against all practical knowledge and reality, that he or she is the one, the only one? Such moments of enthusiastic fantasies are a great aid to surviving the perpetual letdown of reality. Why does such a journey not last? Is the confrontation of anima and animus—always part of a human, most of the time resembling an unbridled wild horse—impossible to tame? The dismal truth is that these collective figures of the unconscious will find other victims when we realize that none of us is particularly unique, despite having been persuaded otherwise. Lovers cannot stop talking to everyone about how life has taken on a new radiance for them. How we wish that those words and intentions would be infinite. But what began so well, often takes a different path. Satiety, disillusionment, and contempt tell us that only a human's *needs* are infinite!

Hafiz, the most beloved poet of the Persians, wrote, "The heart is a thousand stringed instrument that can only be tuned with love."[1]

True love and compassion are expressed more forcefully in the language of gesture and glance, coming naturally to an extravert intuitive like *Phosphorus*, a mute exchange between herself and others, but profoundly felt by anyone in her presence. It is not pity she feels, which is only a perversion of compassion, and would only restore the psychic distance between humans. She feels a genuine solidarity with suffering people who share a common world with her, although she is a person who always remains optimistic, not caught in the monotonous bandwagon of life, always finding an off-ramp to escape falling down a rabbit hole where other people prefer to sacrifice everyone else, family and friends included. For those, to give guidance is lust and power. It is indeed innate to humans to throw up a veil of appearances, behind which lurks suspicious and obstructive motives. But true love and compassion must be part of a fully human life, and can even be expressed through silence, when lovers remain silent as they devote themselves to each other. And it is kind and soft eyes that fire the arrows of Cupid.

True love adapts itself to the contours of any vessel that it fills. True love, piercing all hearts, wants to know who the individual is—always a mixture of pure gold and pure nonsense, but hopefully both sides are accepted with much understanding and observation, besides feeling. It is not the same as Eros, the principle of relationship, the main element in women's psychology, which can contain even hatred and indifference. True love is the infinite love dwelling in a finite heart. It is a sturdy bridge, built one stone at a time, day upon day, year upon year, between two human beings who are accepting each other as ordinary beings—a bridge built with diligence and ease and pleasing to the eye, because to understand each other no words need to be spoken as both end up in a world of synchronicity. There is no danger of the bridge collapsing, as both lovers never cease to put effort and devotion into the artwork called "true love." True love does not allow selfishness to triumph and is where our heart is not corroded by the shallow fashionable egotism of our times. True love *expects* nothing, *accepts* everything. True love is also when a man still loves that elderly woman, transformed by aging from a joyous, leaping composition to a stiff, wilting person with cheese-grater texture to the heels of her feet. The art of true love washes the dirt of our daily life. It is as French philosopher Albert Camus wrote in *The Plague*, "a happiness that forgets nothing" (1947). It carves out a form of freedom, a form of imaginative freedom that does not ignore realities and frivolities of life. Why then are so few permanent bridges to be found in human relationships?

Pains and pangs of the heart seem to find a way to oppress man's sweetest human pleasure, when losing the object of his worship. Reason and desire are usually at war with each other. Marriage is not just a delicious bouquet of fragrant roses, but more often is a business full of thorns. Most human love stories reflect a rose garden where the petals fall, and the briars remain. Unfortunately, the time a marriage lasts—and even more, how pleasant, passionate, and joyous it was—remains for many to be a period of all too short duration of unbridled ecstasy, as the field of roses is strewn with landmines. With the terrible blindness that passion brings upon its servants, they fail to notice, or are not interested in, the elaborate tricks the "Persona-In-Love" projects. This kind of married life—while expecting fierce, fiery-colored joys—always has a short lifespan as such a cornucopia of happiness is bound to expire on account of the realities of life and the lack of true love. Then the evil twins Deception and Jealousy take the place of the angelic twins Happiness and Romance. Too numerous are the deserters of the principle of true love, succumbing to a delirious fanciful world full of unobtainable delusionary wishes far from the true realism of what love stands for: honest conversation, equal relationship, and a life where jealousy and envy and lust for power as well as classical stereotypes that know nothing about true love are delegated to the unconscious tomb, never to be visited or honored. Where and why do relationships take this sad turn—why do so many turn from the life of true love? Is there a guide or understanding to the shifting sands of romantic love? Or is non-true love like light, in that it can fade with the passing years?

Paradise Lost

After a while, it looks like the basis for many marriages is misunderstanding. As years go by—on average about seven—thunderstorms and lightning make their appearance, while explosive lovemaking and intimacy has already left through the door of the dream house like a silent robber. Love seems to be more akin to hate than devotion. Most find out that they do not know whether they hate or love. And most couples swing violently and irresolutely between these two poles, often leading to tragedies that reach the deepest corners of the human heart. Love seems to always be only a hairbreadth away from hate, unexpectedly befalling one of the parties. Should we call Venus the goddess of love and death? At first, partners still seem passionate about each other in public. But for most, it becomes hard to distinguish sincerity from artifice. The once passionate marriage has become a battleground with icy moments of truce punctuating sustained sniper fire. The pledge to eternal constancy from the time they fell head over heels in love is long gone, furnishing the inevitable broken heart. Both parties, flawed and mortal, are startled to find that they cannot bear disappointment well; it turns them bitter and austere.

And so the story of escapism starts: bewildered by the constant sense of accusations and fright triggered by trifles, either party escapes to a pub, a yoga class, or a tennis game every chance they get, or maybe a fishing party with friends without the wife and kids, as the world in which they live at home after so many years has become a life of undreamed harshness and poverty, both material and especially emotional, and they lament the ugliness of their life. We should look at one of the cornerstones of homeopathy—individuality—to realize that when two unique individuals marry, with their own constitution, dominant miasm, and yes, baggage brought from other relationships or a disturbed childhood, no two marriages will be the same. And working hard to make the other party happy often leads to guilt, anger, excuses, and projections that one has failed in this sacred promise. Such travesty of love is nothing but parasitism, a nestling down in another soul, always at the expense of "the host." True love can be like a ghost; everyone wants it, but few have ever seen it.

Rare are the parties willing to bear and meet head-on to work through that suffering, which is part of any enduring marriage. Mostly forgotten is the grace of sweet companionship, the charm of pleasant conversation, the unexpected card with lovely thoughts, and all those gentle humanities that make life lovely and sustainable and balanced, resembling a beautiful melody in tune rather than a screeching composition of tones painful to the ear. Passion in marriage has a finite shelf life, but true love—connection with the partner—is infinite. For me, the only link between two people who truly love one another should be love. Period. Any marriage is made up of problems from the past and the present. The durability of a marriage is hopefully based on flexibility, deep insight and care for the partner, and *not* on resignation of one of the parties. Accepting that there needs to be a change in the partner policies of marriage is one of the most difficult notions to obtain and will be resisted by a multitude of invalid excuses because the last thing desired is change. But refusal to change is a barrier to any growth. Allowing space in togetherness is the key!

Marital love is often cooled by overly continual association and constant devoted attention. Being away from each other in intervals always strengthens love and desire for each other; almost as if both partners have become strangers and therefore attractive to each other again. Does real love keep a couple continually with each other? Not at all, although some spouses exclaim with joy, "We are never apart from each other," convinced that this is the promise of marriage. This really reflects possessiveness, insecurity, and jealousy: if one of the parties is out of sight, or God forbid is late coming home, he/she is thought to be having a steamy affair while the partner bears all life's hardship. A degree of freedom, happily extended to each other, extends life and marriage for both, in which joy and pleasure is shared, even when one of the two parties is absent, as they are present through the joining of souls.

But when that is not the case, either or both parties "by happenstance" meet someone that seems to be better suited to them. They feel that finally, their real soulmate makes his appearance, a duplicate, the kind of person that the other spouse was when they initially got to know each other before marriage. But who was that initial person anyway? Ruled by the dictum "to do all the foolish things that wise (or foolish?) lovers do," he rushes into a rebound relationship, and again has the initial role of flatterer to a thespian beauty, until he will invariably fall anew into a garden full of thorns, feeling love's intolerable pain again. Not learning from his mistakes, he usually repeats them with the same abandon and enthusiasm as the first time. La Rochefoucauld aptly said, "In the human heart one generation of passions follows another; from the ashes of one, springs the spark of the next" (La Rochefoucauld, 2006, p. 50). It does not even stop him from feeling inspired a third time, overtaken by his archaic anima—to be conquered by the loveliness of the next Helena of Troy, when the web is spun and he is caught again, lured by her hair of gold or her crimson lips! As Voltaire in his most acclaimed novel, *Candide*, expressed through the hero, "I too have known love … It's never brought me anything except one kiss and twenty kicks in the rump. How could such a beautiful cause produce such an abominable effect on you?" (Voltaire, 1959, p. 26). For some, the sign above the door of their house should read, "Abandon all hope, ye who enter here."

Divorce is considered one of the most stressful situations we can endure; usually either party becomes sick or suffers a devastating illness, even death by heart attack (a "broken" heart), bleeding in the eye or a stroke, while searching still for that dream partner that he or she knew "they deserved," thinking that "animosity" (the reflection of the unbalanced anima), will never again make its appearance! But true love always unifies, while strife divides! Or should we just accept this advice from the great philosopher Erasmus: "A good marriage needs a blind wife and a deaf husband." Although vices and virtues are not exclusive to either sex, looking truthfully at society, likely characteristics following this dictum are found. A blind wife for infidelities of her man, blind to his contempt and love of power, blind to his insensitivity. And a deaf husband, for who cannot tolerate to be contradicted? One who cannot stand his wife's animus's opinion and only accepts a dwarf's voice? Who cannot accept equality in a relationship?

The question remains: when we start with such great expectations in marriage, why then does the "love boat" capsize so often? Who is the captain of this dream boat?

Projection: Puppet Master of Love

Men and women must understand that every romantic relationship is started by the anima or animus projection. Man, with his archaic anima, his feminine side, which hides in the darkness and is invisible, is attracted to this anima in the woman who seems irresistible. He falls head over heels for the woman who possesses what he does not find in himself, plenty of anima, and vice versa for the woman. He is injecting a perceived seductive love into the heart of his goddess, gazing up at her, hoping it can still the frenzied sexual desire evoked. It is no surprise that an anima possessed man with an ill-equipped feeling function—which is mostly the case—falls in love unconsciously with a domineering animus-ridden woman. And conversely, a woman who is dominated by a negative critical animus (resulting in lack of confidence and self-worth) might wind up with a husband who will accentuate this situation exactly by putting her down and dominating her for the rest of her life. Such a seductive, attractive game played in the theater of life is the real psychological basis of disastrous relationships and misunderstandings in which people make unrealistic demands upon their partners. Not many marriages are made in heaven but instead most fail miserably through entanglement with the primitive anima and animus respectively. Instead of marrying the partner with whom we will climb to heaven, many hellish blunders are made, making life miserable rather than better. And when we meet a content, happy couple we are bewildered, like anthropologists discovering a lost tribe!

Rather than letting the tree grow till it has stable roots and bears fruit, choosing to solve setbacks in love and having the courage to stand frustrations, too many people—when being in-love ends, once the infatuation stage has passed—leave the marriage and depart on an endless search for the God-like divine relationship using the same failed old-trick and hook of projection. Most separate with the haste of people fleeing the plague.

Driven by dark animalistic instincts, something in that other being initially elicited a spark of attraction; contrary to what many believe, it is not a mature mind that makes someone fall in love. It is hard even to describe that tempest of passion which takes possession of the soul. Its journey seems analogous to the initial trickling of water high in the mountain from the icecap, swelling into a stream and converging into a mighty river, where the first signs of struggle appear. Isn't there an expression, "I was swept off my feet?" But these vivid perturbations of the soul, these bewitching moments, either take their toll on our equilibrium, or more surprising, after the initial conquest, can suddenly stop. In the calm eye of the hurricane, we are prompted to ask, "What the hell happened to me? What took me to the sky on wings, and now I don't even know the reason why! What is the name of the spell that came over me?"

Her name is "anima," mostly primitive in man (or animus for women), and possessed by raging thoughts and mounting frenzy, ruling over her owner. A punitive, non-rational entity that has conquered man before he found true love in which unspoken communication passes from soul to soul. Deception and betrayal, wearing a smile as a garment, have suddenly made their entrance, plunging a dagger into the heart and twisting it round in the wound, hurling us as if in a time machine into a world of icy coldness, void of sweet emotion and laced with well-prepared rational speeches, explaining the terms of a contract while tearing the wings off our shoulders. What a hard thumb, to then reminisce about falling in love at first sight and what it really meant: a frigid mockery of love! This could well resemble falling in love with a *Platina* woman, the ice queen of our Materia Medica, who demands to be reconquered every moment as a new mistress. She does not hate mankind. Worse, she has *contempt* for mankind, being exempt from any reflection and indifferent to other people's misfortune (*indifference while in society*), having no inkling of unhappiness in others. She can show disdain with a wave of her hand, an almost aristocratic dismissal of a noisome inferior (*Del, upon entering the room, she is large* and *Delusion, she is very tall*). In her haughtiness, she reveals a soul that can be a waterless desert while she lives remote from humanity (*Delusion, does not belong to this world*). *Platina* loves herself more than anyone else, adoring her own perceived uniqueness and superiority, but aging and fate will eventually cure her of this sore disease.

"Till death do us part," are universal words uttered at the altar. This is probably the only time when death makes its appearance more than once in life! The divorce rate is high in most civilized countries as insight into each other is usually a step never taken by both parties. The frequency of this misfortune ought by now to have reduced its bitter taste, as it has become customary in modern society. One of the more frequent and legitimate reasons for divorce is that one of the partners did not consider marriage as an equal relationship, causing the other person to react against dominance, wanting a healthier balance in the marriage. Refusal to give up excessive control is often the breaking point. What started as a fairy tale that never really was, easily transforms into edgy and caustic bickering where tension is only temporarily relieved by banter and sex (or bantering sex). As La Rochefoucauld expressed, "Judged by its consequences, love is more akin to hate than to affection." And, "No disguise can mask love, nor feign it for long!" (La Rochefoucauld, 2006, p. 9). How did a human go from years of a loving marriage to wanting to blow someone's head off?

If the man's anima or feminine side is utterly undeveloped

—especially in an intellectual—this highly cultivated man may be blindly attracted to the worst sort of woman, a *femme fatale* rather than a soulmate, who represents his immature anima and upon whom he bestows all the fascinating qualities peculiar to the anima. Despite his intellectual prowess, he needs to marry such a woman as she possesses something which he doesn't, always a lure to anyone! Without knowing it, he is under the spell and attack from the anima. There is an Arabic saying, "If you open a window to the right (animus) and another one to the left (anima) don't be surprised if you get caught in the draft" (*author's insertion in parentheses*). As we desire to succeed in the reunion between anima and animus, it is a good idea to not immediately throw the windows wide open (falling in love at first sight), but to open them slowly, investigating what the wind speed is before getting caught in the whirlwinds and hurricanes of marriage, forces that wreck homes in their furious paths.

True love sees the potentialities in others—even those that are not realized yet. It experiences a fascination to search with intent and curiosity before engaging in superficial sexual behavior as an exercise in discovering who that person is. True love should be draped in silk and satin, for it is a luxury. Most dress love in a cloak of falsehoods and deceptions, flattering each other with vanities they both cherish. These falsities bring them only halfway to love. True love shows kindness, a love that has no need for reciprocity and acknowledgment. True love is not only expressed through the noisy clatter of words—all too frequently used in a masterly, lawyerly way during fights and disputes—but more intimately through the soft caress of hands, through a smile filled with tenderness, through infectious laughter cradled in Buddha's belly, imbuing life with lovely patterns of gestures coming from a butterfly uncaged. Love is communication expanding beyond the borders of words, a veritable bridge between two persons in a moment of togetherness, unseen by others, but always recognized by each other as a meaningful expression of true love. Projections have faded away, changing into an intimate melding of two bodies and souls, touching and embracing each other. Modern human beings have the difficult task to accept and understand the reality of the inner world before it begins to malfunction in moods and obstinate opinions. Indifference, a sign of paralysis, is the worst thing in life. We should *stay alive* and accept and deal through love with the ups and downs in marriage. What grades do we get in life?

Straight A's in Academics, C's and D's in Marriage

We must not forget that the anima, being an archetypal figure is not "good" or "bad," but can represent the duality of all archetypal images, a fair and dark anima, appearing as real women in life. The key is the *relationship* we have created towards her. Although we often experience the bad side of the contra-sexual figures first, the anima is also helpful in finding the right marriage partner. This is the case when the man's anima is turned into a trustworthy adviser, allowing him to turn his radio on the right wave, the role of a mediator between the ego and the Self, who puts the breaks on the fall, so that he can tap into deeper, inner values to make a choice that is the result of the marriage of conscious and unconscious. By being real to each other, most likely we will dissolve these magical images from the unconscious placed on each other, so projections—natural occurring events—are therefore an opportunity to understand our invisible archetypal images and to move our inner life forward.

Succumbing to the inferior anima picture is also noticed when the very serious-minded professor, after many years of marriage, elopes with a burlesque queen. As La Rochefoucauld claimed, "Passions often makes idiots of wise men, and clever men of idiots" (Ibid., p. 1). This kind of uncharacteristic behavior is an example of an expression of psychic activity seeking equilibrium through projection of an archaic anima. It is interesting to see, that frequently the duped wife refers to the younger siren as a "witch," a notion that wholeheartedly would have been supported in the Middle Ages and even today leads to much animosity, murder included! Modern language still expresses this in, "He is bewitched," a projection of man's own primitive demonic anima which guided him to the loved one, a trap that is more like the vision of the mythical singing Sirens who lured sailors to shipwreck with enchanting music. Man must accept his anima and woman her animus as another personality, so they can transform them as an ally, not an enemy or someone they are afraid of, as these archetypal figures remain the bridge to the unconscious and to the individual's soul.

That a woman can fall prey even to the projected anima of a man was illustrated by one of my married patients. With her own animus projection, she had fallen in love with a man at work and started a secret relationship with him. When in her dreams this man embraced her and made love to her, she took this as a sign of true love between them. But this is an objective and not a subjective dream analysis, in which she failed to understand that in dreams, sexual union usually represents a part of the dreamer (her animus in this case) to unite itself with her conscious personality. By choosing this unconscious path and following this projection, rather than making realistic changes in her life, she abandoned her husband and child, leading to a disastrous ending when the lover soon after abandoned her. In her case, she fell in love with the animus projection within herself, one that allowed her to be appreciated, loved, and to fulfill the creative energies smoldering within her. She failed to understand that the correct position of the contrasexual figure, anima or animus, is *inward*, not outward. An example of such a dream is the following dream of a 40-year-old male.

Dream

Last night, I had a dream that I was somewhere and tried to reach my wife; I tried to send her a text message, but my phone didn't make connection.

Analysis

Objectively, as it is his wife he cannot reach in this dream, the dreamer needs to investigate the real situation with his wife (objective analysis of the dream). Does he feel that way in conscious life with his wife, on the mental, emotional, or physical plane? More important, subjectively it reflects his disconnection with his female aspect, the duality in him, the yin/yang (only **two** people appear in this dream!). **Two** is therefore also called the number of symmetry and balance. It can represent the coming together of the male and female. It confirms that "She-Who-Must-Be-Obeyed" needs to have a voice. Is there a drive-impulse in his dream-ego towards a *search* for passionate love and greater intimacy? When accepted and properly related to his anima, it will turn out to be a helpful benefactor and guiding light, possibly seen in next dreams. Of course, we need to keep in mind that solving this problem only in a dream is not enough; we need to react responsibly in daily life to these images and messages. At least the dream shows him *where he is*, but now it is up to him to investigate and test this message; otherwise this important dream communication is in vain. How to change the state (identification) of his anima? Is this a classical example of Freudian theory where every dream represents the fulfillment of a repressed wish, censored by the unconscious? I certainly believe that *some, but not all* dreams represent such a secret wish. Is this dream a disguised form of an expression of his ardent desire for his soulmate? What is the purpose of this dream and why can the dream not tell him directly what is wrong? As this must relate to a high feeling-toned constellation, and possible sadness connected to it, the dream rearranges this underlying message in a compensatory way so the dreamer does not have to dwell over an unpleasant event, but nevertheless is able to bring over its dispatch loud and clear.

I have brought our discussion up to the appearance and role of animus as well as the relationship between animus and anima. What happens in man when he does not accept the union of his sygizi? This is addressed in the next chapter.

14

THE DEATH OF A SOUL: NON-ACCEPTANCE OF THE SYGIZI

"He among us who can best carry the joys and sorrows of life in my opinion is the best educated." — Rousseau

The Midlife and Retirement Crisis: Awakening of the Non-Accepted Secret Partner

A 65-year-old woman pronc to manic depressive episodes and insomnia had the following archetypal dream while suffering a "meaning of life" crisis.

She vividly remembered just one small aspect of her dream, not the whole story. But what she remembered told me that this was not an ordinary dream. Due to the archetypal images appearing in the dream, it could be considered a "big dream," touching on an important aspect of her life incomprehensible to her.

Dream

I woke up from this dream very puzzled as I could retain only one image, almost a vision that remained with me. In this dream there was a cat, tan (not white or black), that was sucking a fish out through its tail. Then I woke up.

Analysis

Although there was a paucity of recalled content, the image contained nothing but archetypal images. I knew that she was a very competitive person, rather boyish and harsh—insensitive to others. I do not know anything further of her conscious life (as she was not my patient), but the images of the fish and the tan cat were enough for me to see what was wrong. Their symbolic significance is as follows.

Fish: Contents of the deep unconscious to be drawn up from its waters. A fish is a primitive cold-blooded creature dwelling in the depths of the ocean—a fish is drawn from the deep, or unconscious. Fishing is an attempt to catch unconscious contents and bring them onto land (integrating to consciousness). "The alchemical fish symbol points to an archetype of the order of magnitude of the Self" (Jung, 1978, Vol. 9, Part II, para. 216). Further, "The symbol of the Self appears here as an 'extremely small' fish in the vast ocean of the unconscious ..." (Ibid., para. 219). And, "A fish is also the symbol of Christ, the Christ within all of us" (Ibid., para. 145).

The cat is her fourth undifferentiated or defective feeling function, represented by an animal (undifferentiated conscious functions often appear in animal form). This cat is sucking the fish (the Self) out from behind (an attack from the unconscious by her anima side), an expression of a primitive inferior feeling function (see "Consequences of an Ill-Equipped Inferior Feeling Function," Chap. 8), a battle between consciousness and the primitive anima, the part of her individuation process that is halted. The tan color is brownish or copper, still belonging to the unconscious (where white, or at least a combination of white/black, would indicate the process of integrating her archaic anima). It is an important message that she needs to change and integrate this undifferentiated fourth function side, even at age 65, as it is "eating up" the Self and causing havoc in her life. Interestingly, she was called by others "a man-eater," reflecting her ruthless animus.

While most people accept puberty as a period of transformation and turmoil creating havoc in the mind of the unsuspecting teenager, there are two other periods in life for humans that seem more mysterious, unexpected, baffling, and difficult to overcome: the middle of life or noontide (age 40), and time of retirement (age 65 in most countries), or what is supposed to be the "golden" age. (Note: this "crisis" is mainly a male problem, as men are generally the breadwinners. Of course, it can happen to women too, but more often when children leave the home.) Both crises have the same origin: difficulties in transcending the "morning" of life towards the "afternoon" of life, as Jung called it, creating a kind of depression around middle life when a man thinks he has reached his greatest strength and success. It is the age when the ego purpose fades from life, and an inner sphere in man tries to dictate a different law, one of introspection, away from the external world and from amassing fame and fortune. All of a sudden, man lands in a wasteland, a wilderness of despair, a life—thought to be full of richness—resembling only a mirage! Man feels inert, driven hither and thither by sad thoughts of that moment. No part of him is engaged, except feeling dreadful anguish about his own nothingness.

At this time, we must become a philosopher, undertaking a kind of thinking that expresses an understanding of life. But for many, when looking back on life and reminiscing, an invisible voice questions, "Do you really think anything you did so far had any value?" The origin of this despair is nothing but a standstill on our individuation path, when we are unable to judiciously integrate the elements of the unconscious, especially the sygizi. Often for men a hideous damsel appears in dreams, as a man is unable to deal with the spiritual side of life when caught in a web of success and materialism. Because of all the early energy used to build a career—mainly through the dominant conscious function, without the need to introduce the sygizi—our motor starts sputtering if we do not respond to them (the anima and animus) correctly in middle life. In midlife, idleness appears, the soul is without aim, and as they say, "If you are everywhere you are nowhere." Oscar Wilde in his novel *The Picture of Dorian Gray*, expresses the same idea: "What does it profit a man if he gains the whole world and loses his own soul?" (Wilde, 1966).

Midlife should be a time for reflection and introspection, to construct within us a monastery of silence in order to achieve an authentic life! Although French philosopher Michel de Montaigne[1] called "idleness" and freedom his two favorite qualities, his kind of idleness brought us magnificent reflections in his volumes of *Essays*, showing he was a real Epicurean philosopher for most of his life. His kind of laziness had more to do with the upkeep of his estate, which he was glad to leave to others, not emulating his father in these responsibilities.

The acceptance of the sygizi can also be a problem, or create confusion, for a very feminine woman like a *Phosphorus*, when after menopause she takes on a natural change of becoming more masculine in the sense of listening to her animus, the voice of determination and self-assurance, and taking more responsibilities. Here is a dream from a 67-year-old woman that illustrates this.

Dream

I dream that I am a young, gay female and that society didn't like the fact that I am gay. I am long and thin (tubercular), with mild, feminine gestures, with a shock of longish dark hair, dark eyes, and pale skin. An operation of some kind is forced on me, but it doesn't change my mannerisms. I am very artistic and creative. At what? It isn't indicated in the dream. Despite the physical operation, I am outgoing, creative, but not very happy. I am sent to psychologists to see if my way of thinking can be changed. In spite of suppression to my being, I try to go on with my life in my art. In the dream I can see myself, but there is no one around me or near me. I am alone and lonely. Besides seeing myself as young, I can see that I am naïve and feeling out of sorts with the world. I feel I am being controlled and cannot understand what all the fuss is about and there is nothing I can do about it. I want to be the me of whoever I am meant to be. I don't feel secure or grounded. And I am not sure if anyone even liked me. The questions I have are why is this happening to me and why can't people leave me in peace?

Analysis

The dream reflects her conscious life in general. This woman is still a *Phosphorus* with all her artistic talents, but she also has become more secure in voicing her opinion and taking care of financial matters, as usually happens. When becoming older, a woman takes more care of the daily business, to be prepared if her husband dies before her—which is often the case. This change in family dynamics is not always received with enthusiasm by the husband who is still attached to the free spirit his wife used to be, while he had the animus in the house—being nourished by the warm feminine *Phosphorus* characteristics.

What is expressed in this dream: "Why do people (husband,

mother) force me to be different when I feel secure and happy?" Also expressed is the isolation she feels (friendless), although she does have a lot of real friends (not just sycophants). An operation (intervention) was done against her will, like the constant tugging at her to change back to her old persona (convenient for others), the warm-hearted, creative, and somewhat naïve and willing person who spread the doctrine of empathy, love, and hospitality with an overflowing conscious feeling function and burning anima. But the acceptance of her animus, the decision maker, the one who no longer has a silent voice and opinion, is desirable for her and should be followed by any woman older than 45. A change in personality—even if it is good for her and an example for others—is often frowned upon, and most likely resisted by those who have not achieved the acceptance of their own sygizi. Her mother may say, "You are my daughter, I am your mom," trying to procure and maintain her authority, while the husband, still struggling with the acceptance of his anima, might deplore the sudden emergence of her animus—an animus that cannot be silenced but must find an outlet, yearning to join the daylight with her endlessly burning anima, a union most glorious for her afternoon of life.

So middle life does not necessarily mean a watershed moment that divides interest and vigor from inactivity and idleness in one's life decline. There is a possibility of a reset by having the courage to take a different road, paved with unexplored avenues and stimulating new possibilities, with growing maturity and knowledge. Learning, exploring, writing, studying, and culture are avenues that remain available till the end of life.

It is typical for a *Lycopodium* type to avoid the introduction of a balanced anima and refuse to heed the urgent message to finally accept her. Consequently, he keeps exchanging in real life one woman for another (*discontented; libertinism; lascivious; nymphomania; duty, aversion to domestic duty*). His world suddenly becomes one of boredom, as he lives a lifeless life, a life previously governed by his one-sided, dominant conscious thinking function. Of course the woman is not exempt from such turmoil when children leave the home ("empty nest syndrome") and her animus starts acting like a demon, telling her that her life "was a waste of time and does not really add up to anything." This is an invitation for her to change course and expand into the world of Logos with constructive and positive choices, before she might change into a cruel, destructive, and judgmental person, tyrannized by the negative animus. What to do? The following text applies to both sexes (although I use the male gender throughout).

First off, where does the dreaded melancholy associated with midlife come from? Often, guided by the "love and goodwill" of parents—in reality, their choice of profession—a man has been forced to operate in his primitive conscious function and is now overcome with the thought that he has worked for so long with empty motivation. It is like living the existence of an ant, simply working, or like being on a restless voyage with no port in sight; exertions made without rationale or sense of satisfaction, a man who so far has found no "home." By first of all recognizing the problem, he can realize that there is a need to switch over to another conscious function by simply asking himself what activity he would still enjoy, as it would prove that the activity would belong to an auxiliary function. Otherwise, he is caught in a territory where he is neither an individual, nor belonging to the conformity of the masses or the safety of the collective unconscious of the newborn. "Midlife crisis" is a real phenomenon. One of the reasons for this fall into a dark abyss is not having followed one's true vocational choice, but an imposed one—usually of patriarchal desire. In order to rise from the abyss, a revitalization is needed, an irresistible impetus translating into a meaning of life that comes from the heart. If this call to change is not followed, stagnation and decay of the soul is the result. Can a man be the scriptwriter of the screenplay called *My Life*? Courage, miasmatic forces, constitution, flexibility, and self-discipline will give the answer!

When life poses the question "Why am I here?" and life seems to be boring, it is time to give one of our auxiliary conscious functions the primary seat. Shedding the possession of the old dominant function and approaching life and its situations with this expanded secondary function should now become the primary goal. Staying with such an auxiliary function for a good amount of time can change the whole psychological structure of one's personality and put new impetus and libido into a stagnant life. Some dissatisfied people try to ward off melancholy by traveling to a sunnier country, but they forget that it is their soul that needs to change, not the climate. They still carry with them the unhappiness they try to leave behind; melancholy is like glue to them, and only when the soul is at peace can they start realizing that happiness, and the good life, is available everywhere.

If our primary conscious function was obstructed at a young age and someone else's dominant conscious function imposed, that becomes an additional and important factor behind midlife crisis. Certainly, middle life and retirement are often a wake-up call and a severe test for us to see where we have arrived in our life journey—whether we have emerged or remain entangled in the twists and turns of our individuation process. To what extent have we synthesized conscious and unconscious elements in our personality, and how well have we allowed an inferior conscious function to be a guiding light in our life? To what extent have we been able to shift the center of our personality from the ego to the Self? We must realize that the final and ultimate purpose of our individuation path is the synthesis of the Self. This is achieved more easily by the born introvert, while the innate extravert finds an easier way in the first half of his life. We are best helped to reach self-realization by turning towards the anima and animus, rather than turning away from them, or the question that everyone in his life experiences at least once will surface: "What is life all about?"

Meaning of Life

Everyone has either witnessed or experienced "the midlife crisis" in his friends or himself. It seems like a second puberty with chaos, as precarious questions arise, and changes take place. There are not only changes in the physiognomy, but also a bruising of the soul. The most baffling and unexpected things happen. The floodgates open, and now appear divorces, childish behavior, depression, periods of living beyond one's means, and yes, more visits to the physician to put a name (besides "midlife crisis") on the many ailments that seem to suddenly overwhelm their victim. Physical symptoms such as palpitations, heartburn, weight gain, and hypertension are not nearly as incapacitating as a profound sense of loss of life, or more adequately, a sense of loss of "the meaning of life." "I have everything," this person says. "I reached the golden years; I am successful in my business, I have a great wife, two wonderful children; I am living in a beautiful home, and yet I feel I am sinking in quicksand, unable to pull myself up." While this is surprising to him, those closest to him—his wife and family—are pulled into the abyss with him, and more often than not, think they do this person a favor by telling him to "get over it," or worse, by berating him for not helping with house chores once he comes home. Such a mental state of sadness or depression is often the source of degeneration and discord, as it can be a landmark in individual souls. In reality, such depression is an illness with origins in trauma and isolation, in deprivation of touch, in violence and neglect, in the loss of home and belonging, and often in the lack of a well-created Self based on the four conscious functions.

There are more mishaps in the afternoon of life! Consequences and compensations are numerous, besides illness. Divorce, and marrying a much younger partner (who is often keen on having a sugar daddy), may provide a man the illusion that he is still virile and a force to reckon with, as she suddenly transforms the older sophisticated man into a crazy teenager going through a second puberty, which is nothing other than the desire for immortal life. Or he might suddenly be caught in a religious conversion, trying to be a mana personality in "guiding" others to self-realization, something he himself has no clue of. Some might even try a totally different profession, as I have seen in several physicians who changed their calling to do something like running a pet store. This is because they are burned-out in their aimless monotone profession. But this sudden conversion, so contrary to their previous life, often creates the same unstable state as before, and what is "hot" today becomes "cold" the next day.

For women—especially before women's emancipation—a transition to the afternoon of life seems strewn with nothing but difficulties and emptiness. I refer here to those women who "only lived for their children," and were therefore unconsciously selfish. They think they were living the life of a saint, but really, never experienced their own inner being. The "empty nest syndrome," an identification with the persona, is a familiar occurrence, leaving women stranded in the journey of life, falling into a vacant, monotone existence.

Remedies like *Aurum*, *Arg-n*, and *Calc-c* can help the person preserve previous values and add newfound ones, to avoid what commonly results otherwise—narrow-mindedness, rigidity, and ultra-censorious behavior. Such remedies will keep people from the fear of becoming pillars of the past or dead wooden sticks. Midlife crises need a different approach than what helped in the past when younger. This is the time when we need to experience the images of the collective unconscious, that unvisited terrain, neglected and feared and yet the door to further spirituality, a world full of images experienced by our ancestors. This unconscious world is full of joy, sorrow, love, and pain; all that which stands for life—*true* life, not only in thought but put into deeds. Isolation brings danger to those who have avoided a true life by keeping busy, which at the end was nothing but a life full of disappointment and melancholy: "What could I have been?"

How to avoid the unoccupied mind's descent into gloom and doom and directionless avenues? Are daydreams and escaping in fancies the solution? We might avoid boredom this way, but it does not resemble real life, a life of existential and intellectual growth. Is it not the physician's task to illuminate the patient's choice to resurrect the phoenix from its ashes? Is finding the meaning of life, as short and perilous as life is, only obtained by personal devotion to society in the best possible way?

"The Proper Response to Life is Applause" — Anonymous

It is usually not the doctor who asks this question of the meaning of life, but the patient. And the homeopath is in a perfect position to pursue the answer to this question, as his role as a psychologist cannot be underestimated. Anyone at some point has asked himself that question: some get stuck in it; some move on. It is certainly the most human principle since no animal in the world worries about the meaning of existence. The activity of an anthill or beehive can be called purposeful but not meaningful. My dog Jami is fiercely loyal, kisses out of gratitude, and lies by my side because I walk and feed her. Our relationship serves a purpose for us both—I supply her with the necessities that a master should for a dependent, loving creature —but it does not reflect the great meaning of life (nor does it mean that she, autonomous and loving as she is, questions the meaning of existence). However, I do appreciate her getting me off my sofa or away from my computer for her daily walks, which let me relish the wonders of Nature. Maybe Descartes, with his motto of the first principle of philosophy, "*Cogito, ergo sum,*" "I think, therefore I exist" (Descartes, 1988, p. 36), would not agree with me, but my dog is a living being with an "I" and a "Self," full of personality with plenty of feelings, emotions, and desires. I rather believe, as Plato said in Book II of *The Republic*, that "A dog is the most philosophical beast in the world." Jami is a pacifist putting the carnation in the rifle: she wants to make love, not war. "I am a bundle of love and loyalty," she says. She pretends to obey me, but when the rose-colored glasses fall from my eyes, I see that she is fully in charge, telling *me* what to do. And when I don't pay attention right away, she kisses me, gives me a paw, and of course a strong bark in final attempt, telling me with a voice of command—which is part of her nature—what she wants.

As mentioned before, if patients don't ask you the question of the meaning of life directly, they will seek help to resolve it indirectly by showing up with physical problems, and even more, in states of melancholy and subdued depression, which at first don't seem to need acute intervention. Yet for that person, life feels like swimming upstream: everything is a chore, every situation seems to have more challenges to resolve than solutions to be found. It is mainly a *spiritual disease.* This spiritual disease can be more devastating than any disease on other planes because it isolates the patient, who often *reproaches himself* and thinks he is the only one to ever face this crisis. I can think of people in a *Nat-m*, *Sepia*, or *Calc-c* state—the latter remedy being close to the number one depressed remedy, *Aurum* (besides *Arg-n*), which often comes to the rescue of one descended into an abyss of darkness.

For too many, death arrives without the individual ever having touched the roots of their own existence. Several delusions creep into the minds of such drifters, sailing as they are in a rudderless ship. They may have *Delusions:* of being *unfit for this world* and of *not being appreciated;* of having *lost the affections of his friends*, as well as *his friends have lost all confidence in him* and *he has done wrong.* These are all delusions belonging to an *Aurum* patient, and no matter that family and friends claim the contrary, it falls on deaf ears for the depressed person. *Aurum* can victimize himself by announcing that he has not achieved enough, that he has not put out enough effort, and that he has let down his friends (*Del, he has neglected his duty*). Rather than berating life with "Why did life not give what I asked for," this is rather the time to ask, "What do I owe life and where did I fail to live up to my potential?" How did such a person come this far—how did he sink to such a low point?

Traditional Chinese Medicine teaches a precise time that women and men go through this crisis, although men seem to suffer more from it. The reason for this is that men's lives are geared more towards success and performance, while most women, even despite having a job on the outside, will rarely neglect their nourishing role in the family. The magic numbers in TCM indicate the 7 and 8-year cycles for women and men, respectively: for women, the magic number is 7, and 35 (5x7), when she starts looking more inward, as the latter corresponds with the time limit when pregnancy is still optimal (see footnote 1, Ch. 11, on p. 671). Not uncommonly, women who had only a career and no children up to this point, yearn for a little one, and this is easily seen in what TCM would call late pregnancies: from age 35 till 50 in present times. With men, the magic number is 8, and 40 (5x8), 40 being the age of maximum strength, when a small voice within starts questioning his existence. Or is it, his essence? As Sartre said, "*existence before essence*," a later call for meditation and reflection on what life is all about. Suddenly, there is a quest for "how to continue living" without having to look back with a mournful soul. To take an existential stand is to accept to some extent the meaningless of life, the absurd and the irrational element. Failure to do so is to neglect the total picture of man. But the meaning of life remains alive as can be seen in the situation of contact between each other. Is the midlife crisis the only obstruction in our individuation path, or is there another one, even more tragic to overcome?

The Tragic Sense of Life

Alas! Midlife is not the only time we are confronted with such a dilemma. There is another call for those who identify with their persona, when retirement is near or entered. Preoccupied with earning money, raising a family, and enjoying the power of position during adult life while receiving accolades for hard work, one may have forgotten to look inward and now becomes a petrified pillar, cast aside by young people as old and done with life, with nothing more to offer. In this suddenly appearing depression upon retiring, every warm color in the person has faded into a somber grey; any desire in life has left the person (*indifference to pleasurable things* and *to everything*). The man has lost, along with everything else, all motivation; day after day he does nothing, or as close to nothing as humanly possible. He feels like quietly fading away, waiting for the end of life. He might not always openly express it, but often hears that powerful inner animus voice: "You are not needed anymore!" Obliged to carry on through life, he realizes he does not know how, overcome by irrelevance. Suddenly he feels like he has fallen into a world where people are strangers, having nothing in common with even the most familiar and dearest (*Delusion, forsaken by friends and family*). The world has become the most unthinkably frightful desert, a desert paved with streets but without friends and family, where the perceived climate is worse than hostile and indifferent. At this point, an *Aurum* depressed person makes a wager with himself—weighing the balance of his life. If the positive events supersede the negative ones, he decides to struggle further for some time; if the balance is negative, he might as well throw himself from a height (*suicidal disposition, throwing himself from a height, from a window*), turning off the lights for good in his dark somber life.

The inner man has no more relations and interests. He is enveloped in a dark cloud and hears the greatest collective question facing man in his life history: "What was it all about?" Additionally, we do not usually find the answer to this fundamental question of life because we never stopped to examine it. It is only when a cog stops the rotating wheels of a busy life that fills the hours with work, sleep, eating, and other common necessities, that we start questioning the purpose of it all, and either carry on with increasing squeaks, or we reject the flaws and absurdity of life.

We are at the doorstep of a new life when we hear the loud animus voice: *"Here are the souls of men; which one will you choose?"* Are we choosing to do something purposeful, or do we get sidetracked with idleness or navel-gazing? Is there place for a divine act to create a human masterpiece, which requires honest and hard work, maybe for the first time in our life? The lesson is always the same. All is made more precious, not less, by the impermanence of life. Loss is a kind of external conscience, urging us to make better use of our finite days. Disappearance and loss remind us to notice the transience to cherish, the fragility to defend.

But our cry may come: "No one needs me anymore!" Of course just before retirement, the successful businessman who dedicated his whole life to the glory of his company thinks about his well-deserved retirement: plush vacations, maybe acquiring a second home in a warmer place, playing more tennis or golf, and offering extensive parties for his friends. Is this the answer? It is amazing how many fail to find the same kind of satisfaction in retirement as during their working period. There is *reproaching himself; confusion after mental exertion; want of confidence and thinks others have none in him, making him unhappy; with apprehension of heart disease*—not a stable peace of mind to resurrect from this tsunami. These are symptoms of *Aurum metallicum*, or gold. Gold is a symbol of energy, consciousness, God, libido, and a male or yang radiating force, related to the sun; of consciousness beyond destruction, as it always keeps its color even if unearthed after many centuries (contrary to copper, silver, etc.), and is therefore associated with incorruptibility and immortality. It seems indeed that the sun has set in his life, just as the sun loses its strength once it passes its zenith at noon.

The *Aurum* person is initially strong on the mental and physical plane, but weak and fragile on the emotional plane. It is a house of cards ready to crumble at the slightest contradiction. Obviously, when one tries as hard in life as the *Aurum* person does, he expects to be respected, understood, and not criticized. We therefore understand his reaction to criticism: *he is excessively disposed to take offense; even the least thing seems offensive to him and affects him deeply and causes resentment. The least contradiction excites him to the greatest anger and he becomes choleric and quarrelsome. He is extremely affected and provoked by the least circumstances, which had the appearance of hurting his feelings; and suffers therefore from Ailments from contradiction.* It is not uncommon that many *Aurum* people hesitate to retire and find all kinds of excuses to keep working way past the official retirement time: "I am still needed. I can't be replaced." The real reason is of course that they are afraid to be lost, to have no purpose, as everything in their life was based on performance, honor, and power, which all disappear when they are relegated to their home and own thoughts—a created vacuum that nothing seems to fill. For them, the end of a successful career is the end of the line.

Often, I have seen when they finally take the plunge that

they are struck with a debilitating illness, as if the wind was taken out of their sails, making it impossible for them to at long last take another look at life. I truly believe that this illness is almost a death wish, as only vaguely in their mind was there still a meaning of life, but in reality they were not convinced at all, as they feared the isolation away from the previous morning life full of bright sun, which seemed would never disappear. The gate to the unconscious—so well-guarded throughout life—is bursting under the pressure of dark forces and instincts, which need relief after such a long imprisonment. Of course, there is also the possibility that the person, because of illness, feels he has not been able to fulfill his role and duty as a father. The following story told by one man, expresses this insidious battle of the soul:

> "I have been feeling a **sadness over my condition** more than in a long time, with a **restlessness** and not knowing what to do with it. I have been, since beginning January, very **self-critical**; because I don't know who I am and what I want to do with my life. In short—a 'loser' that didn't succeed in anything so far in life. I am concerned and disappointed with myself and my career, concerned with my own and my family's future since I am so weak and don't know how I will be able to provide for my kids and their security in the future. I am concerned about the state of the world, and how the natives once again are treated at Standing Rock, etc. I see things through the eye of a pessimist at this point, like I am a sponge for negativity, and it is clear I am very sensitive right now to horrible or sad stories. I long for and am better from stability, continuity, and predictability, but neither world—politics nor the weather—gives me any reassurance, and soon, I will be contacted by the social security again as the three years I had financial support is coming to an end, and I most likely will have to go a new 'round' with them to

> convince them of my state, to what hinders me, and my bodily disposition is always a difficult one when asked to reveal what I can and cannot do.
>
> "When thinking back on the last months I see this longing for something. I don't know what, and a sense of being lost again, and irritability and frustration and feeling stuck in a (dark) place and very short days with little daylight, coupled with sadness over my condition and a sentimental mood and nostalgia. I also have felt a longing to connect deeper to people, friends and family, maybe from a realization I have more superficial bonds to people than I thought and I want it to be more heartfelt, and also I think a longing to have the security I would get from being connected to more people in a deeper way. Maybe I just want more family around me?"

We see many *Aurum* rubrics in this patient: *irritability; Del, neglected his duty; Del, he is unfit for this world; Del, is not appreciated; Del, friends have lost confidence in him,* and *has lost the affection of friends; Delusion, melancholy; self-reproach; Delusion, does nothing right; desires death* and his extreme *chilliness* all point to *Aurum*. A dose of 30C came quickly to the rescue. Such a state of depression, and we could say also of boredom, is a syphilitic state because at the end one feels nothing and there is indifference to joy and to pleasurable things. It is a path of being everywhere and nowhere. As this patient is sad, he still feels *something*, and *Aurum* will rescue him from sliding down into the abyss. Of course, this is only the start of the journey!

Reaction to the remedy dose:

> "I started with the 30c before going to bed yesterday and so far, it feels good I must say. A stillness and calmness entering I have not felt in a long time. There are many things in *Aurum* that I see fit, I even said to my wife the other day,

> without noticing or realizing till I read about it yesterday, 'I don't have what it takes to be in this world, I seem to be unfit for it' (***Del, unfit for the world***). I've felt a lot lately like a 'Friday car' (***Del, worthless***). I even have been thinking my wife and the kids would be better off if I was replaced by someone else. I know that is a tricky thought of questionable truth and one that for many ended in suicide. I do not go down that road of thinking I want to end my life, but sometimes when things are heavy I have the thought that **death would be a relief** (*also in the proving symptoms of Aurum*) as I then would be able to rest and have a break from this world that I seem to be unfit for." (*Author's notes in italics.*)

Dreams after *Aurum* LM showed that this man was still doing well, but now returning to the previous situation somewhat. Another dose of *Aurum* LM was advised, and after this next dose, his response was: "I remembered two very interesting dreams, yesterday and the day before."

Dream one

A dead man is found close to a spring or a well. He is my age and looks healthy. It looks like he has been walking in the desert and has a white (clean looking) cloth wrapped around his head. It is a dry Mediterranean-like landscape. A village is on the hillside in the background. He is found dehydrated just four meters from the well, and it is a surprise he did not find it or did not rehydrate from it.

Dreamer's analysis

I have been taking this dream seriously. What is the well (source) in my life, and why am I not seeing it or hydrating from it? Possibly I am on track with what I have been writing above, but I am still looking for more answers. My individual freedom counters the restraints family life brings, and could also be lying in the way (possibly imagined), from *too much sense of responsibility or Del, neglected duty*; maybe I am just in front of the well?

Author's analysis

This dream refers to the untapped good, productive and creative side of the shadow. Indeed, the well, his salvation, is close by, yet he did not drink. As usual, death in a dream (every person/animal in a dream is a reflection or aspect of the dreamer) indicates that something must die, something must change! (If another male dies in the dream of a male patient, it means that a change in his shadow side needs to be integrated.)

Dream two

Similar theme: I have a car that I converted from being fueled by petrol to natural gas. Since converting to the CNG I must go much longer to refill and fuel up and I think this is a nuisance and takes a lot of my time and energy. I go to a store to see if they sell some sort of containers or petrol can for CNG. It turns out I need three different devices or advanced cans and when I ask the price it is 4000 euros. I comment that this is about the same as the remaining value of the car (the same we have in real life). And the sum is huge to me, more than double what we have saved away for emergencies. The salesman proposes I can take it home for free to think about the offer and look at it back home before making my decision. When I get home with the stuff my wife had a call from the salesman saying he wanted me to return it already if I did not buy it. I just got home, it is 5:30 a.m., we live in a bigger city and no way will I be back in time with the goods before closing hour. I try to find the receipt from the store to call them and say I cannot get back today and ask why he changed his mind. But I fail to find any number when looking through the receipts and find no way to get in touch with him before I wake up from a disturbance in the middle of the dream.

Dreamer's analysis

So, I changed "source" of energy, and where I live I cannot easily, or without energy and time output, refuel very well. Changed from an old system to a newer one, albeit maybe not established enough, maybe a premature choice of conversion. I better change back to gasoline or I have to present a lot of money/energy to facilitate the refueling? I parallel this to the move from a more populated and diversified place to this place. What I fuel from here for little money (nature, and I live more or less right in it) will not be in reach as easily in a big town, but will be the other way around: an expensive project in both time and money and energy to get out of the big city, for example to get some nature or hunting. Here, that is virtually just around the corner or outside my house.

Author's analysis

Indeed, same message as before: needs more energy, but from a source easier to tap into.

Guided by a balanced presence and acceptance of the sygizi, and putting the unconscious in front of us to pull us forward, to transfer the previous exuberant energy to a cause or worthwhile object, we will become who we *truly can be*, a more complete person, the person we want to be and can be, a philanthropist or lover of mankind (not necessarily exhibited with money). As an old Chinese master said, "Worldly people lose the roots and cling to the tree-tops."

To be concerned about the meaning of life is not always a reflection of a disease state. We can ask ourselves that question to change direction, to make our life more meaningful. And not just for us, but especially for others, which in turn will reward us as the benefactor. We might use our talents and money to now bring spiritual and material help to less fortunate beings in this world. Posing the question in this context is not a reflection of a neurosis, but rather of a soul-searching quest to improve our quality of life. After all, each person must find his/her life task, an "independent" responsibility. Those immortal words of John Kennedy ring in my ears: "Ask not what your country can do for you—ask what you can do for your country." In this context, the answer to the dilemma of the "meaning of life" was simple for me: *"Do not ask what life has done for you—ask what you have done for life!"* And perhaps more relevant, and true for any individual, *"What kind of world am I creating with my daily actions, and would I want to live in it if someone else was creating it?"*

It should be clear to us all that life is expecting something from us, that man himself is being questioned. And no man is ever too poor or incapacitated to not be able to *give* to life. Do we need great equipment to make ourselves happy? Fortune and prosperity, and misfortune and adversity are just two sides of the same coin of life. More than we realize, we can make ourselves happy, instead of bobbing up and down on the waves of euphoria and depression. Tranquility in the face of the ups and downs of life should be sought after, while at the same time exercising a degree of alertness so as not to be surprised by life's fickleness, to be able to parry an initial attack and keep steadfastness of mind. Accidents, injuries, functional losses, and crippling diseases defy us to find a meaning of life. People who face pain and death without flinching have achieved the greatest gift granted to humankind. There are also plenty of people who start life with a biological handicap, and their defiance towards an apparent bad start makes them achieve great things. Think of Professor Hawkins. His body crippled by ALS (a syphilitic miasmatic condition), he has been able to produce ground-breaking mental work, admired all over the world. Through his work, the clarity of his ideas, and the grace of his being, he was a bearer of light. He was a prime example that a healthy mind can endure any physical hardship, while a sick, unbalanced mind is tortured by the slightest physical discomfort.

One of the reasons people might face the eternal question of life is that they are locked in a job which seems either meaningless, or more frequently, not financially rewarding enough to fulfill all their useless whims and hopes. I was reminded of this when I lectured in China about homeopathy to a group of medical doctors. One of them told me he gave up being a TCM physician, "Because it did not pay enough nor give the stature that being a medical doctor provided." That certainly struck home for me, as from the beginning of my career I made the conscious choice between becoming a physician in a fashionable and profitable private practice, or becoming an outcast as a homeopathic and alternative physician, who all my life had to endure the wrath and cynicism, not to mention the name-calling, of my colleagues. But it was an easy choice, as I chose inner fulfillment above an ensured successful financial life. In remaining faithful to my vocation, I will never have to confess when looking in the mirror, "The man I am greets mournfully the man I might have been."

If a person does not feel a sense of fulfillment in his job, the fault is in the person and not in the work. Work itself does not make the person indispensable; it only gives him the chance to be so. When I did my internship in neurology to become a medical doctor in the US, I started at the lowest level. But my love for the patients and respect for the dedication of the nurses made me irreplaceable to the point that the visiting professor on his rounds thought I was a third-year resident, not a first-year resident. I felt fulfillment in the small role I was assigned: I received no financial compensation for the whole year, but plenty of human fulfillment by being close to the patients and dulling the merciless sting of the hospital environment for them. I did not follow all the mandates and words of my supervisor, as they would have become like the iron bars of a cage, entombing me in the world of others. I also chose to immerse myself in and become one with the world of the nurses and patients, relegating my doctor's status and benefits. I cared as an invisible but omnipresent shadow—not asking for appreciation—and was amply rewarded with love, rather than being imprisoned in the coldness of the hospital and the gang of physicians who, while doing rounds, would discuss the most personal and intimate aspects of the patient's disease in front of the ill person, not noticing the despair on his face when hearing the "bad news."

The true work of a doctor and homeopath lies in what he does beyond the purely medical duties of blood taking, ordering tests, providing the homeopathic remedy, giving orders to nurses, etc., and beyond approaching patients on an entirely intellectual level. The art of medicine is much more than a cold-blooded diagnosis and therapeutic protocol, so often executed by allopaths and homeopaths alike. A physician can do his work as a well-functioning robot, or as a physician who brings his great personality to work, who excels in the manner with which he does his job. Which physician as a patient do you want? We can agree with the German philosopher, poet, and dramatist Christian Friedrich Hebbel (1813-1863): "Life is not anything; it is only the opportunity for something!"

That my profession worked out to a satisfied end may surprise you, when informed about its beginning. I had not chosen my profession; it was my scheming father who imposed it on me, based on the principle of father authority. At age 13, my appointment had been confirmed. I was going to be a physician in the Belgian army. Not out of patriotic love for his country, but because the education was free—monetarily at least, but not free of cost to my soul and wellbeing. Contractually, I was obliged to stay in the army till age 55. Yet I never could integrate into this military world. I was a solitary person out of necessity: punished constantly for lack of military "spotlessness," for being contemptuous of order, and for military subordination, I spent most of my weekends locked up in the vast military compound, a sole inhabitant with the works of Schopenhauer and Greek and Roman classics. I secretly loathed my father's future plans. Had I asked to become a physician? I had to renounce my own burgeoning Self, at least initially.

Being an avid reader, I happened to read about Dr. Schweitzer's medical work in the Belgian Congo (now Zaire). One year before, I was an aspiring soccer player, hoping to get fortune and fame worldwide. That was over! I then felt called upon to become Schweitzer's assistant, and the next three lonely years in the military cadet school only fostered this dream. This vocation was real! My father, the high priest, vouched for it. The poor Africans were awaiting my arrival. Of course, I did not know that Africa had to wait for another forty years, as I was side-tracked in a course that bound me to marriage, children, ignorance and youth, and so-called "sense of duty." The sole object of my passion was heroism for those poor exploited people by my own government. They needed my presence. But is everyone so lucky as to find a solution, or does the fear of death become the focus of some?

Acceptance of Death

The choice of Greek philosopher and poet Titus Lucretius Carus (ca. 99 BC-ca. 55 BC), author of *On the Nature of*

Things, an Epicurean at heart, was to accept that a human has a transitory existence. His advice was to embrace real life, rather than letting life slip away from you in an overwhelming ocean of fear and anticipation. Doors open and doors close, and we must prepare to leave when fate (mostly self-fabricated) calls upon us. If we are enduring continual torment by obsessive thoughts about death and try to find a million ways to avoid it (in the sense of an *Arg-nit* personality who is terrorized by "What if ...?" situations), we are paralyzed and stop living, unable to put one step forward without deep anguish. It is fear that accompanies hope, a mind hanging on to what the future might bring. A mind like this fails to adjust to the present. It is only focused on the future and the past, as memory recalls the fears of the past and foresight anticipates them. The *Arg-nit* and *Arsenicum* personalities, with the help of great imagination, can even turn health into disease, an illness not yet discovered by any diligent physician he has visited. They paint a tortured Self with many diseases that will never really visit them (*Del, his body will putrefy; Del, contaminates everything she touches; Del, time has come to die*). What an unhappy existence—killing the person while he is alive—losing the present through anticipation anxiety about the future. I think we will be miserable enough in time without having to bring so many cares upon ourselves. Many are suffering before it is necessary to suffer! And the future always comes soon enough!

No matter where we hide, death can find us. Oliver Wendell Holmes (American physician, essayist, and poet, 1809-1894) said, "We are all sentenced to death for the crime of living." The problem is, we know nothing of the day or means of execution! Death sometimes comes upon us with such swiftness that we do not know how it came. Life is but a venture. No one can prophesy the time and means whereby the curtain shall close (except the *Aconite* personality who predicts his death). And no one should prefer to know all that is ahead of him; he should choose the venture! It is for most of us the vitality, hope, and joy as we live life that keeps our mind from dwelling upon the day of our demise. Make the most of what you have! Each day should count. We must learn how to live as if we would die tomorrow, and at the same time, as if we would live forever. In general, people die the way they lived: the brave die bravely; the peaceful peacefully; the fearful in terror! Each in their own way will settle the struggle for control to take a last breath—an inevitable outcome—with the tools Nature provided. Witnessing death as bystanders, we hope to show more courage when dying than others were able to find, and hopefully we can help a dying person maintain his courage. True love from others can reduce death anxiety, both by providing a space for people to share and voice their fears, and by contributing to a well-lived life free of regrets. We should try to school ourselves to take life as it comes—a frame of mind almost impossible for most to achieve.

After all, what we are, what we have become, is the result of the past that molded and modified our being. The wise human adjusts to all the inevitable experiences that happened to him—to fit even the worst experience within his life. An *Arg-nit* personality would do well to follow Epicurus's advice to transfer his thoughts from unpleasant to pleasant ones! Such exchange unfortunately is not always a constancy. Everyone at some point can be overcome by the stings of unpleasant thoughts when he thought he armed himself with great intentions. We should not be called an extraordinary human being if we wrestled with the fidgetiness of fortune instead of accepting it. Not everyone is like Socrates, an individual of exceptional moral integrity, who when condemned to death did not seek diversion but fixed his gaze on it, as a true stoic, considering death a familiar part of his life.

Above all, in death we are entombed in other people's memory and perception and there is nothing we can do anymore to change it! Death is the great robber, depriving us of all new creations, pleasures, and projects we might experience, a place where there is no more road. So let's not die while we live! Too many reach their zenith early and then start to fossilize, afraid to start new directions of life and to be influenced by new thoughts. And others are alive so little as to be forgotten; the purpose of their life is simply to make the pass over to the other side where calmness and silence reign.

As I write these words, people daily—myself included—will lose their grip, and some sink to eternal sleep, mingling soon with the elements that combine to make our earth, and soon are known no more. I sometimes wonder why I am still writing about desires, disappointments, worries, and despair that have moved me in my brief stay on earth. But while I am still alive, I not only detest boredom, but even fear it. I write and create just to prove that I still have emotions and appetites, even with the mist gathering about my head reflecting that my stormy journey draws to a close. I write to help pass the time that remains. There are many books out there that teach us "how to live," happier and especially longer, but I think anyone who teaches us how to die teaches us also how to live.

Unfortunately, when many hapless people undergo terrible and painful illness, they seem to have contempt for life since they can no longer enjoy the pleasures of life. Life and death are not two separate entities; they are part of the same undetermined rope—a short or long one—but there is no discontinuity. When approaching death, we can have many thoughts: anger, despair, relief, acceptance, and sorrow, just to name a few strong and fleeting emotions. But it is not a matter of dying as opposed to living. We can only hope that we joined the collective destiny when we were born; death is inevitable, death started when we were born. There is no denying that when we are born, we join the fellowship of the uncertainty of life that will end in death. To begin to exist is the start of proceeding to non-existence; it is a race towards the end, when that cord will be cut—after the cutting of the umbilical cord that gives us that first cry and breath, the second cutting will be our last breath. No one can predict who will be the most memorable after meeting this maligned fate. I must confess, I have felt bewildered and surprised to see that some of the most noble souls, that lived life to the fullest, never complained! Is it because they surpassed dilettantism and became true professionals at how to live?

Boredom in life is equal to not having a use for life. And yet such idle people are the first ones to complain they are losing life. What does it matter, what would they still want it for? Of course, there are some people who feel both ways. I think about the philosopher *Sulphur* who always will tell us that he is not in a hurry to visit the antechamber of the dead, to wave a white flag, a coming to terms with extinction; there is also the eternal lover of adventure, *Phosphorus*; and the family-loving *Calc-carb* —the latter who, till the end, or when going through a near-death experience, would love to fantasize (or create false epiphanies) that they saw "a wonderful blinding heavenly light, feeling themselves floating towards it." The *Calc-carb* would love to see his family members and beloved pets bounding across the rainbow bridge (count me out for the first group, but lovingly I would accept the second one if possible), while the *Phosphorus* person wants to see pearly gates with undiscovered countries to which she flies on her golden Turkish carpet and meets mystical heroic figures from history that were spellbinding to her during her real life. If it makes their lives more meaningful and approaching death more tolerable, so be it.

Of course, emotionally, following the instinct and will to live, I will no doubt act as anyone else at the last moment of my existence. But intellectually, I only must look back and know that life can be a serious burden, a mixture of some pleasure and a lot more sorrows. Many believe in immortality, a future life on the other side of the curtain, but in my view this is more based on fear than belief, hoping that no one will ask them for clear evidence as no scrap of such proof will be found. Rather, we should accept that death is the great destroyer of all human illusions and delusions. This way we will not be dead while still alive. Even those who believe in an afterlife don't seem to be in a hurry to go there, as most prefer senility above ascending to the heavenly abode and exploring the promised land. Life as a whole is pure theater!

So why do most people fail to find courage and dignity at the time of death?

Mishaps at Inopportune Moments

I here list some misfortunes in life, mishaps that people suffer. Of course, these are not all of them, as the reader might have other considerations that he finds more important. But some of these are of a collective nature and occur at the morning of our life.

- Not trying to activate and increase their auxiliary, and above all, inferior conscious functions, letting their dominant function dictate their life journey while often hurting themselves and others.
- Not looking into the shadow side as if they never had one, or just considering it a hostile abode—an ice-cold tomb never to be visited or investigated.
- Using projection and suppression at the slightest trouble within themselves—two defense mechanisms that are destructive in the end and the cause of many disagreements and foolish behavior.
- Not choosing to follow "the road less traveled," the hard journey to self-realization, and getting lost on minor side-tracks, congested with materialism,

egotism, misplaced pride and delusional approaches to life.

- Living only in the world of consciousness, making it the monotheism that guides their limited existence —not descending like Dante into the underworld.
- Concentrating on what disease they will develop (and consequently, living in a world of fear and anxiety) rather than being pro-active and following the advice of the *Organon*. Look at Aphorism 77, in which lifestyle plays a primary role and produces many *non-true* chronic diseases. It is here that modern countries suffer more than Third World countries. Allopathy does not know real "preventive medicine," as it concentrates on finding the first stages of pathology, as with heart tests, cancer research, MRI's and x-rays, etc. Any minor complaint is addressed with suppressive medications, allowing the patient's disease to travel from psora to sycosis to syphilis, ending with sudden destruction or self-destruction. Many claim that allopathy is the supreme science, but it is neither supreme nor science! It is normal, of course, that children should outlive their parents. However, the family miasmatic overload (Aphorisms 74 and 78) produces defective children early in life, not to mention other unfortunate events like accidents, murder, and yes, aggressive allopathic treatment.

We should take the advice of the nobleman and writer, Michel de Montaigne, in his *Essays*, where in the essay entitled, "That to Philosophize is to Learn to Die" (de Montaigne, 1987, p. 17) he sheds some ideas about the prevailing excruciating fear of death. Get "busy," is his short answer! Don't be preoccupied with the possibility of dying from one of the thousands of diseases (and present medical science has added plenty more), but rather spend your time contently as each day can be the last day to shine on you. Anything that you can do another day can be done now, especially those acts and deeds that not only give pleasure to your heart but seem to spread goodwill among neighbors and friends. Get busy: read, write, exercise, observe Nature, relate to others, and so many other things you never found time for.

We need to be able to convert losses to gain, by focusing on a topic or subject previously unknown. Such restoration on a different plane creates an inner strength and newfound joy, to do some things we were not able to find or to call upon when we were in possession of our previous capacities. It is the result of our willingness to not let our soul dwell in the desert. The duration of life is not the all-important and final goal of a human; what is more useful is what we made of life. Death should be as familiar as living. Ancient Egyptians had a rather macabre way of getting used to the idea of death: during their banquets, they brought in a mummified corpse to serve as a reminder that death is a common sight and occurrence. Michel de Montaigne would have fully agreed with this custom as he was all for "depriving death of its strangeness, to have nothing more often in mind than death," so that each day of life becomes more meaningful. We should get used to using the word death, rather than diluting it through periphrases like, "He passed away," or "He lived a good and full life," where we prefer the word "life" over death, even for the one who passed. I am reminded of death once in a while when (besides accidents) I find in my yard near the bird feeders, a bird dead from old age, surrounded by plenty of food and water provided by my loving *Phosphorus* wife, who greets them every morning with "hello my little darlings." (After doing her "precious" yardwork she watches them with love and pride from a rocking chair, because even when sitting she likes to feel as if she were still in motion, evoking the soul of an eternal traveler.)

So many questions should be asked: Have you lived your own life, or that of a family member? Have you followed your desired career path and vocation? If not, why not? Was it the lure of an easy job or a well-paid one? Did you fill a family job you were expected to? Why do you have to ask these questions, if everything seems to be right, but then again, is it right more in the eyes of others than in your own heart? Why does the sun come up every day, but darkness seems to occupy most of your soul? Have you tried to listen to the message of your dreams, inviting new possibilities, new identities and new attitudes (personified in dreams as a young child)? Have these dreams shown the restoration of an old persona, a step forward in self-actualization?

It is possible that a person has had those convincing wishes of having created a "glorious, fulfilling life," but dreams will express with force the opposite message—that renewal of a new Self is necessary in order to grow in the afternoon of life. Too often, the insult of having lived in oblivion is added to our final departure.

A special chapter needs to clarify the meaning of the cyber delusion, or CD, omnipresent in most of us—a hindering or nourishing factor? Remember that a dream takes the compensating form of a conscious one-sided thought, and the CD, as we will see, is a thought that will occupy most of the ego of the patient, preoccupying him fully. It therefore deserves our attention and is addressed in the next chapter.

SECTION FOUR

Birth of the Cyber Delusion (CD) and Direction of Cure

15

THE BIRTH OF THE CYBER DELUSION

"Everything new comes from within." — *C. G. Jung*

Deceived we may be,
but harboring hope,
we dwell in a corner of our conscious,
suppressing the torrential cries
that we must deny,
quelling the voices that remind us
of the reality we must spurn,
squirming to avoid,
in order to smile as though we are whole.

The years, covered in dust,
pursuing a life smothered in lies,
concealing the truth, we so
zealously guard from ourselves.

The truth, veiled beneath my smile,
so carefully painted upon the rigid

statue of my core.
No one can guess the treacherous
secrets of my heart.
I am so deaf that the
increasing echoes of my God
remain unheard.

My friend time has taught me
to be still,
as my smile belies
the crumbling within.

I suspect my shattered Self
will permit the ceaseless cries
to be heard as a whisper
or even as a glimpse
of my shadow, hidden and yet,
threatening to claim its
rebellious independence.

Finally, with my brittle façade,
the day has come
and I surrender to my reflection.
My tormented thoughts are
spurting out of my broken smile.

I am naked and all is visible
to every passerby.
Funny, I never knew
what I resembled.
Could it perhaps be you?

(Seta Araz Shahinian, 2004, inspired by and dedicated to Dr. Luc)

Definition

Cyber delusion (CD) comes from the Greek *cybernetes*, meaning "the helmsman," he who steers the ship and constantly adjusts the tiller of the ship in response to information obtained from the environment. The helmsman within is the cyber delusion or fixed idea that steers one's "ship," the sum of the personal unconscious and conscious. Most people are only partially aware of the conscious part of their life and completely unaware of their unconscious forces, so the CD, hidden and roaming in the vast unconscious darkness, steers and dictates the ego, master (the tiller) of the conscious. In other words, it is in the unconscious that the CD hides in the shadow side, the dark and neglected side of each person that steers man's consciousness! This is quite a frightening thought, considering that this CD is repressed and unacknowledged by most, and therefore remains primitive and archaic. Therefore, a rather primitive and unsophisticated entity is the orchestrator and conductor of our life. It is obvious that a human must be silent sometimes, because not to talk shows that he is ready to listen, ready for soul-searching, a prerequisite of spiritual growth. The perfect road to individuation, to becoming a psychologically balanced individual, would progress in a straight line; this, however, is never possible, even for those few who have the introspection and the courage to investigate their shadow side. Even individuals who are truly spiritual will often fall off the proverbial wagon when circumstances force them to operate in their natural inferior conscious function (see Chap. 8).

This forceful entity, the CD, dictates everything we think (mental), everything we feel (emotional), and everything our body feels (physical); in other words, the CD is the director of our holistic mind-body being. The cyber delusion is the impetus of our every thought and action and becomes part of the shadow, an archetype hidden in our unconscious. The CD can result in the unbroken permanence of one mood or emotion, indicating a serious disorder of the psyche—the Self under attack of a numinous and autonomous entity. In this case, the CD creates a permanent fixed thought, occupying a major part of the conscious, where the human runs around in circles, trapped and searching for an exit in vain and in desperation, lost in a suffocating labyrinth.

We can also be dominated by a false cyber delusion. Many people cling to dreams that they lack the talent to achieve, and therefore waste their entire lives chasing them. Many people, in the grips of their CD, get goose bumps when they announce their big plans to become the next famous actor, author, athlete, or singer. They are convinced that they have extraordinary talents that they don't see in other people but that others will surely recognize in them. When this is not the case, it is the task of the homeopath to help such a person fall softly—but not far, and land, but not hard—on the comforting, carpeted floor called the truth. It is homeopathy's goal to make clear to the patient his hidden contents (his shadow) to be integrated into consciousness, rather than putting the shining light solely on the part visible to others: the mask, or persona, which is only one quarter and often even less than that of a person's real existence! How is such a CD created?

Birth of the CD

Every emotional state produces an alteration of consciousness. Which is to say, a certain decrease of consciousness is produced, as well as a corresponding strengthening of the unconscious. Jung's work on dementia praecox, as published in *The Psychogenesis of Mental Disease*, presents a useful definition of delusion as well as a further approach to its understanding. As René Masselon, a contemporary of Carl Jung, pointed out in *Psychology of Dementia Praecox*, we can clearly see that:

> Certain memories once intimately connected with important events of the patient's life (such as heartbreak, great fear, and strong incidences of indignation like that caused by rape, etc.), tend to reproduce themselves and occupy the patient's conscious mind continually. By continually reproducing themselves, such thoughts tend to coagulate and there is the formation of emotional impoverishment. (Jung, 1960, p. 12)

In Jungian terms, this is the perfect definition of delusions, stereotyped ideas, or *idées fixes*. One extreme situation is the schizophrenic person's coagulation of his mental life with the passive registration of events in his immediate environment: an *abaissement du niveau mental* (literally, a "lowering of the mental level"), a term coined by Pierre Janet in *L'Automatisme Psychologique* 1889 (Ibid., p. 16), or what Jung called a consciousness disintegration.

We might have the feeling at some point in our lives that we are all alone in this world and that no one cares about us—isolation through betrayal by a spouse or best friend, the loneliness of an immigrant, or the differences and frustrations that accompany a physical handicap, to name a few examples—but this is most often a fleeting moment, not a delusion but an illusion. A delusion is an illusion in an advanced state. In our homeopathic Repertory, we often find the same remedies under both rubrics (*delusion* and *illusion*), and it is really a matter of intensity. If, months or even years after the fact, a psychological trauma still evokes the sentiment that "I am all alone in the world and no one cares about me," and if all of my actions and thoughts are driven by this notion, then it can be defined as a delusion. Such a fixed idea dominates the life of the patient; everything he thinks, does, and plans is fueled by that delusion. It is this state of distracted attention that creates a sort of consciousness vacuum in which certain ideas, especially fixed ones, can penetrate more easily than in periods of full attention when many stimuli are stored in the conscious. This creates a vicious cycle for the patient who is already submerged in his cyber delusion. The patient's psychic activity tends to turn inwards, driving an unending elaboration of the same thought, building up the dominance of the cyber delusion. This process takes place in very much the same fashion as a tropical storm gains strength blowing over the sea (a relative fixed symbol that equates to unconscious life) and attains the status of a class five hurricane unless it downgrades when landfall occurs (equating to the return of consciousness, when the ferocity of the psychic thought process decreases).

For example, the strong delusion of being unloved hinders concentration; the patient is unable to tear himself away from it and to funnel his activity and interest into other, more positive and productive channels. Once there is consciousness lowering and disintegration, delusions are created and then freed from all restraint; they are, therefore, able to occupy the ego-consciousness. As the delusional ideas obstruct the patient's rational thoughts, he becomes unable to exert control over his ideas. Thus, the delusions can no longer be eliminated from the conscious process. They remain fully operative and prevent further personality development as well as keeping the patient from fully understanding and enjoying life. This process shows how the patient becomes a prisoner of his delusional thoughts, especially the cyber delusion, over and over.

These fixed thoughts, which are often morbid, overcome the patient and have powers of their own that are hard to control. We will observe that most delusions or fixed ideas come from fixed emotions. Recurrent or long-lasting unresolved emotions are apt to create patterns in our brains, memories that will be triggered by the slightest, even innocent insinuation (*easily offended*). Eventually, we maintain these particular emotions—anger that flares up easily, involuntary weeping, a sense of anguish and foreboding, obsessive-compulsive behavior, etc.—

because we have become addicted to them and they have become part of our personality (in the language of our repertory —*thoughts, persistent*)!

The psychological trauma that can create, amongst other conditions, OCD, autism, and a host of other behavioral disturbances such as violence, *intolerance to contradiction*, and *dictatorial behavior*, often originates at a very young age. The extent to which the word "young" is used here should not be underestimated as it can include intrauterine emotional events. Allopathy still has not linked the emotions of the pregnant mother to the unborn fetus, even though we see the results of unfortunate intrauterine trauma in many of our young patients. As a result, for many diseases, such as OCD or violent (even murderous) behavior in children, the homeopath can answer the two most important questions that allopathy always fails to address: "What is the cause of this behavior?" and "Is there an effective therapy for my child?" These questions also hold true for many adults with similar conditions.

We must keep in mind, that in order to preserve human health, a small quantity of sorrow, fear, anger, or want is always required—just as a ship needs a ballast to maintain stability. This is well known in Traditional Chinese Medicine but is even now confirmed by allopathic studies: that encounters with tiny portions of emotions erect a set of primitive defensive mechanisms starting in utero and teach the fetus about cause and effect. And suppressed emotions in adults always cause more damage to our defense systems than honestly expressed emotions. Repressed emotions fester, creating painful fixed ideas. What is the importance of the CD in a patient's life?

Importance of Early Treatment of the CD

Like a good homeopath, Jung recognized that *abaissement du niveau mental* (consciousness's slow disintegration) may be caused by various triggers like fatigue, fever, intoxication, anemia, religious fanaticism, intense affects, or mental shocks like hearing bad news. It may also be caused by constitutional and hereditary factors (miasms). Recognizing these triggers reveals both the danger and the necessity of homeopathic and psychotherapeutic intervention in any neurosis and "homeopathic delusional state" in order to prevent its progression into a full-blown psychosis. The neurotic and (homeopathically speaking) delusional patient is approaching a dangerous divide: as long as he can hold out on the neurotic side, he remains somewhat in control. As cancer can be a sign of our true feelings and therefore be considered a true friend who is trying to warn us to change our lifestyle and protect our boundaries, so we should accept neurosis as our truest and most precious counselor. Instead of attempting to eliminate the neurosis through suppression with allopathic drugs, we should find out what the neurosis is trying to tell us about ourselves. In this way, we don't cure the neurosis, but the neurosis cures us!

Unfortunately, many neurotic patients, under the continual strain of an unresolved, persistent, and intensified delusion, cross over the danger line. They are no longer considered neurotic and must now be identified as psychotic. Many psychotic patients have struggled as unrecognized neurotics before finally succumbing and drowning in the overwhelming tsunami of schizophrenia, a mixture of mysticism and emotional inferno, of God and the devil or Prince of Darkness, and of insanity and the highest degree of genius! Several of the same negative forces (delusions, neuroses) can be found in the unconscious of normal people, appearing in countless dreams where the neuroses have found a safe haven. People often remain blissfully ignorant of these forces until a trigger induces a dangerous deepening of the problem, leading to a psychotic break. In the clinic we often see that people on the eve of a psychotic outburst are upset by things they have never minded before; now suddenly these matters have become stumbling blocks and obsessions. Here again, without knowing it, Jung touches on the homeopathic miasmatic theory, in which a trigger is seen to produce a flare-up of the dominant miasmatic numerous expressions.

In treating most psychosomatic diseases, one should concentrate more than anything on the psychological traumas that have led to the patient's fixed ideas or delusions. But why, as a homeopath, give so much importance to delusions? In general, in the homeopathic practice, delusion rubrics are scarcely used and frequently misunderstood. When homeopaths attempt to find the simillimum, we must take in account the rubrics of Aphorism 153: "Rare, strange, and peculiar symptoms," and there is no doubt that delusions belong in this category. Let's not forget that there is a second important requirement for selecting the simillimum: symptoms must have remained permanent over some time! Since a delusion is a fixed idea, it is, by definition, permanent. Therefore, a delusion should be considered among the most valuable symptoms for the determination of the simillimum, since it clearly belongs to the Aphorism153 rubrics and syphilitic symptoms (loss of control). The delusion, in the homeopathic sense, always contains some grain of truth, but the quality of life of the individual and of the people around him is affected by the patient's inability to let go of this fixed idea.

The feeling-tone (intensity/character) of delusional thoughts (especially the CD) is so strong that no matter what the emotional excitation or trigger is, only the delusional thought is re-lived over and over. Memories with a strong feeling-tone form complexes of associations, which are very powerful and remain in the patient's unconscious. Take, for example, the psoric phase of *Aurum's Delusion, he neglected his duty*. No matter how much praise and acknowledgment he receives from others, all incoming positive thoughts are consumed by the negative thought "I did not do enough" (*imagines he is neglectful and deserves reproach in consequence*). Homeopathically prepared *Aurum* in such a case will be able to release this person from his delusional fetters, allowing him to take up the task of finding some sort of existential meaning that will enable him to continue living; some sense of self-worth that can replace his resignation and mournful retrospection. Being imprisoned by a delusion destroys a person's capacity to feel joy and compassion and leads to the patient's emotional isolation, as expressed in *Aurum's* delusional proving symptoms: *he imagines he cannot succeed in anything; he does everything wrong; he is in disunion with himself; he thinks he is not fit for this world and longs for death; he sees obstacles everywhere; he imagines he lost his friends' affection*. Eventually, in *Aurum's* syphilitic phase, the emotional alienation parallels the intellectual estrangement (*mental dullness, feels stupid; loss of memory*) and, when physical pathology sets in, heart troubles and hypertension commence. How can we measure the strength of this autonomous force in order to help the patient overcome its destruction of body and mind?

Measuring the Strength of the CD

Is the presence of this CD a new phenomenon? Not at all! It is certainly as old as humankind, but as civilization took root, the prevalence of the CD increased dramatically—and the higher the civilization, the more delusions emerge. When it comes to rational science, entities like Vital Force, Qi, and the CD are in the realm of the immeasurable (although they can be described and therefore do come under the umbrella of the empirical sciences). Because measurement is the foundation of modern science though, science will not concede the existence of anything unless it can measure it. But entities like the CD and the "nothings" hiding away in the subconscious are always measured by the discomfort and suffering they cause and the diseases they will eventually yield. In that aspect, every day of human existence is a measurement of the incredible power of the CD, the invisible rudder which, despite our conscious belief and objections, is the master of life's ship.

Indeed, how could we measure the depth at which we have released the demon (the CD), the beast in the cage (shadow side)? We only know how much of the pain, the grief, or the jealousy is left in the subconscious when we stumble on a trigger that points to the old high feeling-toned complex (Never Well Since or *Ailments from*). All of a sudden, the complex that we thought had been exorcized and removed from the cage, or at least domesticated, comes to consciousness with a viciousness and biting growl that wounds us again and again, and makes us doubt our progress on the journey of our individuation. It is yet again the raw emotion we feel, and as a result, the self-assuredness of our persona is shattered like a mirror into a thousand pieces. We might react with the most incredibly primitive emotions—emotions we may have denied ever existed in us. Of course, it is always easier to deny the existence of evil rather than to accept the necessity of reckoning with it. How to help the homeopath find a patient's demonic power?

How to Find the CD?

In the Materia Medica

I will restate here in brief some of the criteria I used to determine a delusion to be the cyber, or core, delusion of a specific remedy (described fully in the *Advanced Guide for the Professional Homeopath*, De Schepper, 2004).

For me, the first obvious criterion was that, among the many different delusions of a remedy, the CD should be either black type (3) or italics (2). In other words, the fixed idea was present among most of the provers of the remedy. One example is the delusion of *Aconite: he is about to die. Aconite* is a well-known remedy for pregnant women with their first child who may be paralyzed by fear of the impending delivery. Among all its delusions, *Aconite* has only this delusion in bold type. Additionally, *Aconite* is the only bold type remedy in this rubric, and no other remedy has the same intention or meaning as other remedies in this rubric!

If all delusions of a specific remedy are graded "1," that is, are listed in plain type, we can try to determine a delusion in which only this remedy is found. For example, in the *Silicea* proving we find the delusion *left half* (anima) *does not belong to the right* (animus) *one*, which expresses the dual nature of *Silicea* —who is timid in public and, often, a tyrant at home. Only *Silicea* is found in the repertory under the rubric *Del, body, left half does not belong to her*. Another example is *Kali-c*, with the *Del, an abyss is behind him*, pointing to the continuous concern of doom.

Often, the essence of the CD is also expressed by other delusions found in the provings of the same remedy. For example, *Lac caninum* has the CD *he is dirty*, which is also expressed in the delusions *he is small, he is looked down upon, he is despised, he is short*, and *he is insulted*. When many delusions express the same theme, that theme points clearly to the CD.

The CD gives birth to secondary delusions. The CD of *Lachesis* is *he is about to be injured by his surroundings* and *he has suffered wrong*, which leads to further suspicious behavior and secondary delusions such as *he will be sent to the asylum* and *the medicine is poison*.

Last, but not least, a person needing a remedy with a specific CD will always return to his CD after executing a series of defensive compensations and displacements. In other words, the remedy story begins and ends with the CD. For instance, no matter how many positive or negative compensations *Aurum* executes, he always will come back to his CD, I *neglected my duty*, unless the homeopathic remedy frees this victim from his chains. How to recognize the CD in the clinic, during the patient's interview?

In the Clinical Setting

A cyber delusion is the expression of the dominant, ruling emotion. It is the driving force behind the actions, thoughts, and plans of the patient, and it will create secondary delusions along the way. Therefore, all compensations and secondary delusions have their origin in the cyber delusion. It is imperative for everyone (as we all have a cyber delusion) to execute compensations, which can be regarded as defense mechanisms that enable us to flee from the cyber delusion (when it is negative) or to work with it to become a better person. The patient will try hard to compensate, to stay away from his inevitable fate, but he will have to face this cyber delusion at some point in his life. The patient's good delusion, obviously, is also bad for him as it impedes his Self's growth. If we don't ask enough about the motivations behind the psychological behavior of the patient, she will express compensations far away from the cyber delusion, therefore leading the homeopath to prescribe for the mask rather than the shadow side, a mask that is formed by all these compensations. *The mask represents the simile (compensations), but the shadow side is the simillimum (the cyber delusion)!* An ancient Chinese proverb expresses the same: "Confucius says that to return to the root is to find the meaning, but to pursue appearance is to miss the source"! When I find the cyber delusion, the lightbulb goes on: I see the essence of my patient. All his mental/emotional and physical compensations are determined and guided by this primary delusion.

Another hint is that, during the case taking, the patient

often betrays his CD when a very painful issue is touched upon, by even a small hint, reference or thought. At this point, the patient may react with telltale indicators such as silence, anger, irritability, crying, hesitation, or stuttering. When this happens, the homeopath must realize that his words or gestures have evoked the memory of a painful Never Well Since (NWS) event in the patient's homeopathic history. Be sure to record such a reaction during the consult, along with the source of the reaction, so you can know how the CD was touched upon. How does the patient react to the presence of his CD?

Compensations

As a physician, I have observed that the number one regret dying people have is that they lacked the courage to live life true to themselves, and instead according to what others expected of them (social and professional persona). By investigating the shadow side and integrating its contents into consciousness, people can live unbound by fear of failure or disapproval. They can become individuals ready to accept setbacks; with courage they continue to go forward, to try a little more. These are people who adopt the attitude "I will" rather than thinking "I should have." Unfortunately, most people continually resort to compensations rather than taking the opportunity to become more complete individuals.

In the blessings as well as the calamities of life, less depends upon what befalls us than upon the way in which it is met: *how do we react to and compensate for pleasures and misfortunes in life?* Compensations are an attempt to reorganize the chaos inflicted by the CD, a process of continuous rehabilitation on an unstable basis, an attempt to reach homeostasis and to regain and preserve identity. The portraits in my Materia Medica, *Discovering Life, Homeopathic Portraits* (De Schepper, 2013), are to be studied as phenomena of health and disease found in the endless forms of individual adaptations by which human organisms (individuals) adapt and reconstruct themselves when faced with the challenges and ceaseless inconstancies of life, which in reality can be called, "to exist." And a human being hopefully looks diversely upon himself—an entity in constant motion, tasting different fruits from the cornucopia of emotions and passions—reflecting on the inner life of the Self, his natural form.

Depending on the judiciously administered remedy, for some, such reorganization transforms the dark and negative side of the CD into the plus of positive compensation. For others, caught in a vicious cycle, the attempt might only lead to more disorganization until they are finally liberated by the homeopathic remedy that is their simillimum. We must remember that it is not the existence of the problem itself (the NWS), but the patient's attitude towards it (compensation) that gives it the power for good and evil. Out of grief may come determination and undaunted courage, or degradation, meanness, and spiritual apathy. Out of riches and power may come selfishness, self-gratification, and materialism (as with *Nux-v*) or the understanding that it is important to *be*, not to *have*, presenting us with the opportunity to serve and to practice the art of giving—like a balanced *Aurum*! The miasmatic overload and the response to triggers are interwoven, but above all, the miasmatic inheritance must be reached, softened, and corrected by the simillimum in order to reach a stage of renewal.

Using all the elements in previous chapters (persona, shadow, animus, anima, and CD), I now proceed to discuss how to recognize the direction of healing through dream analysis.

16

DETERMINING THE DIRECTION OF HEALING THROUGH DREAM ANALYSIS

"Every one of us is like a man who sees things in a dream and thinks that he knows them perfectly and then wakes up to find that he knows nothing." — *Plato*

The Individuation Path of the Patient

The question can be asked: at the time of consult, using his dreams, where is the patient in his healing process or where does he need to go? Remember there is no need for a dream when the patient sees the conscious situation correctly; the dream does not need to restate what he already knows! I already have shown in many examples how the direction of cure under the action of the simillimum will change the dream from a recurrent dream (no lysis) to a series of dreams, indicating a forward movement, like reading the next chapter of a book. Also, the change from destructive syphilitic dreams, to seize-the-day sycotic dreams with sex, drugs, and rock and roll, to psoric dreams (food, friends, love, support, festivities), show a beneficial working of the simillimum. And as indicated in the chapter on the shadow, whenever a personal figure appears—be it as anima, animus, or shadow—the dreamer can be sure that the unconscious is becoming active, that the unconscious is inclined to form a connection with consciousness. Usually the shadow makes the first appearance in dreams, followed by the animus (for women) or anima (for men). Appearance of these archetypal figures in our dreams is another way of seeing progression on the ladder to self-actualization, and where the patient is in his healing phase. We must not forget that these archetypes are personifications of psychic energy that cannot be killed but only transformed.

The question arises: What different steps does the patient need to accomplish in his individuation path? Everyone who has the courage and has the hero and heroine's quest to follow the individuation path to self-realization, will have to encounter different battles and stages in order to achieve the desired goal. These stages have a kind of hierarchical position, in which the difficulty to the person becomes more and more elaborate and challenging. Initially, the direction of cure might show that the dreamer's conscious life may grow more barren (not always appreciated by family and friends), which is a first sign that old opinions and attitudes need to die, while being replaced by a more burgeoning vivid unconscious life, the "going within," setting the tone to start the individuation process—the rebirth—undertaken with courage and struggle, helped through analysis and the simillimum.

In this rebirth, there is first of all the adaptation to the outer and inner worlds (the psychological types), followed by the acknowledgment of the right use of the persona, before a humble meeting with the unaccepted and repressed part of our personality or shadow can happen. As we have wiggled through this bottleneck of the psyche (the shadow)—already suggesting an anxious journey—the task at hand becomes more difficult as the person is now confronted with the mystical archetypes, the necessity to establish a good relationship with the contra-sexual figures (anima and animus) before reaching that golden goal, the encounter with the Self, so evasive to most. Let's recapitulate each of these steps and how they can enlighten the patient and the homeopath where the patient has arrived in his individuation and healing journey. There is one aspect to remember: depending on our willingness to become conscious, these great archetypal images *will* appear but one can never predict *when* they will appear—their appearance will simply tell us where we are and where we need to be going in order to become more complete (self-realization).

Step one in our healing is to use the mask or persona in an acceptable, adequate way, namely using our different personas at the right time, just as we dress for certain occasions in the right attire. Providing we don't have a malformation (excessive, inadequate, or identification), we use our persona properly in daily life. Of course, many among us are caught in the tangles of one of these malformations! Dreams, through symbols (clothes, diplomas, apparel like a wig or stethoscope, uniforms, and the health of the skin), make us aware from the beginning what persona dominates or is malformed.

Part of step one is also trying to *exercise/activate* three conscious functions: the dominant function + 2 subordinate conscious functions. When our dreams cover the adequate persona and two to three conscious functions appear (appearance from one person to an additional two people), we have made a huge step in our healing, or realization of the Self, but it is only the beginning!

Step two is the task of integrating the contents of the shadow into consciousness, commonly during the first phases of the analysis. Usually people don't have too much difficulty understanding and even somewhat accepting that there is something as a shadow: who is perfect? Jung expresses it very well:

> With the shadow we have the advantage of being prepared in some sort by our education, parents, friends and strangers, which always has convinced people that they are not one hundred percent gold. And if forgotten there is always your spouse, the tax collector or a Sunday sermon for the Catholics to refresh your memory. (Jung, 1958, p. 16)

Except maybe for *Platina*, the white gold, who does not belong to this world and her family. The shadow is an aspect of the personal unconscious that most people are *somewhat* conscious of. Another advantage of more readily accepting the shadow is that it is the figure closest to consciousness—the least mysterious one, and often the first one appearing in dreams during analysis or under homeopathic treatment, the first advanced step on the journey to individuation.

In order to accept the shadow and *de-potentiate it through integration*, we must *resist two temptations*! First, we must avoid *projecting* our own shadow onto others. Disowning it is not the same as integrating it. The second temptation to resist, upon viewing it for the first time, is to *suppress* the shadow, putting it back into the cellars of the unconscious, locking it behind closed doors and throwing away the key. That is like "curing" a headache by beheading someone! No wonder so many people are afraid of their own shadow and even deny its existence!

Although the shadow is the uppermost layer of the unconscious, and therefore has more visible collective traits than the other, deeper, archetypes (anima and animus) and is thus easiest to perceive as it can often be raised to full consciousness, Jung states: "The shadow is a tight passage, a narrow door, whose painful constriction no one is spared who goes down to the deep well" (Jung, 1990, CW Vol. 9, Part I, para. 45). This makes me think of the Hillary Steps on Mount Everest, the tight passage or bottleneck, where people get bogged down for hours because of heavy traffic before reaching the top. Yes, it is a very distressing passage, followed by reaching the top, a temporary triumph, analogous to finally integrating some of the shadow's contents. But as every climber knows, it is the descent of the mountain that is more dangerous, and so is the road on the further torturous descent of the personal unconscious, when we must integrate animus and anima, and realize how much influence these archetypes exert on our conscious life—to achieve our own true survival from the mountain! Such a road is never a straight one, as one challenge after another can be encountered.

Step three: As much as the shadow cannot be accepted without an immense struggle, experiencing the roots which feed the personal unconscious is certainly another challenge: anima, animus, and the Self! When the natural productions of the unconscious, anima and animus, appear in dreams we can be sure that the deepest level of the unconscious (the collective unconscious) has been reached! But if we thought that gaining insight into our shadow side was difficult and a huge step forward in knowing ourselves, it is far more difficult to come to terms with the animus and anima and understand what they are —as they can never be raised to full consciousness—and how they are responsible for many entanglements, compulsive actions, Greek tragedies, and fateful outcomes in men's and women's lives. Even when with much difficulty and panic their effects can be made conscious, they retain their autonomous character, ever playing the role of the rear guard who steers and guides the troops ahead of them, and informs them what path to take to remain safe. They make sure that an overly one-sided conscious attitude is complemented and compensated, so that neuroses can be kept on the safer side of the danger line with psychosis, as long as these sygizi don't burst into the front of the army to create chaos or what would be a psychosis, mainly paranoid forms of schizophrenia.

The whole process is not as easy as it might appear, even starting with the integration of the shadow side, but above all, exploring deeper into the unconscious (personal and collective) poses difficulties. In a further stage we meet the "mana personalities." This is the stage where a human being meets the archetypes of the wise old man, personification of the animus, and the Divine or Great Mother, personification of the anima. These archetypes are symbols of power and wisdom, and primitive people considered anyone having extraordinary power or wisdom to be filled with *mana* (a word meaning "holiness or the divine"). Jung warns us that to be *possessed* by these mana personalities is dangerous, as it commonly results in megalomania or delusions of grandeur.

For instance, a man who allows himself to be taken over by the wise old man is likely to become convinced that he is either some sort of superman or a great guru with superior insight. Copying or parroting a guru is an evil spirit of imitation, as we need to keep our individuality with devotion to our life. The right way to deal with mana personalities is the same way we should handle our shadow side: neither project them on others (and indirectly give them the power and wisdom), nor keep them suppressed, as doing so will stop our healing process. By integrating, assimilating, and giving the contents or archetypes (which are part of the Self) a relative but not absolute autonomy, rather than projecting or repressing them forever, we can expect to expand our ego consciousness tremendously, a vast and important jump to self-realization—a never-ending process. Progress is made when we are ready to see conscious and unconscious not as opposites but as cooperating and complementary parts of our psyche. The two separate parts work together to create homeostasis in the psyche, incorporating what is lacking and discharging what exists in excess, echoing the law of compensation in dreams.

We physicians have all seen the great disturbances in humans when the ego is assimilated and overwhelmed by the unconscious contents, leading to deep psychological states such as schizophrenia and other psychological disturbances like inflation of the ego, where a lack of modesty reigns. It is easily seen in the personalities suffering from an excessive persona like *Lycopodium* and *Lachesis*, where *Lycopodium* trusts himself as little as others (*suspicion in the highest degree*) and where *Lachesis*, in a further diseased state, thinks he is influenced by "the will of God," as he is under direct communication with a superior being (*Delusion, under the influence of a superior being*). The ego must remain the master and captain of the ship of consciousness, and integration of unconsciousness should be a carefully guided process, something homeopaths with carefully and judiciously adjusted doses and adequate repetition of their remedies should assist, analogous to the psycho-analytical process. The last stage of individuation—and few people ever reach it—is the stage of *self-realization*. Another way of putting it, is that you are fully conscious of your body and your body is fully conscious. You feel completely at ease in your body and you feel loving and joyful. But what about an existing CD, as we all have one?

What to Do with the CD? Where is Its Place?

Throughout the process, the *dissolution* and *de-potentiating* (*not integration*) of the CD takes place—the severance of the single, painful high feeling-toned complex which harbors the CD of the patient! Remember, the CD originates from the conscious where a vacuum was created by a high feeling-toned complex, which is then repressed to the unconscious. The more it is denied, the greater the risk for its possessor that it will disturb the ego with its compulsive power. So, this process of dissolution of the CD can be seen from the first step of healing, throughout the process of integration of the shadow side, anima, and animus. The CD is an *overall present* factor, represented by archetypes and associated with each level of the individuation path, and as such shows—through its number of characteristics and intensity—where the level of healing takes place. In other words, as the healing process progresses, the intensity or level of suffering through the action of this CD diminishes, going from a burning flame or bright light blinding and paralyzing us at the moment of the birth of the CD, to a smaller flame as we are healing on the deeper levels of the archetypes. Jung postulated that the high feeling-toned complex can never totally be dissolved but its imprint can be *weakened.* Of course, he did not know homeopathy, so we can probably draw a different conclusion using remedies.

We can conclude that the CD is like the *red line running throughout the entire healing process* and its dissolution starts as soon as the process of step one is initiated. It is not finished when much of the shadow has been integrated (a difficult process to begin with!) but when it is handed over to the sygizi (anima and animus). This explains why we see the impact of the CD throughout the healing process, an impact on the archetypal figures of the unconscious! As the archetypes get integrated, the CD loses steam and strength. It will always leave some scar, so even with little strength it can resurface when it triggers the high feeling-toned complex, warning us there is still some work to do as the healing process is not finished!

To summarize:

After differentiating the persona first, then having analyzed and integrated the contents of the personal unconscious (the shadow and *undifferentiated* conscious functions), we come up against mythological fantasies that stem from the collective unconscious. At this point we come to terms with activated residue of our ancestral history, and the next step of the individuation road is to integrate the anima for men and animus for women. "The personal unconscious corresponds to the figure of the shadow, so frequently met with in dreams" (Jung, 1966, para. 103).

The dissolution of the CD takes place especially in the first three steps of direction of cure. Here is the caveat: when these symbols appear in our dream (shadow, anima, animus, mana persons), they don't necessarily always tell us where we *are* but where we *should be going*. It is impossible to know *when* these images will appear. This would also explain why some people turn away from homeopathic treatment even though their symptoms get better—if someone is not ready to jump the unconscious fence, he or she will turn away from the possibility of cure. So, do I have the simillimum if the patient is not ready to jump the fence when faced with the ugly shadow side (shock and protest of the family who does not like the "new" person, who really is the true person), or is it a question of increasing potencies and good management? Of course, it is the latter! But what will happen if patients turn away from the right homeopathic treatment? They will be plagued by the same recurrent nightmare for the rest of their life! In general, we can say that the shadow side is a lake, a river, or pond, but still somewhat in reach of the conscious, while the animus and anima are the ocean or images of the collective unconscious, their full understanding forever escaping us as they cannot be raised to full consciousness.

Here is another dream of a male, expressing the right direction of cure.

Dream

I am going to run a race with many people. We will start very early in the morning while it is still dark. First, I start alone, it is very dark, and I start running. But soon I am accompanied by a young male runner I recognize. He is not warmly dressed but he is not worried and says he is going to get warmer. Then a woman, pushing a carriage with a baby, joins us and tells us she is happy to join us. Then I wake up with a very calm feeling.

Analysis

This is a very revealing dream telling us the patient is on the right track. First it is a message representing a communication from the collective unconscious as this is a race with many people—hence representing the journey of individuation, not only belonging to the dreamer but to mankind. There are **three** people plus a baby in this dream. First we can see that integration of unconscious elements from the unconscious is taking place: the young male accompanying him, his shadow, not repressed but acknowledged and accompanying him in this race, and they are joined by his anima (the female in him) who is pushing a carriage with a baby in it, representing new potentialities on his way to a new Self. The meeting with the anima is a happy one and the journey to becoming more complete is in full swing. Excellent lysis of the dream, and themes in further dreams will possibly progress.

Here is a dream under the influence of the simillimum which expresses the progress of a 50-year-old *Phosphorus* lady, revealing where she is as she has met the wise old man in this dream.

Dream

I find myself standing on the corner of a sidewalk and the sidewalk is four feet above the street below where cars pass by. All of a sudden, a man and his daughter appear on the street below. And before you can blink your eyes, they appear in front of me on the sidewalk and he says with a deep voice, "Why are you blocking the sidewalk?" I tell him I am not blocking the sidewalk because there is no one else here but me. Then I ask him,

"How did you get up onto the sidewalk from down there?" He said he would tell me another time. He is a large, burly, heavyset man in his 50s with dark, short hair and a scruffy beard. Then I speak to his daughter and ask her where Nomads is? Nomad means wanderer and this shop has crafts, rugs, and clothing from Morocco and other parts of the world. She takes me to where she thinks it is. We walk together and her father walks behind us. We arrive at a shop that is not Nomads, but the daughter asks the shopkeeper where it is. The shopkeeper tells her how to find it and the dream ends there. The daughter in the dream is either 19 years old or in her early 20s, and built like a *Phosphorus* and compared to her father she is much more attractive.

Analysis

Apparently, with the simillimum this patient has already been able to make some progress on her individuation journey as we find her walking on a sidewalk above the street (higher up means some elucidation has already taken place). Then suddenly an old man (the wise old man) and his young daughter (the dreamer's shadow: still young and with the possibility to form a better renewed shadow, or more likely a renewed anima, as she is too much of a wanderer, a dissatisfied person led by an imbalanced anima), jump in front of her to guide her further on her path to self-actualization. Indeed, she asks the daughter where this store "Nomads" is, which is appropriately indicating the wanderlust of this *Phosphorus* dreamer. She needs further guidance on her journey, not only from the young shadow (possibility of renewal) but also from the wise old man who follows them. And finally, the shopkeeper of another store tells them where to find the Nomads store.

Another dreamer goes from a recurrent dream to a series of dreams, confirming the right choice of the homeopathic remedy. Before, he had a recurrent dream of failing exams, indicating that he was not prepared to deal with the challenges and vicissitudes of life. Then he had the following dream.

Dream

I am walking nervously through the city. I am in the military and have to present myself in my unit the next day where I am starting a new year in the university. I realize my hair is too long and even as my clothes are not always perfect, long hair would be a definite no. Previously I had met a colleague and his hair was cut perfectly according to military standards. He told me I should definitely cut my hair. I am looking for a barbershop throughout the town. I am walking because I have parked my red car somewhere and I do not know where precisely. But I am not too concerned; my priority is cutting my hair. I do not have notebooks to start the university either, but that too is not an immediate concern. I know where a discount store is with old books and I have enough money. I cannot see any barbershop but when I come to a student house, I see a row of students sitting at small tables next to each other, eating. But I look carefully and see that one has scissors and comb and I ask him to cut my hair. He seemed to have met me before, so he agrees. Another guy and one female are looking on during this process. I implore him not to cut too much off although the other man insists on it while the female seems more concerned. But the student listens to me. At one point he lifts my hair and shows me that a part of the skin, a flap that has replaced the hair, is woven in the hair. I just tell him to put it back and leave it alone and concentrate on the front and the back. While he is cutting, I am thinking how much money to give to him as compensation: five dollars or five euros? I think, I can't give him too much, although I have a lot. I get stuck on the number 5. At the end I stroke my hair and feel a good job was done.

Analysis

Locale: Dreamer, friend, **three** other people (**two** males, **one** female). City, student house.

Exposition: Looking for a barbershop to cut my hair.

Peripateia: Finding the place with students and seeing someone who had scissors and comb.

Lysis: Satisfied with haircut. Car not found and no notebooks bought yet.

Discussion: What is the central theme? What problem does the dream pose? The cutting of the hair!

- **Hair** stands for extraordinary and magical strength —the lion's mane, and Samson's hair (who lost his strength after Delilah cut off his hair), and the pelt of the werewolf legend representing enormous strength. Abundant hair means virility or male sexuality and is often used as a sign of protection as seen in African tribes who refuse to cut their hair (when I visited the Masai in Kenya, hair meant supernatural power protecting them on their wanderings in the savanna). Hair also represents attractiveness, such as having much and long hair— so self-image is important. Cutting the hair may symbolize loss of perceived virility, so definitely a step forward that he wants to change his persona or self-image! (People often want a haircut when they want "a new me.") Changing hairstyle or cutting hair is like changing attitudes. So going to the barber symbolizes the ability to change attitudes, thoughts, and opinions. It depicts change of mind and image. A *military* haircut reflects conscious discipline. Long white beard: may symbolize wisdom. (Wisdom shows up with age. Of course, with some, like *Lycopodium*, age just shows up by itself.) Idioms: "Letting one's hair down; Hair-raising; Splitting hairs."

- **Car:** He parked it somewhere. Parking lot: a sociably acceptable place to rest, to relax or to make some change. Momentarily he stops the "desire to go forward, to get somewhere or anywhere," to grow further as an individual making personal choices and freedom (he was the driver of the car); right now he is not very concerned about where the car is, as other more urgent things are on his mind. But he starts walking now instead: getting somewhere through personal effort!
- The **red** car: **Red** stands for: passion, sexuality or sexual arousal, emotion, the feeling function, the color of blood, anger, danger, revolution, instinct, and anything fiery in general; Eros; it is also the symbol of life and principle of union and involvement, which binds together (Chinese brides wear red!); excitement but also attractiveness, something that draws attention like red hair (again the importance of image). That he is not concerned where his car is means progress, as he is less concerned about his image, being in the red car with long hair! Red also stands for pulsating life and is the color of the vital instincts and of the overwhelming emotional turmoil they bring about (puberty!). It reflects a sense of energy and vitality. Because of its modern association with traffic lights and warning, such as brake lights on cars, it may sometimes be used as a warning, or a way of saying "stop" or "no." Red can also stand for honoring people: "the red carpet" for the Academy Awards, and the CNN Heroes.

- **New year in university/college:** Individual potential and learning ability; something important you are learning; What do we need to learn there? Obviously, the dreamer has not graduated yet, not reached the sense of achieving adulthood yet! Going from high school to college is for most young people the separation from home and new steps of independence and adulthood.
- The male **friend** he met: His shadow side; secret wish to be more conformed to the rules, but this was difficult since he was cloaked in image and power, hesitating when someone else tells him how to dress or look. This wish was still stronger, so he suppressed conformity to his shadow side! Especially cutting the hair would decrease his attractiveness and power.
- **Books:** Things you have learned or are learning from experience; attitude towards learning; other people's opinions. Old books: inherited wisdom; learning greater awareness.
- Money, and the **number 5:** Can be the number of relationship (4+1=5) but here in this dream there is no question of a relationship. It is all about his hair; he is not whole yet, so **five** indicates to count back **five** years. When I asked him to count back **five** years, he told me he had taken a new job that year to earn more money: again, prestige and money and power, not because he liked the job.
- **Students eating: Students:** In process of gaining insight, not professionals yet. **Eating:** satisfying your needs, any area of need, emotional, mental, or sexual depending on the dream context. To eat is to continue involvement in the fundamental process of

life, to grow; taking in what society has to offer. Not eating is an avoidance of growth and change.

- **The other man insisting his hair be cut more:** His shadow side or alter ego.
- **The concerned female:** His anima.
- **A flap, wig:** False attitudes or thoughts; an assumed social front; the dreamer still wants to leave it there, so not a complete change yet.
- **Front and back:** Front=future or conscious; the more public or expressed part of one's nature or attitudes to meet the world, in other words the persona! Back=past or unconscious; the more private and intimate, out of sight or obscure part (shadow and other archetypes).

Favorable or unfavorable dream? All in all, this was a favorable dream, showing progression from the previous recurrent dream of failing exams. There was a partial lysis with the haircut (in other words, giving some of his power away, realizing that he put too much accent on power and image), so a partial step to improvement was taken in the dream. Provided the patient recognized it, this was favorable. Contrary to the previous dreams, which always ended unsatisfactorily, here part of the goal was achieved. He stroked his hair and it felt good! But he has a long way to go still: finding the car (following his true passions and path of individuation and growth), getting paper to be able to write notes down (part of the journey he has to undertake, to graduate from university, keeping a journal about the trip of his individuation), and money still seems to be important: he was frugal with it although he had a lot.

Why students, and not finding a professional barber? This represents where the dreamer is: he has not reached the level of a successful man but is still a student when it comes to living life, not having become psychologically an individual.

Was there other progress to be seen in comparison to the previous dreams? Yes. In previous dreams he never had paper to write on when he took exams and always had to borrow little scraps of paper from others. Now he knows where there is a shop where he can buy discount and he had plenty of money. Although this part also shows how much he values money. Sounds like a *Sulphur* guy with his *Del, coming to want*!

What is the remedy? Still the previous one, as this is part of a series of dreams, the next chapter of his book.

Dream following the next dose

I am walking in the street accompanied by an old man and two young dogs. I am on my way to a physician's consult and once I arrive at a building that I recognize as the place I was before for a consult, I bid farewell to the old man and two dogs although the old man wanted to accompany me. I take an elevator and arrive in a very spacious room where I meet a physician in a very white uniform. He tells me to take my place and wait. I wake up in a relaxed mood.

Analysis

Locale: Street, building; old man, dogs, doctor.

Exposition: Walking down the street and finding the building.

Peripateia: Bidding goodbye to the old man and dogs. Taking the elevator and meeting the physician in a spacious room.

Lysis: I need to wait, but wake up relaxed.

Explanation

- **The old man, two dogs, the dreamer, and a physician: three** people, but of course they are all a part of the dreamer. The old man could be the old shadow side, the one with the baggage, representing past experiences; old people can represent wisdom too. But here most likely it was a symbol of the wise old man who he bids farewell to as he seeks out a new wise man (the physician, another representation for this archetype). He also let the **two** young dogs go: he is trying to form a new animus to replace the defective natural animus in him and these two young dogs are not fused yet, so he let them go too.
- **Three figures** belonging to the dreamer: **three** functions of consciousness somewhat explored. **What else is seen?** However, no female figure is present (the feeling function), so the dreamer is still too much in the male or thinking mode and his archaic feeling function has not developed yet or doesn't show any sign of change.
- But the dreamer is on his way to a **physician** (*the new archetypal symbol of the wise old man*)—in other words he wants to investigate, he wants to change. He wants to know what is going on, how to go further on the individuation path. *A healer appearing in dreams symbolizes something you desperately need in your life in order to move forward towards greater wholeness (individuation path).* He leaves the old man and dogs behind: at least a good evolution, not wanting to take the old with him, seeking more spiritual guidance from a new source.

- He takes an **elevator/lift: A.** This is escaping the unconscious, and now going to the light or conscious, attempting to bring elements from the unconscious to conscious mind, where you obviously want to look at these elements you bring up. **B.** It can also mean becoming more "heady," more rational but less in touch with instinct and intuition. **C.** Being trapped in an elevator: frustration; feelings of restriction or trying to make change, being stuck. **A** most likely represents the significance here.
- He meets a physician all in **white** (reflecting the absolute truth): again, reflecting consciousness but also pureness, happiness, innocence, joy, truth, and "He-Who-Has-All-The-Answers"!

The whole dream feels like it is a good dream, an attempt to change. And the appearance of a mana personality at this point (the wise old man, then the physician), shows good progress as there is acceptance of this mana person for changes in his life. **Lysis?** There is not much lysis yet except that he takes his place in the room and patiently waits. At least the fact that he wakes up not in terror (like previous dreams in which he missed the airplane, lost his car, or failed an exam), but relaxed tells us that this dose of the simillimum has worked again. We can only hope for more messages from the unconscious with the next dose.

Next dream after another dose of the same remedy

I am in the barbershop and waiting my turn. Suddenly another man comes in and the barber says, "I will take him first as he is my good client." However, I protest loudly and insist on going before him, to which the barber finally agrees.

Analysis

Good lysis. He stands up for himself and goes before the "good client"—the shadow side has a chance to go first! And he allows the cutting of his hair, so excellent movement forward as he rejects/stops the old shadow side and lets the "glorious" persona (the hair) be cut off!

Next dream (three months after the previous dream, and after the fourth dose of the same remedy)

I am living next to a Mexican family, waiting for a tennis tourney to go to. I am working in the yard when the man next door asks me to remove stones that were somewhat hindering the entrance to his garage. Before, he had asked my wife to remove them, but she refused saying he had to buy the removal of those rocks. But when he asks again, now I take them and put them in my yard above the objections of my wife. I tell him, I'd rather be good neighbors with you. He embraces me, and my wife starts speaking Spanish to him. I thought I understood one word but when I repeated it in Spanish, he said no, "It is not death, it means feelings." Then he proceeds to give a gift to my two children, a boy and a girl. I say thank you and look at my clock. It is 4:10 p.m. and I say I have to leave as my tennis match is at 4:30 p.m. and it is a very important match. I have a good feeling about this dream.

Analysis

- **The neighbor:** His shadow side: he is considering his shadow side a friend now, not an enemy—a favorable prognosis!
- **Garden/yard work:** To plant seeds for personal

growth; any disorder (weeds instead of flowers) in the yard would represent one's own disordered psyche; a garden might represent one's true Self particularly if the garden is symmetrical—a square, rectangle, or circular shape and with a central point like a mandala. So, it is an archetype for fertility and fruitfulness and a symbol for individuation and wholeness.

- **Removing some blocks of stone from my neighbor's garage: Stones:** Ossified memories and suppressed emotions (rock=permanency and antiquity). **Garage entry:** A quiet place to go to, so the entry to his unconscious was blocked by these stones, so now he removed them and an investigation of his shadow side is possible.
- **His wife** (his anima) gives in and speaks to the neighbor: it was about feelings; it shows that finally the previous initial archaic feeling function is maturing. This is confirmed by the fact that where before money was demanded by his wife (his anima), now he does it for free as he has a good relationship with his neighbor or shadow side.
- **Gift** to his two children: a newly formed anima and animus. Receiving a gift: consider what is received, to define what one is accepting. A gift: What is received in a relationship, such as support, sense of worth.
- **Clock:** 4:10 p.m.: past 4, which is **four** conscious functions—a more complete person and on his way to 5:00 p.m. (4+1=5 or a relationship with his unconscious or shadow side). At 4:30 p.m. is an important match: a new test for him to see if he is still proceeding on his way to individuation. He will have to pass this test, as it brings him closer to 5:00.

> It is not as close as 5 minutes to the hour, which would always imply that when the 5 minutes are up there is growing tension to do something. When a clock appears in a dream showing the time, the dreamer is pestered by the unconscious and the tension created is heightened by the clock, by waiting for something to happen.

No new remedy is needed, only repetition!

Next dreams, two months later

Dream, part one

I am with my brother on a trip and take an elevator that at first goes too high, but after a few seconds comes down to the right floor and stops to arrive in an apartment. Then I tell my brother I only have shorts and a T-shirt, and I need to give a lecture. But I am not worried as I have plenty of money and I am thinking of buying casual slacks. When we are trying to leave the apartment, I am going to leave my money behind, but my brother is not able to lock the apartment with the key he has. So, I am afraid to leave my money (foreign currency) behind.

The second part of the dream happened the same night—when dreams happen the same night, usually it reflects that these dreams are connected theme-wise.

Dream, part two

I am sitting at a dinner table with my brother and a woman I love very much. She asks me what kind of food I want, and I answer, "What you have on your plate." She only gives me a small portion of food from her plate. When I wake up, I have a pleasant feeling.

Analysis, first part

- **His brother:** His shadow side; not leaving him behind, as we can never do this, but not threatening either, more accepted.
- **Elevator:** Becoming conscious, making conscious unconscious contents; journey of individuation. First too high but coming down to the right apartment: enough and right amount of unconscious contents released. Going up in a lift symbolizes attaining a more spiritual attitude, or becoming more "heady," but less in touch with instinct and intuition. Going down: conscious ego descending into the unconscious to look around, to investigate.
- **Shorts/T-shirt/casual slacks:** Less importance placed on image or persona (the clothes!). If one is dressed in inappropriate clothes: rebellious against authority or society.
- Not leaving his **money** behind: Still too much importance on money/power. Money=what we value; being valued by others; or having power, even over someone else but also to advance on our journey; opportunity, because money buys time to explore or try the new. **Foreign** money: an aspect of himself that is unknown, unfamiliar, foreign; belonging to the unconscious. One needs "money" to be able to grow up, to become an adult. Money also means power to change things, to do things. For Schopenhauer, who inherited much money

from his family to the point he never had to work for a living, money was the means to stay away from all the nuisances of life, to have freedom from pain and annoyance. He considered someone born into riches but remaining a mere idler and thief of time a contemptible fellow. He says inherited wealth reaches its greatest value when it falls to the individual endowed with mental powers of a high order, who is resolved to pursue a life of genius by producing a work which contributes to the general good. He was of the same opinion as Socrates, who said upon seeing many luxury articles spread in front of him, "How much is there that I do not want!" Money might also mean **excrement or feces**, something you need to get rid of, something from your past that has been poisoning your psyche (he is "stinking rich").

Analysis, second part

- **Brother and woman:** Reunion with secondary conscious function/shadow side and anima. Three people present in this dream: excellent progression. There is food for the mind, food for thought, food for the body, and nourishment that gives a sense of connection with something eternal; we can digest information or experience, the latter being food for growth. This is food in connection with the anima, so the dreamer is being nourished by the relationship with his anima. This is satisfying the dreamer's emotional hunger. His anima wants to feed him (emotional nourishment) and he is open to it as he wants the food on her plate. She just gives him a small part: indication that further connection with his anima is needed, but an excellent start.

Dream two months later

I am on my way to give a lecture. While going to the lecture hall I pass a lawn where people are sitting. They seem to recognize me as they are calling my name. In this crowd, in front, is a small girl sitting and I take her in my arms and tell her how beautiful she is. As I enter the lecture building, one side of this building is inaccessible as water was surrounding it going to the top of the building. I enter on the other side and come into a room but feel somewhat confused as to what direction to go. Then one of my more experienced male students comes in and I follow him to the room where the elevator is. I take the elevator with him to the 13th floor where the lecture takes place. Once I am there I am somewhat confused as what to teach but I assure them I have a lot of interesting things to teach. I also notice that far fewer students are present than I had expected. I am still hesitating about what to teach when my male student who entered with me tells me to go on with it. I wake up at that point.

Analysis

- **Lecturing:** Still a person with a dominant thinking function. This is possibly used as a convenient metaphor to convey its message, which is to try to connect more to the feeling function. It is also someone who is working on knowledge. (The dreamer should ask himself, "What am I ready to acknowledge or share?")
- **Lawn:** Part of the dreamer that possibly needs much

attention, as any lawn; but also, feelings of relaxation or family life.

- **Small girl (always refers to under age 13):** He connects with his immature anima and tells her how much he loves her. In male dreams this reflects his emotions. The child in the dreamer is the growing part in him, his anima. It can be the possibility of a new beginning. However, he does not take her to the lecture hall (we hope he will in later dreams!), so again dominance of thinking, but at least there is recognition of the beauty and special attractive characteristics of this girl, confirming the willingness to connect to his female side or anima, a beginning of a good Eros connection (relationship).
- **Tall building surrounded on one side by water:** Stands for the dreamer, the Self. We can see the two worlds of every person: conscious and unconscious. One side surrounded by water to the top (=unconscious), the other one he enters through a door (the conscious half of the person), but then is confused about what direction to go. In other words, he is in the lower part of the building—not the cellar but lower floor (start of consciousness), and knows he has to go to the upper part (13th floor), to become more enlightened, to make conscious unconscious things. The number **13** usually stands for calamity, evil or misfortune, or bad luck (Friday the 13th). Does it indicate the hesitance of the dreamer?
- **Experienced male student:** His shadow side which still stimulates him and guides him, as it has more experience and wisdom than the conscious, even at the end of the dream telling him to get on with the lecture. His insecurities were placed in the

> unconscious and now they become conscious and the shadow side encourages him on. That there were not as many students as expected points to a disappointment, creating some more confusion and doubt although he tries to convince everyone he has nice things to teach.

These consecutive dreams are all part of a favorable evolving series of dreams. There is more desire to throw off his excessive persona, and guidance from mana personalities and a desire to connect with his anima are demonstrated. This is not the end of the "book," as hopefully many chapters will follow under the influence of the simillimum.

To finish this chapter, here is a dream of a 70-year-old woman who discovered a hard lump in her left breast. She refused biopsy as she did not want to follow the allopathic treatments. Here is her dream, an archetypal dream—so an important one—after taking one dose of *Carcinosin* 30C, ½ tsp from the RSB directly.

Dream

We (my husband, I, and my dog) are in a large living room, much like the one we have. On one wall is a shelf where a snake is coiled up above our (black) dog. She is on a long divan with lots of pillows and fast asleep, unaware of the danger above her. I feel great fear for her as I do not want the snake to kill her with one bite. I cannot tell if the snake is poisonous or not but feel I must kill it to save the dog and us. On the opposite wall hangs my long saber, but there is another snake coiled on the shelf just below the saber. I now feel terrified. We are now standing in the middle of the room between 2 snakes. I tell my husband to bring my tall leather boots, to make snake bites impenetrable. I somehow have the saber in my hands. The snake above our dog comes down on top of our dog. It is a big, long, heavy looking snake. I fear it will bite her. Our dog does not move; her eyes are now open. She stays calm. The snake slithers over her body and once it is away from her, it stops long enough for me to cut it near the neck and then I hack it a few times to disable and kill it. Then there is the question of the other snake. I look for it. It is still on the shelf. We look at each other eye to eye, locked in a gaze. It leaves, sliding over the dog, which does not react. Nothing happens to it. And I don't know where it went when it left. End of dream.

Analysis

Living room: Part of the Self of the dreamer.

Black dog: In reality, she has a middle-aged dog, a very vivacious and strong dog. A dog is her animus (her husband appearing was her real husband). The interesting thing is that the dreamer is more concerned about her dog being killed, rather than her or her husband. Black: representing her animus in the unconscious. In this dream, one snake is not killed, and neither the husband nor the dog reacts to this snake, even when it slides over the dog. Why would that be? The answer lies in the snake symbol. Like any archetypal symbol, there is a duality, two sides of a coin, opposite each other. As seen before (Chap. 2), in certain aspects it is the symbol for supreme wisdom and the great healer or redeemer. On the other hand, it is the tempter to evil, to poison—the devil himself. Whenever a snake appears in dreams, it symbolizes a piece of the instinctive psychology in us, something of tremendous and fiery power. It represents the vital and the instinctual stirring in us, our unconscious dark side. These **two** snakes represent the duality, a unification of the opposites, as seen in the caduceus of medical doctors. So the dreamer, concerned with the killing of her dog, her well-balanced animus, tries to preserve the dog and orders her husband (representing the good balance between anima and animus in this dreamer, which she possessed in real life too) to get her boots for protection and then she takes a saber that hung on the wall (in reality too). We can again see in this whole dream the good animus/anima balance the dreamer had, as she does not call on her husband for help, but takes all the decisions and actions herself, pointing to a commanding animus. She kills one snake (the bad one) and looks the other in the eye. It slid over the dog, which does not react at all, as it is the good snake (who can prepare for the idea of healing), and then that snake is gone, and she wakes up. This is a good lysis.

Although this is only one dream, immediately occurring after the first intake of *Carc* 30C, in my opinion it shows the curative action of this remedy as the dream follows the direction of cure. Hopefully, following dreams will tell us more, but this single dream, instead of a series, already provides the patient and the homeopath with a very positive healing message, a communication from the Inner Healer, the dream.

EPILOGUE

As a child I was looking for pretty shells on the seashore; as an adult, I realize that the real treasures lay in the depth of the ocean.

After completion of this book, you should not be overcome with shame or despair of not having yet attained the level of self-realization. Even despite our most heroic attempts we can never reach perfection. The reader should be "moved" in the two meanings of this word. Moved to begin the journey to happiness, but also moved to the soul, to realize that while we all are troubled and flawed persons, no one should hesitate to start sailing to a port of self-knowledge, atonement, and liberation. Even the greatest philosophers (the lovers of wisdom), especially the existentialists and phenomenologists who examined a life of freedom, were not always "super humans." Look at the lives of Jean Paul Sartre and Simone de Beauvoir, two intellectual icons of the 20th century. The first died from exhaustion brought on by abusing uppers and downers, alcohol (whiskey and vodka), and excessive smoking, followed by kidney failure. Simone died six years later from liver cirrhosis. In her book *The*

Existential Café, Sarah Bakewell describes the "easily offended" Sartre and his different political stances during his life, unforgiving to those who did not agree with him (Bakewell, 2016). Close friendships with Karl Jaspers, Raymond Aron, Maurice Merleau-Ponty, and Albert Camus could not be sustained because of differences in political and philosophical opinions, and he walked away from them without regret. As Simone de Beauvoir quotes in her book about Sartre: "Breaking off a relationship doesn't affect me in the least. A thing is dead—that's all" (de Beauvoir, 1984, p. 275). But at least Sartre, a diminutive 5 feet 2 inches in size, was always "moving," never at a loss of opinions, even when bringing danger to his life, bursting forward till the end of his life with energy until his light resembled a little candle flame because of exhaustion and illness, remaining an anarchist convicted of his thoughts and ideas until the end. Sartre might have been a flawed man as we all are, but when he tensed his muscles for the good, as when he aided Franz Faron, French psychiatrist, humanist, and revolutionary, in supporting the cause of the native Algerians against the oppressor or settler (France), he used his intellect and heart to support the defenseless in their rights to self-determination and dignity. Who will ever be able to heal the ontological psychosis of the restless animal, Homo sapiens?

About myself, if I could start again from zero, I think I'd try to fill my life with more adventure, in a *Sulphur-Phosphorus* way. The combination of decisiveness and a sense of adventure and travel, of genius and chaos, of philosophy and romanticism, would be moving in every sense of the word—moving forward relentlessly and moving others to tempt the same. This mixture of salt and pepper would provide a life with more passion, less worry, and living more courageously! And, if anything more—when everyone is laughing at me—then I would choose the best thing: laughing at myself, abject surrender, which is better than being pissed off or being all too easily offended. I should have decided much earlier to strip away my mask and display what lay hidden beneath. It is not that I think that whatever I would have shown would be magnificent and heroic, but that whatever would have been exposed is what really matters—that every human bears the stamp of the ordinary human condition. Sometimes we laugh from pure enjoyment, but sometimes laughter is driven by our own reflection on what fools we mortals are.

I can see that I was often ruled by the combination of a melancholic-sanguine temperament, with one superseding the other in a changeable, often uncontrollable way. At a later age, dreams helped me to discover the dark side of my Self, the changeability that often governed my spirit (also being controlled by Taurus-Gemini), and the fight against demons that now disappear step-by-step; there is Self-discovery, coupled to some regrets and astonishment, in discovering that, as most ordinary people, I could be two trying to fuse into one, often in a painful way, fighting against memories that haunt me, but at the same time push me forward.

Where is it going to end? Is there enough time to ever come closer to self-realization? Forget the philosopher king and Nietzsche's superman. But such utopia can bring a smile to my face, as it continues to give me some direction while dreams never fail to educate me and others. I have a great thirst for continuous self-exploration and desire to keep the individuation process alive at optimal speed, scanning the depth of my human passion, frailty, and folly. The goal is always the same, but I might change the means from time to time if I am to stay true to myself. I have to find room for the fun in life too, not only for self-exploration through ascetic life, and neglecting principles, but as much through sports, dance, and literature—or every expression my Vital Force wants to use to find its way to self-expression, and to find and awaken what still lies dormant in my unconscious or in my shadow. After a dream, even more after a disturbing one, I am not afraid to analyze it, seeing what other part of my life needs still illumination. So, I must embrace the imperfection and ceaseless changes of my life because they *are* my life.

For too long, with youthful exuberance while it lasted, I took the road leading to pleasure—an alluring and inviting course—making the same blunders as others that made up my fate. So, it is not my task to forcefully point out to someone else what road to follow, but only to hope that consciousness and elucidation will come sooner to my fellow man than it did to me. Far too often I was overcome with ambition, which today I find distasteful, even revolting. I have the same questions as most humans: "Why?" "How was it possible?" I am not even sure if a second life could give me the answers. The ordinary human—and most of us are—is driven by innate urges and animalistic instincts along the highway of life. There is a certain dull uniformity in human destiny where dreams seldom come true. Yet pleasure can be found in small steps forward and hopefully we can hold on to the achieved higher rung of the ladder to self-actualization, as it matters a great deal more to us than it matters to others, till finally the night falls and obscures the view. It is these short-lived delights that dull the sting of the immutable laws that form our human destiny. I am not sure how much or little I have accomplished for my fellow beings, as many lived as my neighbors for some time and then were seen no more. I have tried to help them as best as I could, tried to understand their suffering, to the point of transference to some degree. Why I did it I could not help, as my Self was shaped that way. At the end of my life, I was simply a fellow traveler upon life's road, not a guru or prophet. I was always interested in the study of humanity and continued to study the motives that controlled life.

Chateaubriand declared, "I should like not to be born rather than be forever forgotten." Alas! Only a few like Ataturk, the father of Turkey (Mustafa Kemal), can put a claim on this aphorism, as most of us are not remembered at all. If I would live again, I would only live the life suggested in this Epilogue sooner! At the end, few can transcend the rat race with sustained elegance, leaving the fake ephemeral world behind and becoming a *Sulphur* philanthropist and maybe a hermit. Allow me to tell you: be true to yourself, be firm in your convictions from the start, cherish and enjoy every day as a gift of life, be as far advanced as possible in your itinerary by accepting and exploring the unconscious, by trying to grasp the meaning of those "foolish" dreams and practices. Hard as it might be, if you do, you are further forward and have won! Dreams are to be mined for insight, to be treated as portals to a hidden world. Increase your field of vision wide enough for you to glimpse a landscape that can hold direction for your next step in life.

As far as I am concerned, when dying, I don't want to say anything prosaic to someone else like: "I feel now I'm standing at the pastures of peace, or elevated in the high clouds, that I can now fully forgive my father…" No! Is it time to sum up life with a resolution of encouragement and inspiration? Who knows! I certainly must allow other people to express the convoluted labyrinths of their own lives. Regarding myself, I hope my last whisper is nothing verbose and grandiloquent; just a gentle human interaction for which my wife hopefully tenderly remembers me, forgiving me for unnecessary battles, misunderstandings of my own making, and mood swings—a collective human trait, which were part of the internal tempest reigning my world too often.

Are my last words eloquent and introspective enough to be attached to historical archives? It is the least thing on my mind, as soon I will journey to the land of ghosts and the forgotten. Did I contradict myself in life? So be it, I am human and contain multitudes. Imperfections are the truest acceptance of the human condition. We all have them. Unfortunately, humility and being honest with ourselves are not traits as widespread! In the end, I hope to have made a possible difference to those who came to me as patients and to those who have read my books. But all in all, it was my life, I was responsible for it, and now it is too late to change anything and it may well remain an enigma to even the closest of my friends and myself —possibly resembling a hundred shades of scintillating grey—quoting Sartre, *the shifting nuances of being and nothingness*, a course into the midst of the unknown. A last farewell, coming from my last breath, would be words by Hafiz, the beloved Persian poet and mystical, to my dear wife Yolanda, and to life in general: "One regret that I am determined not to have when I am lying on my deathbed, is that I did not kiss you enough," from the poem, "I am determined" (Ladensky, 1996, p. 85). And don't expect me to make elaborate plans for my funeral although that is one evening I'd love to attend! If I had been carving the epitaph for my own tombstone, I would choose nothing more than the simple phrase, "The Individual," or maybe, "The Rebel." As for myself, I echo Edith Piaf's immortal song, "Non, Je ne regrette rien!" I have lived!

INDEX: BASIC HOMEOPATHY TERMS

The *Organon*: fundamental book establishing the principles and directing the practice of the science of Homeopathy
Aph (Aphorism): numbered sections of the *Organon*
Provings: experiments to discover what symptoms specific natural substances can cause in healthy people, hence cure in homeopathic dosage
Repertory: compilation of proving symptoms and remedies that can cure
Rubric: symptom listing in the Repertory
Materia Medica: collection of all knowledge about homeopathic remedies and their therapeutic properties
Delusion: term for a person's subjective reality
Simillimum: most perfect dynamic remedy matched to a patient
Miasm: dynamic, inherited predisposition to all/any disease. The three main miasms are Psora, Sycosis, and Syphilitic.

(To learn more about Homeopathy, see *Hahnemann Revisited*, by Luc De Schepper.)

INDEX: HOMEOPATHIC REMEDY NAMES

List of remedies as used throughout the book: abbreviations and full names

Aconite — *Aconite*
Alum. — *Alumina*
Ars. — *Arsenicum album*
Bar-carb. — *Baryta carbonica*
Calc-carb. — *Calcarea carbonica*
Calc-phos. — *Calcarea phosphorica*
Carc. — *Carcinosinum*
Fl-ac. — *Fluoricum acidum*
Hell. — *Helleborus*
Hura — *Hura brasiliensis*
Ign. — *Ignatia*
Kali-brom. — *Kali bromatum*
Kali-carb. — *Kali carbonicum*
Lac-c. — *Lac caninum*
Lach. — *Lachesis*
Lyc. — *Lycopodium*

Med. — Medorrhinum
Merc. — Mercurius
Nat-mur. — Natrum muriaticum
Nit-ac. — Nitric acidum
Nux-v. — Nux vomica
Op. — Opium
Phos. — Phosphorus
Plat. — Platinum
Puls. — Pulsatilla
Sep. — Sepia
Sil. — Silicea
Spig. — Spigelia
Staph. — Staphysagria
Sulph. — Sulphur
Tarent. — Tarentula hispanica
Thuja — Thuja
Verat-a. — Veratrum album
Viola-tric. —Viola tricolor

APPENDIX: RELATIVE FIXED SYMBOLS

No excellent dictionary of relative fixed symbols presently exists. The Dream section of the Repertory is useless to really understand dream symbols because dreams are unique compensated expressions from the unconscious towards a one-sided conscious position. So, for example, even *Dreams, falling* will have a unique translation depending on the *individual* personal conscious. And, one's culture can affect the meaning of symbols; for instance, according to Eastern or Western philosophy, colors (red, white) can have a different meaning in dreams, still dependent on the content of the dream.

That is why dream interpretation, because it is so individual, should be resonating with the homeopath looking for the simillimum.

To understand the possible meanings of symbols in dreams, much depends on the reader's erudition, his desire to study mythology, philology, philosophy, psychology, fairy tales, Traditional Chinese Medicine, comparative religion, archeology, and alchemy. Derived from my education, reading, and personal study, here is a list of a few relative fixed symbols.

Abdomen or Belly: relates to the unconscious, the oven "where children are baked." In TCM it relates to the lower burner, containing the most precious organs, Kidney and Heart, the origin of life.

Angel: from the Greek *angelos*, meaning "envoy, messenger, or courier." The intermediary between man and deity, serving as messenger.

Animals: refer to an instinct drive that wants to be integrated into consciousness. Animals can be helpers but also tricksters, so we need to always pay attention to their appearance in dreams, to what role they play. When walking with an animal in a dream, you are walking with your instincts, rather than just living in consciousness only; pointing to what you are going to do, or what is happening to you. Additionally, different animals have different meanings. For example, an **eagle** is heaven, spirit, yang; he is also a messenger and bringer of salvation; power and leadership; a symbol of the spirit and of self-renewal. Such an aggressive bird (also **ravens, hawks)** in general represents a spiritual uplifting, evolving to awareness (integration). A **snake** is earth, nature, and yin, and represents our psychology that we are afraid of since we cannot understand it. Among the archetypal and recurrent animal figures the **serpent** occupies a unique and ambivalent place. In some respect it is the symbol for supreme wisdom, instinctive knowledge (not intellectual), and the great healer or redeemer. It is the mediator between the conscious and unconscious worlds, forming a bridge between heaven and hell. On the other hand, it is the tempter to evil, to poison—the devil himself. The snake can have different meanings depending on the person and the situation. It can be the symbol of healing/spiritual awakening, healing/transformation, and resurrection, the shedding of the old persona. It stands also for femaleness, sexuality, the darkness, night, yin, death, and fear. Whenever a snake appears in dreams or delusions, it symbolizes a piece of the instinctive psychology in us, something of tremendous power. It represents the vital, the instinctual, the drives stirring in man, his unconscious dark side in contrast to brightness (the conscious side of his nature). The serpent in Oriental psychology symbolizes the treasure of wisdom but also the cunning of the primitive or animal mind of man. It can also be a symbol of danger, of being caught in coils, swallowed, or poisoned. A snake is also an anxiety symbol; monkeys and horses, for instance, are instinctively afraid of snakes. When a snake appears at the sickbed in dreams it can indicate foreboding of death. The snake is also a symbol of time: the idea that the snake represents time is probably connected with the fact that it sheds its skin. Some aboriginal peoples interpret this as a reincarnation and infer from it the snake's immortality. The three most important aspects in snake dreams are that of an earth demon, a savior, and a time symbol. Its duality is seen in the caduceus of MDs. Analogous to this, the greatest poisons in homeopathy are the greatest healers (*Arsenicum* and *Lachesis* being just two examples). **Horse:** represents the non-human or instinctive side or instinctual energy, the unconscious. A horse represents the lower part of the body and the animal impulses that arise from there. A horse with no rider in a dream reflects the uncontrolled instinctive drives erupting from the unconscious. The horse is dynamic, signifies vehicular power, and has to do with sorcery and magic spells, especially the Black Knight horses. **Black horse:** stands for the unruliness of the passions. A **dragon** is the symbol of evil, an evil anima figure, something that must be overcome in order to be liberated; a cold-blooded animal representing the cold-blooded part of man's psychology, although in China it is the symbol of heaven, a figure of light, a symbol of masculine power, happiness, health, and positive energy. Dragons are believed to control rain, and this ability to influence the harvest reinforced their power in China's agrarian society. Often, they are shown clutching a flaming pearl, meant to symbolize wisdom they've captured that will be of use to humankind. A **lion** is destructive, a nuisance and dangerous to human beings, but is also a symbol of strength and courage. **Owl:** sees in the night, so a symbol of understanding of the dark things in the unconscious; Minerva, the goddess of wisdom. A **dove** represents love or Venus. A **mouse** represents an animal of the darkness, of the night and fertility. **Bull:** blind impetuousness of psychic behavior. **Ants:** industrious, with strength exceeding their size; cooperative in a colony with great discipline and order within their community. **Spiders:** teach us patience, weaving a web while waiting for the prey to come. **Elephant:** the wisest being, before humans; very sociable and bonding. **Tiger:** passion, power, stamina. **Pig:** dirty sexuality. **Dog:** loyalty, but also unbridled sexuality, having sex with any female dog. **Beetles:** scarab beetles often appear golden (symbol for the sun) but when they are black it denotes the color of the unconscious, depression, and death. **Cow:** fertility; motherhood; nurturing aspect of the feminine psyche.

Assembly: (or an audience or crowd) represents the collective unconscious, a voice of many.

Bathing: cleansing and transforming.

Blood: genuine life; passion.

Bluff or cliff: where conscious ends and the unconscious begins, similar to the entry to a tunnel or the subway.

Bowels: contents of the unconscious.

Butterfly: expressing a wish to emerge from a confining cocoon, either a cocoon of oppression and dominance or a cocoon of old protective attitudes.

Candle: symbol of consciousness.

City: reflecting the Self. Travelling to another city can be exploring a part of the Self never "visited."

Colors:

- **Black:** unconscious, the unknown; evil; the

unaccepted side of the Self; unawareness; death. **Black animals:** unconscious urges or drives. If in a man's dream two girls appear, one with dark black hair, the other with light hair, it shows the two sides of his anima, the light and the dark undifferentiated side.

- **Blue: Dark blue:** may symbolize the collective unconscious (stormy ocean), or the power of the conscious mind. It may also represent a "dark blue depression" (having "the blues"). Color of the sky, usually the color of the spirit, the heavens and upper world, as God is nearest when arching high over the dark underworld like the blue dome of heaven. The color of the sky can reflect the feeling about life you have: a clear sky versus a grey sky, etc. Idioms: "It is clear as the sky!" The sky is the limit; "out of the blue." It can stand for the essence of masculinity but also the opposite, like in the idiom, "He hasn't got a blue fog of a thing"—meaning he hasn't the foggiest notion of it. Blue stands also for the vertical (the elevator going up and down) as blue means height and depth (blue sky above, the deep blue sea below). **Light blue** stands for Logos or Thinking/Intellect or intellectual clarity: it indicates a cool and calming state; it is the intellectual clarity, the essence of masculinity; it is also the color of water and therefore represents the unconscious—it is also the bluish green sea that houses the spirits of the dead. A blue coat might also indicate spiritual freedom.
- **Brown:** color of the earth: did we stay on earth or were we lifted to the sky (inflation)?
- **Gold** indicates something valuable or of deep significance (an act of "pure gold"); the highest goal

of alchemy (transformation into gold—compare to *Aurum* in homeopathy).

- **Green:** color of spring life. Signifies growth and belongs to the sensation function; the color of Nature, the elements and forces of regeneration, bringing new life from the death of the old (green appearing in spring); the color of life and hope; also the color of envy or jealousy or reflecting naivety as in, "He is green in the job."
- **Grey:** the color of ghosts, grey is semidarkness in which light starts to emerge.
- **Orange:** balance of emotions and intellect; color of fertility, hope, and new beginnings.
- **Pink:** softness; femininity; tender love rather than passionate love.
- **Purple** stands for healing.
- **Red:** passion; blood, energy, fire, living desire, aggressiveness, excitement, fiery passionate nature; masculine. Red and white are a pair of opposites (masculine versus feminine). Blood-red indicates overwhelming emotional turmoil. The Roman generals would hang a red mantle on their tent as a symbol of beginning battle. Chinese brides wear red dresses. Red belongs to the conscious feeling function.
- **White:** purity and childish innocence; also, the garment of youth; before worn by the mother—think about a white wedding dress, showing the virgin state of the woman! It stands for purity and suggests radiance, a sense of wholeness, peace, happiness, and the feminine, also joy, delight, and solace, according to the French Renaissance writer Rabelais. (In the East it is associated with death and mourning.) Cleanliness. Awareness. Light feeling.

The Romans showed their admiration and joy for a victorious general when he was allowed the honors of a triumphal entry into Rome on a chariot drawn by white horses. Also, white stands for "lifeless," as with the expression, "White as a ghost." It is also the color of enlightenment, as white reflects the rays of light. **White light:** absolute truth. **White animals:** urges and sexuality that have been integrated and accepted in consciousness.

- **Yellow:** intuition (also indigo); hopefulness for the future. The sacred color in Buddhism; in the Chinese symbol system, yellow was sacred to the Emperor (*The Yellow Emperor's Classic of Medicine, Essential Questions*, or *Huang Di Nei Jing*, is the classic Chinese internal medicine text) and in dreams it can represent the wise use of authority and power.

Dancing: creation, the idea of something produced.

Earth: collective unconscious.

Father: representing intellect and rationalism.

Fire: the breaking out of a fire can be an emotional outbreak threatening to destroy the psychic equilibrium; a fire destroying the house (the Self) can refer to imminent death of the person or a diminishment of consciousness. The place in the house (Self), attic or cellar, indicates the outburst of passion taking place on that level of the Self. Fire stands for the center of life, where it is warm and light and safe, a place where people like to gather (around the campfire, around the open fire in the living room).

Fish: contents of the deep unconscious to be drawn up from its waters.

Flowers: the growth of flowers represents life's renewal and beauty; they also stand for emotions.

Forest: a place where the collective unconscious is projected, a place full of risks and dangers, where ghosts reside.

Gold: related to the Sun; to consciousness beyond destruction as it always keeps its color even if unearthed after many centuries contrary to copper, silver, etc., and therefore is associated with incorruptibility and immortality and great value.

Heart: symbol for the feeling function, love, and courage. We speak of "a broken heart, a bleeding heart" to express a state of grief and intense love for someone. "My heart goes out to that person" represents compassion and empathy, all appropriate emotions belonging to a well-functioning feeling function. And "when I lost heart in battle," it means I lost courage to fight the challenges in life. Having a "big heart" is symbolic for the largeness and generosity of that person.

Hermaphrodite: the infantile, not-yet differentiated state, the preconscious condition.

High noon: reflects maximum yang changing into a gradual increase of yin, or the beginning of the second half of life.

House (building): symbol of the human personality, the Self.

Kitchen: a place of creative change, a place of nourishment.

Land: "terra firma" of consciousness; an **island:** place of psychic isolation.

Left side: the sphere of the unadapted unconscious reactions; the protective shield or feminine or yin side, but also the "sinister" side, the dark side of the soul, evil that comes from the unconscious; the unintelligible part.

Light: consciousness. **Dim or murky light:** deficiency of understanding.

Lightning: a sudden unexpected and overpowering change of psychic condition.

Mandala: A Sanskrit word meaning a magic circle; a symbol of order, occurring mainly in patients during times of psychic disorientation and reorientation. They are as magic circles, offering protection from the perils of the psyche, and represent wholeness. The circle denotes a holy and inviolable place, even a taboo place where a human can meet the unconscious. Any round object points to the circle of completeness. A circle is also the symbol of totality. The center is the consciousness and around it is the unconscious, containing the archetypes.

Mirror: refers to the intellect, with which we can think, and which persuades us constantly to identify ourselves with its insights and reflections. Our true nature, an allegory of self-reflection.

Money: a symbol of our own energy, our psychic capital (Idiom: "paying one's own way").

Moon: crescent moon refers to the rising power of the world of the feminine, emotions, love, renewal, the mystery of the womb. *Luna* in Latin, it also refers to "lunacy," the world of craziness.

Mother: is also the unconscious. When in a dream we are carried by the mother, it means we are carried by the unconscious.

Mountain: level of intense consciousness.

Ocean: collective unconscious, vastness of unconscious life, the storehouse of the past—the good, bad, and ugly.

Octopus: destructive power of the unconscious, the regressive force which sucks back and destroys individual life.

Phallus: creative mana, power of healing and infertility; as such, a **pen** can have the same meaning also, a sexual symbol but also a reflection of means for creative expressions.

Rainbow: a bridge under which mortals must walk—only for gods is it a road to walk on, mortals will fall to their death; a place of harmony and beautiful colors, a bridge reaching earth and sky, a link between the unconscious and conscious.

Right side: where things become conscious; active or yang or masculine side; the side of adaptation, sword or action side; of "being right"; blinding the right eye means the conscious vision is destroyed.

Sea: collective unconscious versus a lake or stream or river (or the river of energy and life), representing personal unconscious.

Sibling: Older sibling: someone we look up to, our model and anticipation of our own life; the seemingly virtuous child admired and favored by the parent, often held up as a mirror for the younger ones.

Stairs, steps, and ladders: used to go upwards (consciousness) or downwards (investigating the unconscious). The ascent can also be represented by a ladder, or in modern times by an elevator. They point to the process of psychic transformation with its ups and downs.

Star: symbol of individuation and guiding life.

Street: the world of collective unconscious.

Sun: the center of consciousness, yang, and light. For American Indians the sun represented the Great Spirit. It is also a symbol of masculine consciousness, as the moon symbolizes feminine consciousness.

Sunrise at dawn: new life, awakening of consciousness, emergence of the self.

Sword: symbol of masculine libido and destructive power, while **libido** itself is every manifestation of the expression of psychic energy.

Table: sitting around a round table means connectedness and relationship, while "round" stands for the composition of wholeness.

Third eye: symbol of intuition; the **right** eye is the conscious vision, the **left** eye is the unconscious vision.

Toilet: collective unconscious, which is also symbolized by a jungle, forest, bottom of the sea, mud.

Tree: a new form of life appears. A tree makes a connection through its branches growing into the sky, with the life-giving breath of the spirit, while its roots are nourished by the earth. Sucking up all nourishing minerals and water.

Tunnel: symbol for rebirth, going through the birth canal. Deep place in the unconscious which one must pass through to come into the light again, finding a new attitude.

Wave: symbol of power of the unconscious, sweeping in on consciousness.

White dove: Holy Ghost for Christians; peace symbol.

Wind: archetype of a living spirit, the breath of a god.

Window: opening a window is the way to go to consciousness.

REFERENCES

1. Bakewell, S. 2016. *At the Existential Café.* New York: Other Press.
2. Barret, W. 1958. *Irrational Man.* Garden City, New York: Doubleday Anchor Books.
3. Biklen et al. 2005. *Autism and the myth of the person alone.* New York: New York University Press.
4. Cirlot, J.E. 1971. *A Dictionary of Symbols.* New York: Philosophical Library, Inc.
5. de Beauvoir, S. 1984. *Adieux, A Farewell to Sartre.* Translated by P. O'Brian. New York: Pantheon Books, a division of Random House.
6. de Lery, J. 1990. *History of a Voyage to the Land of Brazil.* Translated by J. Whatley. Berkeley & Los Angeles, California: University of California Press.
7. Descartes. 1988. *Selected Philosophical Writings, Discourse on the Method.* Translated by Cottingham & Strothoff. Cambridge University Press.
8. de Montaigne, M. 2014. *Shakespeare's Montaigne. The Florio Translation of the Essays. A selection.*

Edited by S. Greenblatt & P. Blatt. New York: New York Review of Books.

9. de Montaigne, M. 1987. *The Essays: A Selection*. Translated by M.A. Screech. New York: Penguin Classics.
10. De Schepper, L. 2004. *Advanced Guide for the Professional Homeopath*. New Mexico: Full of Life Publishing.
11. De Schepper, L. 2013. *Discovering Life: Homeopathic Portraits*. New Mexico: Full of Life Publishing.
12. Edib, H. 2005. *Memoirs of Halide Edib*. New Jersey: Gorgias Press.
13. Freud, S. 1998. *The Interpretation of Dreams*. New York: Avon Books.
14. Gaugin, P. 1958. *Paul Gaugin's Intimate Journals*. Bloomington/Midland Book. Indiana University Press.
15. Hafiz. 1996. *I Heard God Laughing, Renderings of Hafiz*. Translated by D. Ladensky. Oakland, California.
16. Hahnemann, S. 1982. *Organon of Medicine*. Sixth Edition. Translated by J. Kunzli, A. Naude and P. Pendleton. Washington: Cooper Publishing.
17. Hayman, R. 1980. *A Critical Life, Nietzsche*. New York: Oxford University Press.
18. Hollingdale, R.J. 1977. *A Nietzsche Reader*. New York: Penguin Books, Ltd.
19. Jung, C.G. Reprint 1978. *Collected Works of C.G. Jung, Volume 9, Part II: Anion*. Edited and translated by Gerhard Adler. Edited and translated by R.F.C. Hull. New Jersey: Princeton University Press.
20. Jung, C.G. 1984. *Dream Analysis: Notes of the seminar given in 1928-1930*. Bollingen Series XCIX.

Edited by William McGuire. New Jersey: Princeton University Press.

21. Jung, C.G. 1974. *Collected Works of C.G. Jung, Volumes 4, 8, 12, 16: Dreams.* New Jersey: Princeton University Press.
22. Jung, C.G. 1963. *Memories, Dreams, Reflections.* Recorded and edited by Aniella Jaffe. New York: Vintage Books, a division of Random House.
23. Jung, C.G. 1958. *Psyche and Symbol. A Selection from the Writings of C.G. Jung.* Edited by Violet S. de Laszlo. New York: Bollingen Foundation, Inc. New Jersey: Princeton University Press.
24. Jung, C.G. 1953. *Collected Works of C.G. Jung, Volume 12: Psychology and Alchemy.* New Jersey: Princeton University Press.
25. Jung, C.G. 1989. *Collected Works of C.G. Jung, Volume 3: Psychogenesis of Dementia Praecox.* Bollingen Series XX. Edited and translated by Gerhard Adler. Edited and translated by Sir Herbert Read and R.F.C. Hull. New Jersey: Princeton University Press.
26. Jung, C.G. 2009. *Red Book, Liber Novus. Philemon Series.* Verona, Italy: Foundation for the Works of C.G. Jung.
27. Jung, C.G. 1990. *Collected Works of C.G. Jung, Volume 9, Part I: The Archetypes and the Collective Unconscious.* New Jersey: Princeton University Press.
28. Jung, C.G. 1990.*Collected Works of C.G. Jung, Volume 6: The Psychological Types.* New Jersey: Princeton University Press.
29. Jung, C.G. 1966. *Collected Works of C.G. Jung, Volume 7: Two Essays on Analytical Psychology.* New Jersey: Princeton University Press.

30. Kaplan, C. 2011. Diogenes. Brookline, Massachusetts: International Authors.
31. La Rochefoucauld. 2006. *Maxims.* New York: Dover Publications.
32. Lincoln, F. & White, C. 2001. *The Confessions of St. Augustine.* London: Frances Lincoln Ltd.
33. Maciocia, G. 1989. *The Foundations of Chinese Medicine.* London: Churchill Livingstone. Medical Division of Longman Group UK Ltd.
34. Nietzsche, F. 1967. *Basic Writings of Nietzsche.* Walter Kaufman. New York: Random House, Inc.
35. Nietzsche, F. 1954. *The Portable Nietzsche.* Walter Kaufman. The Viking Portable Library. Viking Press Inc.
36. Plato. 2015. *Phaedrus.* Sheppard Publications.
37. Plato. 1955. *The Republic.* Translated by Desmond Lee. New York: Penguin Books.
38. Plato. 1984. *Great Dialogues of Plato, The Republic.* Book VII (517C-519C). Translated by W.H.D. Rouse. A Mentor Book. New York: Penguin Group.
39. Powers, T. 2010. *The Killing of Crazy Horse.* New York: Vintage Books. Random House Inc.
40. Redmond, A. 1996. *The Epigrams of Oscar Wilde.* London: Senate, an imprint of Random House UK, Ltd.
41. Schopenhauer, A. 1970. *Essays and Aphorisms.* R.J. Hollingdale. Middlesex, England: Penguin Books, Ltd.
42. Schroyens, F. 2007. *Essential Synthesis.* London: Homeopathic Book Publishers.
43. Voltaire. 1959. *Candide.* Translated by Lowell Bair. New York: Bantam Books.
44. von Franz, M.L. 1985. *Dreams.* Boston, Massachusetts: Shamballa Publications.

45. Whitmont, E. 1969. *The Symbolic Quest*. New Jersey: Princeton University Press.
46. Whitmont, E. & Perera, S. B. 1991. *Dreams, a Portal to the Source*. London: Routledge.
47. Wilde, O. 1966. *Stories, Plays, Poems, and Essays*. "Lady Windermere's Fan." New York: Collins Sons & Co. Ltd, Harper Collins Publishers, Inc.
48. Wilde, O. 1966. *Stories, Plays, Poems, and Essays*. "The Picture of Dorian Gray." New York: Collins Sons & Co. Ltd, Harper Collins Publishers, Inc.
49. Wilhelm, R./Baynes. 1977. *I Ching*. New York: Bollingen Foundation. Princeton University Press.
50. Wilhelm, R./Baynes. 1962. *The Secret of the Golden Flower*. Translated and explained by Richard Wilhelm. San Diego: A Harvest Book; Harcourt Brace and Company.

NOTES

2. The Language of Dreams

1. Taken from Greek mythology, the term psychopomp means a spirit-guide of the soul.
2. Hermes was the official messenger of the gods and his symbol was the caduceus, a long-winged wand around which two serpents intertwine, surmounted by two small wings or a winged helm. It is a very ancient symbol. For the Romans, the caduceus served as a symbol of moral equilibrium and of good conduct. The wand represents power and the two snakes, wisdom. It also signifies the integration of the four elements; the wand corresponds to earth, the wings to air, the serpents to fire and water. (Cirlot, 1971)
3. Homeostasis comes from the Greek *homoios* or "similar" and *stasis* or "stillness." It is the capacity to sustain internal constancy, an essential feature of an organism, sustaining life (even psychological life). As the French physiologist Claude Bernard wrote: "The constancy of the interior environment is the condition of a free and independent life." Homeostasis does not occur by chance but is the result of organized self-government.

3. Important Dreams During a Human's Lifetime

1. Lucien Lévy-Brühl (1857-1939) was a French scholar trained in philosophy, whose primary field of study involved primitive mentality. His work, especially the concepts of "collective representation" and "participation mystique," influenced the psychology theory of C. G. Jung.
2. According to a study by the CDC, 20% of American children ages 3-17 experience mental disorders each year. Among the most common emotions/behavior that engulf these children are social problems (9.1%), ADHD (8.4%), and separation anxiety (7.6%).
3. William Hazlitt (1778-1830) was an English essayist, drama and literary critic, painter, and philosopher.

4. Common Themes in Dreams

1. Pierre Janet (1859-1947) was a French psychologist and neurologist. C.G. Jung was a student of Janet, who came to use this term also.
2. Arthur Schopenhauer (1788-1860), German philosopher, had an independent spirit, writing with little respect for authority. In 1809 he inherited

great wealth from his father Heinrich, one of the wealthiest businessmen of his time. He preferred to be alone even when with others, for fear of losing his integrity. He was influenced by the works of Plato and Kant. Despite his work going virtually unnoticed for many years after publication, he continued believing in the supreme value of his work, confirmed after his death when he became one of the most influential writers of Europe.

5. Different Classes of Dreams

1. Disease Levels: **1.** Ectoderm **2.** Endoderm **3.** Connective tissues **4.** Mesodermal organs **5.** Neuro-endocrine system **6.** Neural plate **7.** Cell neural plate (Vijayakar, 2000.)

6. The Ego Formation

1. At 9 weeks, neurons in the spinal cord develop, from week 12 on, the brain is developing and releasing hormones, and from week 12-18 bones and muscles grow, the lungs develop, the female and male genitalia differentiate and fat stores are formed to give energy to the baby.

7. Persona: The Masked Individual

1. Fata Morgana is the Italian name for "Morgan the Fairy," a sorceress of medieval legends. Among her powers was the ability to change shape. The term has come to be used for a mirage that significantly distorts an object to the point where the object on which it is based is completely unrecognizable.
2. Arthur Schopenhauer (1788–1860) was a German philosopher known for his atheistic pessimism and philosophical clarity. At age 25, he published his doctoral dissertation, *On the Fourfold Root of the Principle of Sufficient Reason*, which examined the fundamental question of whether reason alone can unlock answers about the world.
3. Dr. Samuel Hahnemann (1755-1843), discoverer of Homeopathy, acclaimed as the "Leader of the Great Medical Reformation," was homeschooled as a boy by his father. His education consisted primarily of being given a problem to solve each day. No doubt his genius, his ability to think scientifically, rationally, and creatively as an individual, was inspired and fostered by this early training.

8. The Four Conscious Functions of Jung and Two Attitude Types

1. Nondifferentiation is failure to recognize, identify, and utilize conscious functions other than one's dominant function. When a function is not called upon in any situation, in other words is the least used, it is not developed and as ready to respond to an event as a well-trained and utilized conscious function (the dominant function).
2. Eros is an archetypal principle, a principle of relation, union, attachment to, attraction to, and involvement. It is *masculine* or yang, according to its definition, an active and powerful Vital Force to reach out to and embrace things, to shoot an arrow into the heart as Cupid did. Anima on the other hand is always *feminine*. They are not the same. We can see in someone who marries a "lifer" in prison that her feeling function is "a mess," but her Eros is present. And in everyday life, many people are in love with Eros, but at the same time don't hesitate to cheat, lie, and have affairs (due to poor feeling function), leading to countless lawyerly debates.

10. The Swampland of Extensive Ghosts: The Shadow Side

1. Sisyphus, in Greek mythology, was the cunning king of Corinth who was punished in Hades for his self-aggrandizing craftiness and deceit by eternally having to roll a huge stone up a hill only to have it roll down again as soon as he had brought it to the summit. This fate is related in Homer's *Odyssey*, Book XI.

11. Anima

1. This formula comes from the *Nei Jing*, the source of Traditional Chinese Medicine, which speaks to women's development in seven-year stages. Five times seven (5x7) starts a weakening of the yang brightness meridians, when the face begins to get dark and hair falls out. At four times seven (4x7), or 28 years old, the body (hair, tendons, and bones) is still strong. A similar process is described for men: 5x8, or 40 years old, is when the Kidney ying is weakened, and hair falls out and teeth become loose. At 4x8, the tendons and bones are the strongest and the flesh is full and strong. For women, menopause sets in at 7x7, or 49, when infertility sets in. For men, at 8x8 andropause sets in, with loss of hair and teeth. (Su wen, Chapter 1, pp. 4-5)
2. Logos is not identical to animus (just as Eros is not identical to anima—see Chap. 8). Logos is the principle of knowledge. Animus is the archetypal personification of masculine psychological characteristics. Anima is the archetypal personification of feminine psychological characteristics.

13. The Human Love Story: Projection of the Sygizi

1. Hafiz (c.1320-1389) was born and lived in Shiraz, a beautiful garden city, where he became a famous spiritual teacher. His collected poems are a classic in the literature of Sufism and mystical verse. His work became known to the West largely through the passion of Goethe.

14. The Death of a Soul: Non-Acceptance of the Sygizi

1. Michel de Montaigne (1533-1592), French philosopher, was born in his father's chateau near Bordeaux. He was taught Latin before he learned French. He was a counselor in the Parliament (1557-1570), and upon retiring devoted himself to writing his *Essays* and became an acknowledged master of world literature.

www.ingramcontent.com/pod-product-compliance
Lightning Source LLC
LaVergne TN
LVHW011534200926
848484LV00001B/261
9780942501162